Praise for *The Body Code*

"I read Dr. Bradley Nelson's *The Emotion Code* book several years ago and started using the information in it to help my patients, family, and friends. Many of my experiences with *The Emotion Code* were amazing and quite beneficial for each of the recipients of that process. When Brad asked me to read his new book *The Body Code* and to write an endorsement, I gladly accepted. *The Emotion Code* was a very good book, but I think *The Body Code* is even better. I really like the methodical way that Dr. Nelson has presented the principles and practice of *The Body Code.* The many life-changing testimonials and case examples in *The Body Code* provide great encouragement and specific, actionable examples for its readers. It is a book that, if the information in it is properly applied, can positively improve not only the reader's life, but also the lives of whoever the reader chooses to help using its information. I highly recommend *The Body Code*!"

—William Lee Cowden, MD, MD(H), chairman of the Scientific Advisory Board, Academy of Comprehensive Integrative Medicine

"In *The Body Code*, Dr. Nelson builds on the work in his bestselling book *The Emotion Code* to create an all-encompassing framework for bringing balance, health, and happiness back into your life. These pages contain knowledge and skills you can immediately put into practice. This book will truly expand your understanding of what it means to listen to your body! Dr. Nelson's work has changed my life for good! This is a powerful book for the ages and I highly recommend it."

—Steven R. Shallenberger, author of the national bestseller *Becoming Your Best: The 12 Principles of Highly Successful Leaders*

"Dr. Bradley Nelson has done it again! *The Body Code* is a true masterpiece. Your body is a pure reflection of your mind. Change your mind, heal your body. This book and Dr. Brad's work are a must for anyone and everyone ready and willing to do the real work when it comes to deep healing change. Simple and full of golden nuggets and practical ways for unlocking the body code so you can live your very best life!"

—Dr. Darren R. Weissman, developer of The LifeLine Technique® and bestselling author of *The Power of Infinite Love & Gratitude*

"I have been fortunate enough to experience the Body Code, and it's tangible the difference I had in my energy levels before and after my session. Having filmed Dr. Brad a few times, I can tell you firsthand he definitely walks his talk." —Frazer Bailey, director of documentary films *E-Motion* and *Root Cause*

"Dr. Bradley Nelson and *The Body Code* book are gifts from Heaven! *The Body Code* is a fantastic healing modality, and along with *The Emotion Code*, it jumpstarted my journey into healing with vibration and energy in a whole new way. *The Body Code* book is beautiful, thorough, and highly accessible to anyone wishing to take charge of their own healing."

—Dr. Karen Kan, doctor of light medicine and founder of the Academy of Light Medicine™

"*The Body Code* is mind-boggling—literally! The theory, easy treatment path, and algorithms are absolute genius, work like gangbusters, and, I believe, are a comprehensive 'do it yourself' health kit for life! If my son needed help in the area of health, Brad is the only person I would recommend to him!" —Alexander Loyd, PhD, ND, *New York Times* bestselling author

"A brilliant, comprehensive, easily understandable system for achieving profound healing results quickly, effectively, and most importantly, safely. This is an inclusive guide for everyone from self-healing newbies to experienced professionals. *The Body Code* will reintroduce you to the most profound healer you could ever encounter: your own precious body."

—Kris Ferraro, author of *Energy Healing* and *Manifesting*

"*The Body Code* is one of the most revolutionary methods of our time. It provides a gateway for emotional freedom, offering a system for releasing and transforming some of the underlying causes of both emotional and physical pain. It includes remarkable testimonials, illustrating the power of the human energy field and subconscious mind. A true gift to both the medical and psychological community." —Sherianna Boyle, author of *Emotional Detox Now*

"Imagine an ally you can always trust and turn to for guidance to improve your health, free yourself from physical and emotional pain, improve your relationships, and create a better future for yourself and your loved ones. That ally is your body, and with *The Body Code*, Brad Nelson teaches you how to access its innate intelligence using the simple yet powerful and effective techniques he has developed over his many years as an acclaimed health expert. Read this book with an open mind, apply what Brad teaches, and get ready to experience results that may astound you!" —Larry Trivieri Jr, author of *No Doctors Required*

"The Kingdom of God is within you. Prayer, meditation, and service provide access to the divine wisdom within our hearts and souls. *The Body Code* offers a key to unlocking the infinite knowledge and healing that is our birthright. Read this book and decode the mystery of your own body, mind, and spirit."

—Michael Alexander, Emmy-nominated host and executive producer, *Conscious Living*

THE BODY CODE

ALSO BY DR. BRADLEY NELSON

The Emotion Code

THE BODY CODE

UNLOCKING YOUR BODY'S ABILITY TO HEAL ITSELF

DR. BRADLEY NELSON

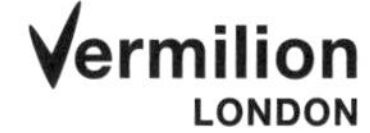

3

Vermilion, an imprint of Ebury Publishing,
20 Vauxhall Bridge Road,
London SW1V 2SA

Vermilion is part of the Penguin Random House group of companies
whose addresses can be found at global.penguinrandomhouse.com

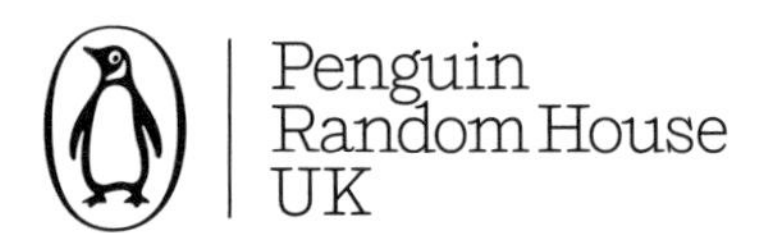

First published in Great Britain by Vermilion in 2023
First published in the United States by St. Martin's Press in 2023

www.penguin.co.uk

A CIP catalogue record for this book is available from the British Library

ISBN 9781785044038

Printed and bound in Italy by Lego S.p.A.

The authorised representative in the EEA is Penguin Random House Ireland,
Morrison Chambers, 32 Nassau Street, Dublin D02 YH68

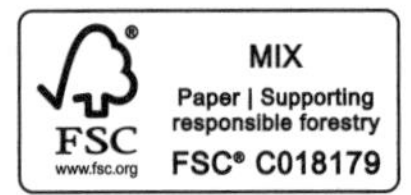

DISCLAIMER

The Body Code System is a self-help method that quite often produces marvelous results and wonderful benefits, both physical and emotional in nature. Nevertheless, it is a relatively new discovery and has not been thoroughly studied.

The information in this book is not intended to replace the advice of the reader's own physician or other medical professional. You should consult a medical professional in matters relating to health, especially if you have existing medical conditions, and before starting, stopping, or changing the dose of any medication you are taking. Any application of the material set forth in the following pages is at the reader's discretion and is his or her sole responsibility.

The information contained in these materials is intended for personal use and not for the practice of any healing art, except where permitted by law. No representation contained in these materials is intended as medical advice and should not be used for diagnosis or medical treatment. For diagnosis or treatment of any medical problem, consult your own physician. The author and the publisher do not accept responsibility for any adverse effects individuals may claim to experience, whether directly or indirectly, from the information contained in this book.

The stories in this book are all true, and permission has been obtained to use people's full names wherever possible, but they have been changed in some circumstances to protect privacy. This book is based on the personal observations and experiences of Dr. Bradley Nelson and others who have experienced this healing method. You, the reader, must take 100 percent responsibility for your own health. The Body Code should not be misconstrued or used to diagnose the presence or absence of any particular mental, physical, or emotional ailment. Neither muscle testing nor the sway test should be used to diagnose the presence or absence of disease.

Individual results may vary, and the author and publisher make no representations or warranties of any kind, nor do they assume liabilities of any kind, with respect to the accuracy or completeness of the contents, and they specifically disclaim any implied warranties of merchantability or fitness of use for a particular purpose. Neither the author nor the publisher shall be held liable or responsible to any person or entity with respect to any loss or to incidental or consequential damages caused or alleged to have been caused, directly or indirectly, by the information or programs contained herein.

The fact that an organization or website is mentioned in the book as a potential source of information does not mean that the author or the publisher endorses any of the information those sources may provide or any recommendations they may make.

This book contains personal experiences that have been submitted by people around the world. To protect their privacy, last names are represented by their initial only.

To Mom, for my love of reading, and for raising me with an open mind. You were the early adopter and healer I have been modeling all my life. Thank you for your amazing example of always seeing the good in people. Thank you for getting me to the right kind of doctors when I was so sick at thirteen. It made all the difference to me and, it turns out, to many others.

To Dad, for your entrepreneurial spirit and example of unconditional love and living without ego. Thank you for asking me that pivotal question on that cold winter day in 1983 that led me to my best path.

To Jean, for being my best companion and friend, for being such an essential part of this work and mission, for all your hard work and constancy, and for your selfless service and sacrifice.

CONTENTS

The body is a self-healing organism.

It knows what is wrong and what it needs.

The Body Code is how we “decode” those needs.

FOREWORD

I'm best known for my exploration of what you can't explain in life. The unknown has been my playground and my career platform. In essence, I've sought to know the unknown. This may be a similar search for you. Perhaps you seek not only to understand our planet, but also your own body, health, and more.

When I first interviewed Dr. Bradley Nelson on my radio show, *Coast to Coast AM*, we discussed his wildly popular first book, *The Emotion Code*, and how emotions get trapped in one's body. Dr. Nelson explained just how these trapped emotions can lead to disease in the body. I was fascinated, and so were my listeners.

Today, more than ten thousand people all over the world, including doctors and medical professionals, are trained in Nelson's work in *The Emotion Code*, and today he's expanded his groundbreaking work further with this book now in your hands, *The Body Code. The Body Code* helps us understand the physical body's manner of holding and processing your emotions in a way that may cause disease, disorder, and other harmful health conditions, and it does so in easy-to-follow language that empowers the reader to intimately glean how the body works as it is integrated along with our emotional condition. The body will inevitably speak to you in all of its mysterious intelligence. Pay attention and become acquainted with what it is saying within the context of symptoms so that you are able to resolve the condition being expressed.

What if you could have insight into what can't be explained about your health? What if you could get direct information from your subconscious? There are many things in the body that still baffle us; however the one thing that we now know for sure is that the brain and body are connected. The fine body of work contained here in *The Body Code* gives you a method to understand your body's coding system. In other words, it gives you the keys to unlock the mysteries that currently baffle you. I'm delighted to see hundreds of thousands of people learning to unlock the mysteries of their bodies with Dr. Bradley Nelson's work. I wish you the same.

Allow yourself the adventure of cracking codes and solving mysteries while giving your body a greater chance of recovering, healing, and staying healthy so that you can live actively and thrive as we are all destined to do. Enjoy the experience this book will give you, and enjoy the journey!

George Noory, host, *Coast to Coast AM*

INVITATION

Things were going great in my life, and a friend said, "Well, one thing you can count on about life—it'll change." I had to laugh, as I realized she was right. Everything can be going along really well, and then suddenly something unexpected can happen, something that really throws you off balance. As much as you plan, prepare, and work toward any substantial goal, there's sure to be a bump or a turn in the road, something you didn't want or couldn't have anticipated. That doesn't mean you shouldn't seek dreams or set goals. It just means that opportunities come with challenges. That's just how life is, and that's how it's meant to be.

Has life handed you something challenging? Are you looking for a solution to regain your health or heal your injured body? Maybe you have loved ones who need help and you lack the ability to help them. Are you suffering from a broken heart? Do you want a deeper or more connected and loving relationship? Maybe you're unable to find success with your work. Is something undefined keeping you from reaching for your dream? Maybe you are still searching for your life's purpose. Often, it's those perceived challenges and difficulties and the desire to do better or have more that can cause you to search for answers in unfamiliar places.

This book is an introduction to a simple and practical method for finding solutions to create balance and function for your body and your life. It is my hope that you don't let the problems of life hold you back or keep you stuck when you could have better health, greater success, and more happiness. I have been teaching, sharing, and finding solutions to intractable problems, using this method or way of thinking, for over thirty years. It has worked very well for me and for countless others. I'd like to help you, too.

Everybody has something that they want to change, something that bothers them or something that causes distress. You probably don't have to think very hard about what that is for you. You might even have a few things in your life that you really want to change in big ways.

We all seek answers from time to time, because life is always changing, bringing its inherent difficulties. I hope to impress upon you the accessibility of the answers so that you know where to turn when you most need help.

Almost anyone can use the Body Code to find answers that make all the difference in how they feel. Others use the Body Code as a tool to help their families and loved ones at home without compensation. Some use it to propel their own lives in a new direction of meaning, purpose, and joy. Some take our online courses and become certified practitioners of The Body Code to truly master the process and create or augment their own healing practice.

Most people who use the Body Code reestablish enough balance to allow for the natural flow of self-healing and progress—to feel better, alleviate pain, reduce doctor visits, improve function, increase creativity, break through mental blocks, improve relationships, and more.

Before you jump into the chapters about what the Body Code is, how it works, and how to use it, I suggest you deeply consider a few basic principles that will greatly increase your opportunity for success:

1. **Open yourself to new information.**
   I'm going to offer concepts that might be new to you. When you're open to new information, you're more likely to get results you've never had before. None of us knows everything there is to know. For example, what do we know about the universe? We are sitting on the edge of a galaxy with billions of stars. Our galaxy sits within trillions of galaxies. With all the possibilities out there, could it be that there are simple, powerful, and effective ways of accessing healing that you've never heard of?

   I'm sure that, in spite of decades of working at it, and though some might consider me an expert in energy healing, I may understand only a fraction of what there is to know about this topic. What I have learned thus far has been life changing for me and for those with whom I have worked. I believe what I know will be valuable to you, too.

   I hope you will be open, even though this information may be new to you. If you admit that there is more for you to know, you will be positioned to be teachable. The things that I will share have been tried and proven to be true many times with many individuals.

   If you are ready to decrease your emotional and physical pain, have more fulfilling relationships, create a better future, help others on their journeys of happiness and success, and do this all by the light of love and gratitude, then you must suspend skepticism and disbelief while reading this book. If you will open your mind to new possibilities and enjoy the journey, it will be a rewarding one.
2. **Have reasons for achieving your desires that are bigger than yourself.**

Without a vision for your future, you may not have a strong enough reason to get well, to get unstuck, and to move forward. Wanting to be free from pain can be a huge motivator, but is it compelling enough? Take a moment to envision the life you want. Imagine how much more joy you might feel. Envision how you are a contribution to the world with your new outlook and energy, to make others' lives better as a peacemaker, or as whatever state of being moves you. Through this work, you will be freed to make that contribution. Start deciding now what that might look like for you.

3. **Choose to work with the energy of love.**

   As you open your heart and mind to the unknown, let me offer a word of caution. Opposites exist in all things—light and dark, health and sickness, love and hate. As you open yourself to learning the Body Code, choose to do so with love, not fear. Trust that love and truth carry enduring transformative power, and that working within the bounds of this light will keep you on a positive path of progress.

   Positive and negative energies swirl around us. Consider that as you work in the positive energy of light, joy, hope, and love, that the darkness automatically retreats. Just like flipping on a light switch, the darkness is instantly gone.

   For this reason, you are invited to draw upon whatever faith tradition you may have. That which you can passionately feel and that which inspires gratitude, peace, and love will guide you through this work.

   The essence of the Body Code is restoration. The body has an innate way of healing itself. The Body Code simply helps you find the causes of imbalance so that they can be addressed and corrected. As you create balance, the way to healing is open for mind, heart, and body.

   This is your invitation to empowerment, to help yourself and others, and to discover the joy that comes with the art of healing.

TERMINOLOGY

Some of the words that I will be using in this book may be substituted with other words if they make you more comfortable or if they fit your own belief system better. For example, when I use the word "God," feel free to substitute "Higher Power," "Source Energy," "Creator," or any other word that might make you more comfortable.

The key terms listed in Appendix 3 are the ones most frequently used in this book. Since there is often no standard definition for each of these that everyone agrees upon, I offer my own definitions in hope of creating some clarity. For example, one particularly puzzling set of terms is "spirit" and "subconscious." While I see them as two separate aspects of the self, with distinct purposes, I use them interchangeably in this book for simplicity.

The philosophical discussion on this topic could fill volumes, but what matters most for our practice of the Body Code is that we can access the answers we need through that intelligence within us all, which I will refer to as the "subconscious mind."

PART I

FOUNDATIONS

Not only is the Universe stranger than we think,
it is stranger than we can think.

—WERNER HEISENBERG

1

INTRODUCTION TO THE BODY CODE

Future medicine will be the medicine of frequencies.

—ALBERT EINSTEIN

I have good news in this age of uncertainty. Seemingly miraculous things are quietly unfolding everywhere. People like you and me are gently lifting their loved ones out of depression, anxiety, chronic illness, pain, and more. We seem to have direct access to light and truth as never before. The art of healing used to be limited to highly educated professionals, but no longer. Over the last few decades, simple and effective methods of natural healing have emerged. These new ways of healing and transforming are not arising from Western medicine. Rather than being based on yet another pharmaceutical drug or a new surgical approach, these innovative methods take advantage of new understandings of quantum physics and neurobiology and epigenetics, to name a few. We are finally beginning to treat the human body for what it actually is, a highly complex energy field.

No matter what you are dealing with, things can change. Maybe you are exhausted from unrelenting physical pain. Maybe you find yourself feeling easily triggered and emotionally drained afterward. Perhaps your relationships are stressful and unfulfilling, or it may be that you are dealing with a diagnosis that seems hopeless. No matter what your issue is, resolution and healing are possible.

I am energized and excited by what has suddenly become available to us. I am humbled and thrilled to see a mother help her child eliminate asthma, or a grandfather teach his grandchildren how to remove anxiety, or a woman help a friend eliminate her knee pain. I've even seen people help their pets return to full health. In this book, I am going to explain how simple it can be to find and eliminate the underlying imbalances that cause stress, pain, and disease, that block fulfilling and loving relationships, and that hold you back from being your best self.

In my first book, *The Emotion Code,* I explained how your subconscious mind, your vastly intelligent inner self, knows all about the "emotional baggage" you are holding on to. The Emotion Code provides a way for you to find and remove your own trapped emotions, the emotional baggage that has been disrupting your life, creating physical, mental, and emotional symptoms.

In the last three decades of working with people of all ages who were suffering from all kinds of diseases, disorders, and symptoms, I have learned repeatedly that the subconscious mind knows the true reasons for a person's suffering. The subconscious knows about the trapped emotions that are causing your physical pain, contributing to disease processes, or blocking your success. It even knows about inherited emotional energies that may have been passed down for generations, sabotaging your life.

The global success of the Emotion Code is largely because it teaches people how to tap into their subconscious minds, ask questions, and easily receive answers, empowering people to take their health into their own hands by finding and releasing their trapped emotions.

The Body Code expands on the Emotion Code, teaching how you can access the subconscious mind to address the other sorts of imbalances you may be dealing with. It's vital to understand that these imbalances are the underlying reasons behind your physical, mental, and emotional symptoms.

Not only does your subconscious mind know about your emotional baggage, it also knows perfectly well about all of the other imbalances in your body. For example, if you are missing a certain nutrient that your body needs to function optimally, your subconscious mind knows it. Your subconscious mind knows if there is a low-grade infection that is draining your body's energy. It knows that a misalignment of a tiny bone in your skull is the secret cause of your migraine headaches. Hidden away in your subconscious mind is the knowledge that your allergies are actually being triggered by the mercury fillings you had as a child, a heavy metal that is now overwhelming your liver.

But while imbalances like these are extremely common, they are also easy to identify and resolve, and when they are corrected, your body has an incredible ability to bounce back and regain its health and vitality.

The Body Code System is designed to help you "decode" and correct the imbalances that are the true underlying causes of your problems. It's a comprehensive knowledge base of all that can go wrong in the body, and it uses the laws of quantum physics to create balance where there is imbalance. When these laws are used with love and intention, they enable you to navigate within the body to discover what is wrong and make the corrections that are needed to restore health.

People just like you have successfully used the Body Code to resolve issues such as migraine headaches, neck pain, back pain, knee pain, carpal tunnel syndrome, asthma, morning sickness, fibromyalgia, chronic fatigue, digestive issues, infertility, depression, anxiety, loneliness, painful memories, relationship struggles, panic attacks, post-traumatic stress disorder (PTSD), eating disorders, phobias, money problems, and self-sabotage—to name just a few. The good news is that overcoming problems like these may be much easier than you think, and it usually doesn't require the use of toxic pharmaceutical drugs or surgery.

My goal with this book is to teach you the fundamentals of a whole new way to take care of yourself. The answers are within you. They are available for the asking. Even if you have been sick for decades and feel that you have exhausted every possible option, the truth has been within you all the while. In this book, I will teach you how to find that truth.

Imagine having direct access to the most advanced medical database in the world, one that could give you the "correct" answer for nearly any health-related question you could think of. Now imagine using those answers to help yourself and your loved ones to overcome the health obstacles you face, improving the condition of your lives, and adding vibrancy to your everyday experience of life. What if you could do all of this from anywhere in the world with no need to be in physical contact with the other person? It's not only possible, it's happening every day with many thousands of people worldwide that have learned this simple method of energy healing.

But why do we need this? Our Western "state-of-the-art" medical system has the best and the brightest medical professionals, with trillions of dollars spent annually to support them. Surely, they would have the best answers to all our ills. But for some reason, we are not only struggling to find mental and physical wellness, we seem to be losing the battle. In fact, a recent study showed that less than 5 percent of the world's population had no health problems whatsoever.

WHY ARE WE STILL STRUGGLING?

Something is not working in our health-care system. As of 2014, an estimated 150 million Americans, 47 percent of the population, were suffering from at least one chronic disease*, and that number was projected to grow to 157 million by 2020.

In the United States, we spend the highest amount of money per year on health care of any country—$9,237 per person annually in 2017.† Yet Americans die younger and suffer higher rates of disease than people in sixteen other developed nations.

Medical errors and prescription-drug misuse or overdose are among the leading causes of death in the United States. Many of the surgeries performed are drastic and unnecessary. The United States spends more on health care as a share of the economy than any other country in the world, yet it has the lowest life expectancy and one of the highest suicide rates among the industrialized nations.

What all this money is buying us is neither good health nor happiness. In one study, the United States ranked seventeenth on a list of seventeen affluent nations for overall health.‡

I believe that Dr. Benjamin Rush, one of the signers of the American Declaration of Independence, was prescient when he reportedly said:

> *Unless we put Medical Freedom into the Constitution, the time will come when medicine will organize into an undercover dictatorship to restrict the art of healing to one class of men and companies, and deny equal privileges to others, and will constitute the Bastille of medical science.*

Unfortunately, his prediction has come to pass, and this is now exactly the situation we find ourselves in, at least in the United States of America.

Why is the health of Americans so poor, even though we're throwing more money at this problem than any other country? What are we doing wrong? One reason is that medicine is largely focused on chasing symptoms. And chasing symptoms is a very ineffective way to take care of the body.

In the minds of most people, symptoms are the problem, and they need to be suppressed. Most of the drugs produced by pharmaceutical companies are designed to suppress symptoms.

---

*https://www.americanactionforum.org/research/chronic-disease-in-the-united-states-a-worsening-health-and-economic-crisis/

†https://www.npr.org/sections/goatsandsoda/2017/04/20/524774195/what-country-spends-the-most-and-least-on-health-care-per-person

‡https://www.theatlantic.com/health/archive/2013/01/new-health-rankings-of-17-nations-us-is-dead-last/267045/

Most people have taken medications to suppress symptoms of one kind or another, which can be very appropriate at times. But suppressing symptoms doesn't solve the underlying causes of those symptoms; it merely masks them.

Chasing symptoms is ultimately ineffective. Because this happens so frequently, it's not unusual for people over sixty years old to be on a dozen or more different medications at the same time. Some of those medications are taken to counteract side effects of other drugs they are already taking, and it's impossible to determine what dangerous drug interactions may be occurring when so many different drugs are being consumed.

But what if we looked at symptoms in another way entirely?

As a practicing doctor of chiropractic, I did not have a license to prescribe medication that would suppress people's symptoms, nor could I perform surgery to remove troublesome organs. So I was faced with the dilemma of having to figure out what was actually causing people's problems.

One particular patient comes to mind. Sheryl had hurt her back lifting one of her children and had come to me for help. As I spoke with her, I could see she was very uncomfortable. It wasn't just her back pain. She was also suffering from a migraine headache that she'd had for the previous two weeks without any break. She was taking potent medications to deal with her symptoms, with little effect.

During her treatment, I found that she had a misaligned bone at the base of her skull. When I realigned that bone through a chiropractic adjustment, suddenly her migraine was gone, instantly and completely. This was totally unexpected and quite baffling to her, but she was grateful for the relief, although she seemed a bit confused.

I saw her again about a week later, and I was surprised by her emotional state. She was angry. At first, I thought she was angry at me, but she explained:

I've had migraine headaches almost every day for the last twenty years. I've been to many different doctors during these last two decades, and all they've done is prescribe drugs for me to treat my migraines. The last twenty years have been like a living hell. I can't tell you how many countless hours I've spent in a dark room with the shades drawn, trying to endure this pain. I can't tell you how much money I've spent on all these medications that have been prescribed for me, some of which have been very expensive and have made me sick. I have not had any headache pain of any kind since I was here and you adjusted me. I'm not angry at you; I'm angry at all those doctors that I saw over all those years, because not one of them ever told me that there might be an underlying cause for my migraines. All they did was give me medication and tell me to live with it, and that there was nothing that could really be done. They should have known. I'm angry because I've lost twenty years of my life that I cannot ever get back.

Sheryl's story is all too common in the Western medical system. Over the years I've seen too many people with stories like hers. And you can't really blame the doctors. They are doing the best they can, but their education and training is slanted toward suppressing people's symptoms instead of finding the root causes of illness.

Until Western medicine can adopt a more holistic approach, people are seeking alternatives that work, and the Body Code fills that need very well. And while I will not be teaching you how to realign bones in this book, I will be helping you to understand how to remove the underlying imbalances that cause many misalignments.

HEROIC MEASURES

The traditional approach to medicine matured on the battlefield in the Civil War and in World Wars I and II. It developed around a concept that I like to call "heroic measures." That means that if you're a soldier and a cannonball comes bouncing along on the battlefield and takes off your leg, you'd better hope your doctor performs heroic measures on you, and fast, because you certainly need urgent help. Of course, there have been many doctors on the battlefields and in the operating rooms who have performed heroic feats and lifesaving surgeries, and there are certainly times when these are absolutely the best choice.

The problem, however, is that this focus on last-minute intervention has created a situation in which we are prone to wait until a crisis erupts before we do anything about it. As a result, modern Western medicine focuses on external causes of disease, on dramatic intervention, and symptomatic relief. I was faced with the dilemma of having to figure out what was actually causing people's problems.

SURGERY—A DRAMATIC INTERVENTION

Surgery is the most common dramatic intervention in Western medicine. Certainly, there are times when surgery is appropriate, after a traumatic accident, for example. Advances in microsurgery have yielded astonishing benefits that have resulted in successful reattachment of fingers and limbs, requiring the incredibly precise reconnecting of tiny blood vessels and even nerves. No one is more grateful for these advances than those who have benefited in their own time of crisis.

Surgery is sometimes perfectly appropriate, but it has proven to be an unnecessary form of treatment in too many cases. It is extremely invasive, and is often ineffective. For example, in 1976, the American Medical Association (AMA) called for a congressional hearing on unnecessary surgery, claiming that there were "2.4 million unnecessary operations performed on Americans at a cost of $3.9 billion, and 11,900 patients had died from unneeded operations." And over forty years later, not much has changed.*

What if those patients had tried the Body Code before having surgery? In this next story, a Body Code practitioner named Norah helped a client do just that.

Back Surgery Averted

I worked with a man who suffered from severe back pain and who had been awaiting surgery for many months. His lumbar spine was deteriorating badly. In our first Body Code session, we corrected imbalances in each one of his lumbar vertebrae. In the second session, we both set an intention to eliminate the pain, so he would no longer need the medications he was currently taking. He did a liver cleanse and stopped eating gluten. Since our Body Code sessions, he now is walking daily, on no medications, and for the most part is free of pain. We continue to work on inflammation energy and releasing trapped emotions as needed. One of many miracles!

—Norah B., British Columbia, Canada

Physical pain is probably the most common symptom that human beings have to deal with. In 2016, it was estimated that approximately 50 million people in the United States were suffering from chronic pain, or about 15 percent of the population.

In the Western world, we tend to rely on drugs and surgery as ways to find relief from our symptoms, rather than working to remain free of the imbalances that are the causes of our symptoms in the first place. It's a very expensive way to conduct a health-care system, or more accurately, a sickness-care system. For the tremendous and often prohibitive cost, it's not surprising that people have looked for alternatives. It not only hits them in their pocketbooks, but robs them of their precious time and quality of life.

In Carmen's story, a dark future full of pain and suffering was changed by a friend who learned to use the Body Code.

A Different Future

A very close friend of mine got vaccinated before a trip, and shortly after, while on holiday in Costa Rica, she started experiencing lots of pain and inflammation through her body, as well as brain fog and paranoia, making it unbearable to be around others. . . . She eventually was diagnosed with lupus, fibromyalgia, and osteoarthritis, and

*Stahel, P. F., VanderHeiden, T. F. and Kim, F. J. "Why Do Surgeons Continue to Perform Unnecessary Surgery?" *Patient Saf Surg* 11, no.1 (2017): https://doi.org/10.1186/s13037-016-0117-6

was hurting from head to toe. Her specialist said she would have to live like this for the rest of her life, managing her discomfort with prescription medication, which made her feel even worse.

At this point I had become certified in the Emotion Code with the Body Code to follow. We addressed her discomfort and inflammation, as well as all the toxicity. It took quite a few sessions addressing these chronic symptoms, but after each session she noticed an improvement! She said I was the answer to her prayers. That was five years ago! Today she lives free of suffering, takes no medication, and her energy levels feel like she's back in her twenties, even though she's sixty-two. I remember all the distress she continually suffered. It was horrible. She said I was her godsend and wished me great success with this incredible technique. Brenda is also now a fellow Emotion Code practitioner, and has also touched so many lives.

—Carmen D., Ontario, Canada

A TURNING POINT IN HEALING

Just a few decades ago, scientific thought denied the existence of any sort of human energy field. Since then, scientists have completely changed their minds. They now know with certainty that an energy field exists.

For example, one device, called the SQUID (superconducting quantum interference device) magnetometer, can detect the biomagnetic fields, that are created by the biochemical and physiological activities of the body.

Biomagnetic fields around the body have been found to give a more accurate reading of a patient's health than traditional electrical measurements, such as EEGs and EKGs. In fact, scientists now know that the heart's electromagnetic field is so powerful that it can be accurately measured three feet away from the body. The reading can be taken from any point on the body and any point in the electromagnetic field, because the field itself contains the information in a three-dimensional, or holographic, way.

Still, the importance of the energy field is not taken into account in conventional Western medical practices. As a result, patients often suffer needlessly due to lack of proper attention to the underlying causes of their illnesses.

Recently, however, many nontraditional healing practices have shifted from being ridiculed to being respected. This is so partly because technology has improved, allowing scientists to test more accurately, and also because these alternative healing methods actually do work. For example, a popular mental health modality called EMDR (Eye Movement Desensitization and Reprocessing) is one of the most effective treatments for PTSD among veterans, according to multiple studies. However, less than twenty years ago, it was considered quackery by accredited institutions. Even at that, EMDR for PTSD is often recommended as a three-month-minimum process, whereas the Body Code and other energy-related methods are frequently effective within days or weeks.

Another example of an effective and widely embraced alternative modality is acupuncture. Wikipedia, as of this writing, reads,

> *Acupuncture is a pseudoscience; the theories and practices of TCM [traditional Chinese medicine] are not based on scientific knowledge, and it has been characterized as quackery.*

However, *Scientific American,* a popular science magazine, in 2014 said:

> *Strong evidence exists that acupuncture is effective for chronic pain conditions. For depression, we have evidence that acupuncture is a useful adjunct to conventional care. In one recent trial patients on antidepressants who received acupuncture did significantly better than those who just took medication.*

Perhaps more compelling are the testimonials of millions of people who have found relief from pain and have improved their health through acupuncture since its beginning thousands of years ago.

The knowledge and understanding of the energy meridians that have long been used and recognized by Chinese medical doctors were once considered mysterious and strange by Westerners. But now that mainstream science is beginning to acknowledge that alternative therapies are actually viable, more people are open to methods that utilize energy. Acupuncture in particular is being recognized for its energetic healing power. Chiropractic adjustments, which remove nerve interference, are also being proven in clinical trials to have long-lasting and significant benefits, something that chiropractic doctors and patients have known for over one hundred years.

Chiropractic was nearly destroyed by a highly organized smear campaign that resulted in a successful lawsuit against the American Medical Association, the American College of Surgeons, and the American College of Radiology. In 1987, federal judge Susan Getzendanner described their conspiracy as "systematic, long-term wrongdoing and the long-term intent to destroy a licensed profession." Judge Getzendanner's decision said the nation's largest physicians' group spearheaded a physicians' boycott designed to "contain and eliminate the chiropractic profession."

Over the last thirty years, there has been an accelerating shift to natural healing methods, including methods of energy healing. People are looking for noninvasive ways to get well, while the medical-pharmaceutical establishment has been doubling down on questionable vaccination practices and chemical therapies.

Abundant evidence exists to prove that the human body is an energetic, vibrant, emotional, and spiritual being. Attempting to treat every illness with drugs and/or surgery is proving to be a primitive approach to the body, in light of what we are learning about the nature of energy and of the universe.

Today, we are at a turning point in medical history. With the discoveries of quantum physics and quantum biology proving that everything is energy and that all things are interrelated, a door has been opened. To relieve suffering, addressing the true underlying imbalances—the actual reasons for the symptoms—is a vastly more efficient and effective way of restoring wholeness and health.

Research will continue to push back the boundaries on what we know about the human energy field. As it does, I am hopeful that energetic imbalances and the damage they cause will eventually be fully recognized by the medical community. Magnetic and energetic healing techniques that alternative practitioners use are beginning to be integrated into conventional medicine to provide the best, most thorough, and most gentle healing possible.

Consider this experience, when Western medicine couldn't help a woman's paralyzed arm, but in one session, a man named Robert used the Body Code to do just that.

A Paralyzed Arm

When first learning to use the Body Code, I'd often go to the students' homes in the treatment program that I ran. I'd do the Body Code with anyone who wanted to. After an evening session was almost over, a female staff member asked me if I'd work on her left arm. She shared that for many years she was unable to lift her arm due to paralysis. She had no feeling in that arm, even though she had been going to a doctor and had accumulated years of doctor bills. Using the Body Code, we found and released some imbalances. Soon after her session, she reported that her arm was starting to tingle. A little later she found out she could lift her arm a little. As I was getting ready to leave, to the amazement of us all, she lifted her arm all the way above her head. Her arm has been fine ever since, and that was a few years ago. When she showed her doctor that she could lift her arm and told him about the energy work, he emphatically announced, "That is impossible!"

—Robert N., Utah, United States

I'm reminded of the quote from the great science-fiction writer Arthur C. Clarke, who said, "Any sufficiently advanced technology is indistinguishable from magic." The Body Code is not magic, but it is very advanced technology indeed.

If you can find the underlying imbalances that cause disease, you can remove them. The Body Code makes it easy.

MY EXPOSURE TO ALTERNATIVE MEDICINE

When I was thirteen years old, I began to suffer from severe pain in my back that would come and go, striking me unexpectedly and taking my breath away. My anxious parents took me to the hospital, where diagnostic tests showed that I was suffering from a form of kidney disease. Many years later, my mother told me that the doctors privately told her and my father that I had a fifty-fifty chance of survival, but that there was no medical treatment available for my condition. Since there was nothing Western medicine had to offer, they were on their own to help me. The doctors had no advice, except to say that I shouldn't run or play, to avoid jostling my kidneys. I didn't need to hear this, as it had become more than self-evident. Sometimes the slightest movements would result in excruciating pain.

Our lives were turned upside down. Suddenly my life was in jeopardy. My parents were deeply concerned, and I was walking on eggshells to avoid the sudden, stabbing pains that would shoot through my body.

When I was a young boy, I can recall making many trips to the health-food store with my mother. She was considered by many to be a "health nut." This was long before it became popular or trendy. Back then, the medical profession seemed to think that anyone who took vitamins was actually a bit crazy and that people who rejected drugs and surgery as their main methods of health care were truly "nuts."

Our shelves at home were stocked with all kinds of vitamin supplements, which my mother doled out to us regularly. She was very interested in health and was constantly studying natural treatments and remedies. She seemed to know just about everything that was related to health. People would often call her and ask her advice on various health topics, and she was never without an answer or a suggestion.

So when my parents were told that Western medicine had nothing to offer their sick son, my mother was undaunted. She and my father took me to see some alternative doctors. In fact, these doctors seemed to me to be an entirely different breed than those in the hospital who had not given my parents much hope. They didn't practice in a hospital. Instead, they practiced out on the edge of town in a trailer house, situated in the middle of a wheat field. I can remember sometimes having to scrape the mud off my shoes when we would go to see them. I can also remember seeing busloads of people who had come from other states to see these alternative doctors, traveling hundreds of miles to get the help that they could not get anywhere else.

These two doctors did not practice Western medicine at all. Instead, they looked at the body as a whole. They began treating me as a whole person, giving me herbal drinks that were bitter tasting, and realigning the bones of my spine.

The result? Immediately, the pain began to be both less frequent and less severe. Within a few weeks I was feeling dramatically better. Before long, I was back to my normal life and had nearly forgotten that I had ever been sick.

Just to be on the safe side, my parents took me back to the clinic to have the same medical doctors run their tests again. As I recall, the tests were run not once more, but twice. They were negative. I was cured, but not by the medical doctors in that big, expensive clinic. I knew that they hadn't actually done anything to help me.

Instead, those holistic doctors practicing out on the edge of town in an old trailer house in a muddy field had saved my life. I knew in my heart, at the core of my being, that what these people had done was exactly what my body needed. It seemed odd to me that the medical profession did not understand what to do for me. In fact, they had offered me nothing whatsoever. It was at that point in my life that I decided I wanted to grow up to be a doctor that knew how to help people get well.

If I needed to practice out on the edge of town in a trailer house in a muddy field, that was okay with me. As far as I could tell, that seemed to be the natural habitat of doctors who got results.

THE FIBROMYALGIA SUPPORT GROUP

Many years ago, I was invited to be the guest speaker for a fibromyalgia support group held at a local hospital. In case you are not familiar with it, fibromyalgia is a very painful and often hopeless condition resulting in widespread and irreversible muscle pain with no known cause. I spoke for about an hour to this group of fifty people. I couldn't help but notice one woman, sitting a couple of rows back, who cried quietly through my entire presentation.

When I finished, she told me that she'd had fibromyalgia for nineteen years. She had been to nine different doctors over those past nineteen years, and all of them had told her the same thing. They said that there really was no hope for her to ever be well again. She'd been told that all she could do was take the medications that they recommended and resign herself to living with the pain. She apologized for crying but said that she cried every day because of her intense pain. She wanted me to know that she cried during my presentation not only due to her pain, but also because it was the first time in all those years that she'd ever heard a doctor say that there might be hope for her to get well.

When she came to my office, I examined her and found that she was imbalanced in all of the six areas that the Body Code addresses. She had a lot of misalignments in her spine, creating poor communication between her brain and the organs and glands and other tissues of her body. She had a Heart-Wall (where emotional energies become wrapped around the heart), along with other trapped emotions. When I checked her for pathogens, I found parasites as well as a number of viral infections. She had multiple nutritional deficiencies, toxicity, and imbalances of her organs and glands. Her subconscious mind indicated all of this through muscle testing. When you know how to ask questions and get answers from the subconscious mind, it's amazing how easily and quickly the answers come.

I started working on her regularly, correcting these imbalances. Within three weeks her fibromyalgia symptoms were entirely gone. In fact, the only pain she had left was from the arthritis that she had been dealing with for many years in her right thumb. She could live with that minor discomfort. Her life was transformed.

During the last ten years of my practice, I saw many patients suffering from chronic and supposedly incurable diseases. The vast majority of them were able to get well, with just a couple of exceptions. Sometimes they got well very rapidly. Some of them got well over the course of just a few weeks, some over months, others over many months. The point is that when you're asking the subconscious mind for the true underlying causes of sickness, it can provide you with the shortest path to wellness.

Navigating the often debilitating challenges of physical, emotional, and mental health can be overwhelming. We need new ways of addressing our problems. Integrating mind and body healing practices is not new. But doing so with a method that anyone can learn and that is relatively quick is revolutionary.

In Mie's story, her entire family was transformed by the impact of just one person using the Body Code to bless and to heal.

Healing a Family

My mom, who is seventy years old, alarmed us when she started to show dementia-like symptoms and mild hallucinations. She was acting as though she'd aged thirty years within a few months. My family was distraught. I felt especially helpless because I left Japan and could not help from afar. All I could do was research her symptoms and her medications and make suggestions. Just some of her medical conditions included insomnia, high blood pressure, irregular heartbeat, and a severe stomachache, each having its own prescribed medication, with side effects.

That's when I happened to read *The Emotion Code* book. I started to apply Emotion Code healing on her as soon as I got the idea. Her Heart-Wall and more than two hundred trapped emotions were removed within a couple of months.

My dad, who had been taking care of her, could not believe the changes he started to see in her. She was communicating just like she used to. She slept through the night without any medication (which she'd been taking for more than fifteen years), and her stomachache disappeared. Her communications became as quick and witty as before, and her hallucinations were gone.

She gained her health and her smile back! My dad thanked me countless times and said, "My loving Seiko has come back! Whatever healing you did for your mom, it worked, and it's amazing!"

When my sister saw the changes my mom went through, she asked me to work on her back pain. After two or three sessions, she called me and said she no longer needed to rest to ease her back pain, even after working on her feet for hours.

She also asked me to work on my eight-year-old nephew, who had been suffering from asthma since he was a baby. After releasing about thirty trapped emotions, he called me and said he could breathe well, and he stopped taking the asthma medication. I can't forget his happy voice saying, "Thank you, Auntie, I can breathe now!" It's been amazing. I can't thank you enough.

—Mie T., Ontario, Canada

It is important to understand that the Emotion Code is a part of the Body Code, the part that enables you to release emotional baggage or trapped emotions that cause dysfunction in the body. In Mie's story, just using the Emotion Code alone was enough to make an enormous difference in the lives of her loved ones.

The Body Code allows anyone with minimal training to fully unlock the vast healing power of the subconscious mind. It is simple yet incredibly powerful and comprehensive, and it enables anyone to practice the art of healing in a spiritual, holistic, and complete way. I have long believed that every person on this planet has the ability to heal themselves and others. It is the birthright of every man, woman, and child to be a healer.

I agree wholeheartedly with Norm Shealy, MD, founding president of the American Holistic Medical Association, who said, "Energy medicine is the future of all medicine." The Body Code is my contribution to that better future.

I believe that all healing will soon revolve around the profound understanding that the answers truly live within each one of us and are available for the asking. This is the simple beauty of the Body Code, and I believe it will change the world.

2

WHAT IS THE BODY CODE?

The day science begins to study non-physical phenomena, it will make more progress in one decade than in all the previous centuries of its existence.

—NIKOLA TESLA

The Body Code offers us a revolution in how we can take care of ourselves and others. People are suddenly finding out that there's an incredible amount they can do themselves for their own health without having to rely on doctors or medications.

The Body Code is a "knowledge base" of imbalances, or things that can go wrong in the body. It gives your subconscious mind a way to reveal the true underlying causes of ailments, whether those imbalances have combined to create symptoms or not. The Body Code can be thought of as a table of contents for the things your subconscious mind is tracking.

The Body Code is the result of deep study of the human body, time-proven ancient practices, meditation, inspiration, and the unlimited power of the subconscious mind. When you access the subconscious mind, you're tapping into the most powerful computer that we know of, a computer that holds all the answers and knows with a perfect understanding what is really needed to create optimum health and wellness. My training and experience as a computer programmer as well as a holistic physician has helped me to make this simple for those who use it.

Most physical, mental, and emotional issues we face can be addressed with the Body Code System, because it comprehends nearly all possible imbalances of the mind, body, and spirit. It's a comprehensive tool that is being used to help people of all ages, from newborns to the elderly. And it's not only for improving your health. It can be used to enhance or repair relationships, uncover blocks to abundance, and help in finding your heart's desire. It can even help you overcome blockages to better performance at school, home, work, or sports. The Body Code makes it simple to remove blocks to success of all sorts.

For those who fully desire to change and are willing to put forth effort, not only will their thoughts and ways of being shift, but their very futures will often transform. The Body Code helps them create a new future—a new reality with less pain, dissatisfaction, and self-sabotage, in which dreams more easily become reality.

DISCOVERY OF THE BODY CODE

Obtaining the knowledge to create what eventually became the Body Code System took many years. As I was learning through experience with my patients, my understanding of many aspects of health and well-being gradually increased, piece by piece. My childhood illnesses and remarkable recoveries instilled a great desire to help others as I had been helped. I had an early understanding of what was really possible, regardless of the conventional wisdom of the day.

Before I knew that I was going to become a doctor, I took a computer class in college. Computer programming ignited a new passion that still serves me today. I took the class on a whim but was entirely captivated. Computers appealed to the perfectionist in me. If a program has an issue, it won't run correctly until it's fixed. For the next few years, I dove into this world with all my heart and soul and loved every minute. I became a self-taught computer programmer and began making a living freelancing as "The Computer Tutor." Little did I know how this experience would affect my future as a healer.

For a time, I had decided that becoming a doctor was only a dream, one that would remain unfulfilled. I had never been particularly good at math, and I found the idea of having to take chemistry and physics courses intimidating. I came to the conclusion that I would forget about becoming a doctor and pursue a degree in business.

I was six months away from going into the MBA program at Brigham Young University in Provo, Utah, when my wife, Jean, and I traveled from Utah to Montana with our little daughter

Natalie to visit my parents for Christmas. As we sat around the fireplace talking, my father suddenly asked me if I was still interested in going to chiropractic school. He said that it seemed like a great career and reminded me that I had always wanted to go into the healing arts. I replied that I had made my career decision, that I was going to get a master's degree in business administration and go to work for a big corporation. I loved working with computers and studying business processes, and I felt that getting an MBA would be a good career path for me.

He said, "Well, why don't you think about it one more time?" After a moment's pause, I replied that I would give it some more thought and consider it again. I had a great deal of respect for my dad. He was wise and had been very successful in business. I knew he had my best interest at heart. He had always enjoyed being his own boss, and I think he felt that I'd be happier being a healer in my own practice than working for someone else. Because of my dad's influence and suggestion, suddenly I had a lot to contemplate.

SEEKING AN ANSWER

Have you ever had a situation in your life in which you went from having everything figured out to suddenly arriving back at a place of uncertainty? My old dream of going into the healing arts had somehow been resurrected. I was now faced with two very different futures. Either could be very rewarding. I wasn't sure any longer what direction my life should take. I had to think. I felt that it was important to figure it out right away.

Jean and I discussed the two options together. We decided to compare them on paper by drawing up a pro-and-con list, one side for the business world and computer programming, the other side for a healing practice of our own. The list was long on both sides. This exercise wasn't enough to solve our dilemma. Both options were compelling. I felt the weight of the decision. My career and the future of my family rested upon it. But was there a right and a wrong about this? Was one decision better than the other? I couldn't tell. I felt that I could go either way and have a good life.

Having learned at a young age that there is a Higher Power I could draw upon, I decided that I really could use some help with this. I believe the Higher Power hears us and is interested in helping us. So that night before bed, I got on my knees and asked for guidance. I said, "Father in Heaven, if it makes any difference to you, please help me to know what direction I should go. I'll do whatever you think I should do." I thought that if it mattered to Him, He would let me know.

A few hours later I was awakened, as if from an unremembered dream, to a mind filled with thoughts of how wonderful it is to help people to heal naturally, to serve people, to serve God and family. I thought to myself, "Well, that's certainly true. But I also love computers, and business, and . . ." With that last thought, I fell back to sleep. After a while, I had the same experience again, and felt those same feelings about health and serving people naturally, just as I'd had before. I countered the impressions with the same conscious thoughts about computers and business, and I went back to sleep. The whole experience was repeated a third time.

At this point, you may be thinking that the answer should have been obvious to me, that the Higher Power was trying to communicate with me, and you'd be right. The next day, I mulled over my experiences of the previous night but still couldn't come to a conclusion about what path to take. I guess I thought I would have to give up computers, and I loved assembling them and programming them. Little did I know then that I would have plenty of time to use computers and incorporate them into my future healing practice.

The next night found me once again on my knees, asking for guidance. And incredibly, I had the same experience that second night. I was again awakened three times, but with a marked difference. Each time I was awakened on that second night, the feelings seemed to be exponentially more powerful than the time before. When I was awakened the third time on that second night, the thoughts of service and healing to the entire world, to all of humanity, were absolutely overwhelming. Just at that moment, I heard a very clear voice that spoke to me and said, "This is a sacred calling." I had received my answer in an unmistakable way. I now knew the road I was to follow, and I never looked back.

I've thought a lot about that experience. I believe that our very existence is sacred, and as a result, anytime we are helping someone to feel better, to function better, to be able to live his or her life more fully, we are doing something special. I believe that each of us has a destiny to fulfill and a mission to perform while we sojourn on this earth. Illness can stop us in our tracks and prevent us from living the life we could be living. I believe it is a sacred calling to help those who are ill to recover, because the ripple effect from their healed lives never ends.

(To learn more about my spiritual beliefs, visit drbradleynelson.com/my-beliefs.)

STAYING OPEN

I can remember lying on my back on a treatment table as a thirteen-year-old boy while those holistic doctors were working on me. I told them several times, "I want to do what you do when I grow up." Their response was always the same. "No, you don't. If you go to some school of natural medicine, you'll become so indoctrinated and so full of fixed ideas about healing that you won't be able to think for yourself."

These people had saved my life. I believed everything they told me. So when I finally enrolled in chiropractic school, I was very much on guard. I questioned anything that was taught as being the "best way" to do this or that. I tried to stay completely open to any alternative that might work. I was always looking for additional insight.

The thing I loved the most was learning all the intricacies of the human body—how it works automatically and does all of the things it needs to do to keep us alive from one moment to the next.

One of the most amazing things that I remember learning is that many of our responses are hardwired into us. For example, if you reach out and touch a hot stove, the pain message travels along the nerves to the brain, and the muscles in your arm respond almost instantly. The result is that, before the fact that you are being burned has even reached your conscious awareness, you are already pulling your hand away from the stove.

I learned about the nervous system in great detail. My classmates and I spent months dissecting human cadavers, truly the best way to learn anatomy. I learned how misaligned vertebrae can irritate or put pressure on the nerve root that has just emerged from the spinal cord on the way to its destination. I learned multiple methods of realigning vertebrae, some forceful, some gentle. I began to appreciate the complexity of the human body and how everything is orchestrated to work together so beautifully.

I was fortunate to attend chiropractic college with my two brothers and my two brothers-in-law, as well as a lot of wonderful and funny people that made the whole experience even more enjoyable. I can remember sitting in classes and hearing my instructors say things like, "The human brain is the most powerful computer in the known universe." The thought fascinated me. I used to wonder, "Will we ever have the technology to access the human computer and get answers from it?" This would be the ultimate way to find out what's really happening within the body.

Little did I know that I would spend the rest of my career doing exactly that, tapping into the subconscious mind—accessing the internal computer that is within each one of us—to find out what was out of balance with my patients and causing their problems.

When I started my private practice, I continued to stay open to any new approach and all possibilities for healing that might help my patients. Whether that meant using some method or some technique that was frowned upon by Western medicine or by anyone else didn't matter to me.

ASKING AND RECEIVING

I learned firsthand that help from above is available. Early on in my private practice I developed a habit of asking for it. Before working on a patient, I would take a moment to direct my thoughts heavenward and ask for help with my patient. This was a completely private, personal effort, which just took a few seconds. I believed that it was important to ask for that help.

I know that the ancient maxim "Ask and you shall receive" is true. On rare occasions, in response to those silent requests, information would suddenly flood into my mind about what my patient needed. Sometimes these downloads would present a completely different way of looking at things than what I'd ever imagined or considered before. It was exciting, and I felt supported and guided in what I was learning.

I didn't care if my treatments were different from what other doctors of my profession were doing, or if my methods seemed a bit out of the ordinary. Interestingly, as my understanding increased over time, things actually became less complicated. The treatments became simpler and faster. Unrelated understandings about the body began to finally fit together like the pieces of an intricate puzzle. The more I learned, the simpler it all became.

I came to understand the cause and effect between various parts of the body and how each part affects the other energetically. With every new understanding, I could see how complex, awe-inspiring, and beautiful the body is, and how simple it is to find the blockages that keep the body from functioning as it was designed.

Before long, my practice grew, and I seemed to attract more complex cases as my knowledge and skills increased.

During the last ten years that I spent in practice, most of my patients were suffering from chronic conditions that were considered incurable by Western medicine. Even so, most of them still held some hope that they could recover.

BELIEF AFFECTS HEALING

Some of my patients, deep down, believed what they had been told—that they'd never get well. I found that when a patient internalized the belief that they couldn't recover, their disbelief stood in the way of their healing. Thought is energy. Belief affects outcome. It became more difficult to work with them because I had to help build their faith in the possibility of recovery. Belief is part of the healing process itself. It's important to want to be well and to believe that getting well and being well are possible.

I consistently told my patients, "I don't treat diseases. I don't claim to cure diseases, but I believe that the symptoms that you are having are because of imbalances that are going on in your body. Imbalances interfere with your body's ability to heal itself. If we can find and remove enough of those imbalances, your body may be better able to heal itself, and perhaps your symptoms may go away." And go away they did. During those years, I saw patients with difficult problems from all over the United States and Canada. The vast majority of them got well, and often did so quite rapidly.

My approach was drastically different from typical Western medical practices. Instead of attempting to suppress my patients' symptoms, I was attempting to address the underlying causes of those symptoms.

I've worked with many different diseases and conditions and have found that they all have underlying causes. When those causes are addressed, the body's natural ability to heal itself is facilitated.

SYMPTOMS ARE YOUR "CHECK ENGINE" LIGHT

If the "check engine" light turns on in your car, you likely have no idea why, but you are being advised that something needs attention—and soon. The symptoms you experience can be thought of as "check engine" lights, alerting you that something is not right in your body.

After more than thirty years practicing the art of natural healing, I have come to the conclusion that almost every symptom we suffer from is a message. Imagine that you have a headache. The pain that you're feeling right now is a message from your subconscious mind. Perhaps you're dehydrated. It may be from a trapped emotion caused by the argument you had with your husband last week, or from your parents' divorce when you were eight years old. Perhaps the headache is a message from your subconscious mind that a bone is out of alignment in your neck or in your skull. That headache may be from a single underlying cause or from several underlying causes. The message—the headache you are experiencing—is designed to get you to seek out and eliminate the underlying causes, whatever they may be.

For example, if you're suffering from depression, please understand that the depression is a symptom. In Western medicine, the depression itself would be seen as the problem. Depression is certainly a difficult state to be in, but in reality, as with every other symptom that we experience, the depression is a message—a message that there are underlying imbalances that need to be addressed. Perhaps you have emotional energies wrapped around your heart causing the depression. Perhaps you are deficient in a certain vitamin or mineral and are unable to make serotonin, which may lead to depression. There may be many underlying causes, but taking medication to address the outward symptoms will not address those causes, as Heather found after trying all sorts of medication.

From Deep Depression to Happiness with the Body Code

In all honesty, I was very skeptical to try this method of healing and only did so because my grandmother gifted me six sessions and encouraged me to try. After living with severe clinical depression for over a decade, I had tried everything from antidepressants, to talk therapy, psychiatry, diet and exercise, medical cannabis, and even sleeping pills, and had little success with any of it.

I lost my mother to cancer, watched my father battle a horrific terminal brain disease, lost a dear friend to cancer, quickly followed by another friend who overdosed. These memories were traumatizing and sent me into a very dark place. I could barely make it through more than a few hours without crying, which was uncharacteristic for me. All of this was compounded by other life-changing circumstances that led me into an even deeper depression, which was relentless.

I gained fifty pounds and found even the simplest tasks daunting. For two years I was barely living, struggling to even get out of bed in the mornings. I was in constant pain and regularly thinking about death, wishing I could leave this world. To be only twenty-five and to have forgotten how it felt to be happy was the most disheartening realization to come to. I remember continuously thinking to myself, "How can I live like this? I can't keep going on feeling this way. . . ." I honestly believed I would never feel truly happy or like myself again. I even decided I didn't want to have kids because I didn't want to pass this horrible mental illness on to anyone. This type of pain and suffering I wouldn't wish on anyone. I was basically a shell of a being, with no joy or excitement in life, constantly "waiting for the other shoe to drop," so to speak.

After my first Body Code session, I felt very heavy; I still felt the depression but in a different way. . . . It took time and reassurance that I was healing. I had to continue to remind myself to be patient and allow my body the time to let these energies go and heal from the weight I was carrying.

During my second Body Code session is when everything changed. We cleared a lot of trapped and inherited emotions. Afterward, I was happy and not drained; I was laughing and enjoying every moment, and I recall thinking to myself that this was the best time I'd had at home since my dad was diagnosed.

Even my sister noticed the change in me. . . . Funnily enough, it wasn't only a change in the way I was feeling: everything else seemed to be falling into place as well. I had been unemployed for six months because I had quit my job due to the depression, and one week after applying, I received a job offer that was better than the job I had left.

I could feel my connection with people in my life becoming stronger; my cravings for bad food began to relinquish, and feelings of abandonment, which I had struggled with for my entire life, seemed to disappear. I felt genuinely happy for the first time in years. . . . I felt like myself. And that is a gift that I will never take for granted.

I am still in awe of how much the Body Code has helped me. It has honestly made me happy to be alive, and that is something I thought I would never feel. I can't wait to explore other areas of my life in which the Emotion Code and Body Code can assist. If you take nothing else from this, all I hope is that you will try at least one session, with an open mind, because it can quite literally change your whole life.

—Heather A., Calgary, Canada

The old saying among holistic doctors is "Anything can cause anything," and for good reason. It's fairly easy to understand that physical symptoms could have underlying causes and emotional symptoms, such as depression and anxiety as well.

What about behavioral symptoms? What about that friend of yours who keeps picking abusive partners to date? Could that also be a symptom? The answer is yes. What about that tendency you have to avoid exercise or eat dessert when you had decided not to? The emotional baggage, traumas, and experiences stored in our energy fields can very readily cause recurring problems like this. Sometimes we behave in ways that are puzzling even to ourselves. Only by finding and releasing the underlying imbalances that are driving these behaviors from the deep subconscious mind can this kind of self-sabotage be fixed.

Because of my undergraduate training in computer programming, I was always trying to combine the use of a computer with the healing work that I was doing. The Body Code was developed in response to my need to figure out, in the shortest time frame possible, what was really causing my patients' suffering.

The system that I ultimately created was a mind map that enabled me to "drill down" through layers of information to find and correct my patients' underlying imbalances very efficiently.

THE DIRECTIVE

One early morning in August of 2008, I woke up to find my mind full of a very specific instruction. As the fog of sleep swept away, the emphatic command was crystal clear. It was not from my own mind. This directive had awakened me. As I came to consciousness, the instruction was already there, perfect in its clarity and solemn emphasis. The instruction was:

> *You need to take everything that you have learned about natural healing and put it into a self-study course that anyone can learn, and make it available to everyone, everywhere.*

These were not my thoughts, that was clear. There was no doubt whatsoever about what I was supposed to do. I'd been given an assignment from above. I remember thinking, "Are you sure about this? This actually sounds like it could be a lot of work."

After some weeks of hesitating to embark on a project this large, I finally began. For many months I essentially did little else but create what I had been instructed to create. I would start working on it before the sun was up and often still be working on it deep into the night.

I had to figure out how to take all of the knowledge I had acquired in my practice and do a brain dump. I had to organize all of the pieces and make a course for people, for anyone and everyone, to learn what I'd learned and to be able to use it effectively. It needed to be easy to use and understand. The result of that directive ultimately became the Body Code System. It took me a year of focused intention to create the first version. There have been several updated versions since then.

I believe that the Body Code System is the most advanced and comprehensive method of natural, energetic healing available on the planet today. My knowledge of computer programming prepared me to make it into a digital product, a software app, that could be made available everywhere.

This book is an introduction to the Body Code and will give you enough information to actually use Body Code concepts yourself and hopefully get great results.

I am so grateful for everything that I have learned and for how I was qualified to share this work. My life's experiences have prepared me to be the teacher and messenger, to bring the Body Code System to the world. I believe the Creator wants to give back to every single one of us our healing birthright and turn us back into the healers that we are capable of becoming.

ON THE SHOULDERS OF GIANTS

The Body Code System is a tool that enables you to find and correct imbalances in six categories, which ultimately encompass all of the aspects of our being, providing an integrated, holistic approach to restore health and wellness. I could not have put together the Body Code System had others before me not brought their contributions to the world, contributions that make up much of the Body Code knowledge base. I feel like Sir Isaac Newton, who once said, "If I have seen further than others, it is by standing upon the shoulders of giants."

Early in my chiropractic practice, I realized that my education did not give me all the answers to all the difficulties my patients were dealing with. Often people would bring me issues that a spinal adjustment would not fix. And sometimes I would find out that they had previously been to many kinds of doctors who also did not know how to help them. Fortunately, I had a passion to find the answers they needed. As an insatiable learner, I devoured new discoveries and approaches to healing, incorporating anything that worked and felt right.

My lifelong thirst for knowledge has repeatedly been quenched by a long list of mentors, friends, family, and frequently by patients themselves. The list is too long to recount here and comprises an entire lifetime of learning everything that I could, from everyone that I could, in any situation that presented itself. My heart swells with gratitude when I think back on all that

I've learned from everyone who touched my life in one way or another. I'm especially grateful for the sudden insights, downloads, intuition, thoughts, and ideas that have come in answer to prayer. That kind of learning is truly the best, clearest, and purest of all.

So I did not come up with everything within this modality. Instead, I organized everything I learned about the body, mind, and spirit into one unified system that anyone can use. Truly, I do stand on the shoulders of giants. For without all the aggregated knowledge of the best thinkers and healers of the last three thousand years and more, the Body Code could not exist.

Most people who are using the Body Code successfully started using it with minimal knowledge of the body, mind, and spirit. The Body Code is unique because it essentially becomes your teacher. As you use it to help yourself and others, you will be taken to underlying imbalances, one at a time, whether you consciously knew anything about them before or not. It doesn't matter. In fact, people who know little about how the body works are often at an advantage because it is easier for them to keep an entirely open mind to any possibility, whereas those who have lots of knowledge sometimes tend to have more rigid thinking.

DOES IT WORK?

The Body Code is remarkably effective. As of the writing of this book, we have received over ten thousand remarkable unsolicited stories from people just like you who confirm it. We have inserted a few of their stories throughout this book—real experiences of ordinary people creating extraordinary results. I've seen all aspects of life improve and miracles unfold through this simple method. Here is a sampling of what people have to say:

> The human body was created with the ability to heal itself. The Body Code was created to unlock those abilities painlessly and with lasting positive effects.
>
> —Marianne B., Washington, United States

> The Body Code assists you in finding freedom from past emotional trauma, getting quick answers to illness, and in experiencing relief from pain using nothing more than intention and an easy-to-follow body map.
>
> —Bobbi Lynn G., California, United States

> Do you want to be able to heal yourself, or do you want to take drugs, mask the symptoms, and deal with the side effects for the rest of your life? It should be a simple answer, and if so—then the Body Code can help you with just about anything. If this

work were covered by insurance in a true health-care system, there would be little need for drug companies.

—Chuck E., Colorado, United States

The Body Code works like a translator of your inner healer for you. It knows everything about your past, all possible connections, even those you can't think of. And it knows what is most important to release and in which order.

—Sabine H., Heiligenthal, Germany

Dr. Bradley Nelson's methods, as taught in the Emotion Code and the Body Code, empower average people to heal themselves, their families, and their neighborhoods with an infinite ripple effect.

—Vera E., Massachusetts, United States

Your body is very intelligent, it knows what is causing your discomfort, symptoms, and disease; it wants and will tell you if you ask, and the Body Code provides the tools to ask, find, and release the imbalances that are there from past unconscious living and trauma so you can thrive and enjoy fresh liberty, joy, and peace.

—Keith B., Utah, United States

After getting to know the Body Code System and its unbelievable potential, I can imagine that we might look back in a few years and say, "Gee, do you remember? In the old times they gave people drugs and cut them in these situations! Now we can heal it with energy!"

—Fiete W., Lüneburg, Germany

UNDERSTANDING IMBALANCE

One of the oldest ideas in the world is that your state of health is dependent on how balanced or imbalanced your body is. The more imbalances you accumulate, the more likely you are to start having symptoms such as physical pain, loss of energy, negative emotional states, and eventual disease.

In the Body Code, an "imbalance" may refer to a deficiency, infection, infestation, toxin, need, negative energy, misalignment, dysfunction, disintegration, disconnection, trapped emotion, or an unhappy body part, to name a few. If enough imbalances exist for a long enough period, noticeable symptoms will arise, and disease may be the eventual result.

The incredible complexity of the body can seem daunting. One example of this is the energetic connections that exist between the organs and glands and the muscles of the body. If your right knee is bothering you, for example, it's very likely that your gallbladder is imbalanced, and the underlying cause of that is probably trapped emotions. If you have low-back pain, you very likely have an unhappy kidney or two, perhaps because of your caffeine habit, or possibly because of the car accident you experienced at age sixteen, or both. Left knee pain is highly related to stress overloading the adrenal glands, which are connected energetically with certain muscles.

If you're suffering from anxiety, a possible cause may be the toxic overload in your liver from your old mercury-amalgam dental fillings. If your neck is feeling particularly stiff, it may be because of your unwillingness to be flexible in your relationships. And so it goes.

How can we possibly figure out such a complex system? How can we even begin to address such a high-level organism and have any hope of making sense of it? The answer is the Body Code. By relying on the intelligence of the subconscious mind and the road map that is the Body Code, your questions can be answered and imbalances relieved, usually quite rapidly.

The Body Code explains the connections for every body part that has relationships. You do not need to learn or memorize any of these relationships because all of that information is found in the Body Code System. Finding imbalances and correcting them is what this system is designed to help you do.

The original versions of the Body Code System consisted of a couple of thick three-ring binders and multiple DVDs and CDs, which have now been compressed into the Body Code System app, putting this massive amount of information in the palm of your hand. In writing this book, I found it was an impossible task to include the entirety of the Body Code System's knowledge base, which in the app includes over a thousand pages and images. What I have attempted to do in this volume is to teach you how the Body Code works by explaining its concepts, and by giving you in these pages some of the most common imbalances that I have found, so that you can find a measure of success using the book alone. Please visit discoverhealing.com/app for more information about the Body Code System software, which is designed to run on both Apple and Android mobile phones and tablets, as well as both Mac and PC desktop computers.

My sincere hope is that this radically different and incredibly powerful way to heal will be easy for you to use and understand, and that through it, your life and the lives you touch will be changed for the better.

3

WHAT MAKES THE BODY CODE WORK?

The ultimate approach to healing will be to remove the abnormalities at the subtle-energy level which led to the manifestation of illness in the first place.

—RICHARD GERBER, MD

Let's explore how the Body Code works.

The Body Code by itself does not "do" anything. It's not a machine or a device. You might call it an interactive knowledge base that serves as a guide to help you form effective questions. The right questions facilitate useful answers, which guide you to know what corrections need to be made. The Body Code includes all the explanations and instructions you will need to correct whatever imbalances you uncover. It is an unequaled tool that will empower you to decode those underlying causes of things, bringing them to the light and enabling you to correct them at last.

KNOWLEDGE IS POWER

When you understand how something works, then you can use those principles to solve problems. Just as an electrician can wire your house to enable you to turn on your lights, you can use true principles to help yourself turn on your metaphorical lights to generate well-being in your body and mind.

The following concepts are foundational to the Body Code. Intentionally working with energy is the engine, if you will, that powers the work, including the following:

- Energy
- Energy body or Spirit
- Subconscious
- Higher Power

BASIC PRINCIPLES

1. ENERGY

To understand why the Body Code is so effective, you must understand energy and how it makes up all life. Energy is the foundation of everything.

Without it, planet Earth would not exist, nor would you. You are a being of pure energy. Your unique vibration is specific to you and makes your body and spirit show up as they do.

Energies vibrating at different frequencies make up each thing you see and touch. So each organ, system, and part of your body has its own frequency. For example, if your head hurts, it's not vibrating at the frequency of when it does not hurt. When you remove whatever is interfering with the normal frequency of any area, that area will naturally return to a healthier state. Sometimes it's not about removing what's in the way, but adding what is missing. Whether the solutions to your challenges are subtle energetic changes or more tangible physical changes, all are ultimately made of energy at the quantum level, and all are affected by energy.

Energy is the master ingredient in the universe. Invisible energy is all around us in the form of radio waves, gamma rays, infrared radiation, thought waves, and emotional energies, to name a few. You can think of our universe as a "LEGO" universe, made up of tiny building blocks called subatomic particles. These are extremely small units of vibrating energy. In the same way that LEGOs can be combined to create anything you like, differing arrangements of these little energies will produce atoms of different elements, such as hydrogen, carbon, and oxygen. Elements are combined to make molecules, which come together to make DNA, which constructs the components of your cells, ultimately becoming your body.

All of the everyday objects in your life that you can touch and see are made of matter, including your own body. Matter is typically thought of as anything that has mass and that takes up space. However, as Albert Einstein reportedly said, "All matter is energy."

If we are made of matter, and all matter is made of energy, then are we not beings of energy?

Our understanding of this is greatly helped by the discoveries of quantum mechanics—the study of atoms and subatomic particles. Albert Einstein and his followers devised ingenious experiments as they attempted to learn more about the nature of these tiny energies. Quantum research revealed that energies behave in different ways depending on what the observer is expecting to see. Our expectations or intentions carry enough energy to influence how particles move and form substances. Many physicists believe that the only explanation for these mysterious behaviors is that the energy within the atom itself is intelligent to some degree, or at least that it is being governed by a supreme intelligence of some sort.

For example, Max Planck, the originator of quantum theory said:

As a man who has devoted his whole life to the most clear headed science, to the study of matter, I can tell you as a result of my research about the atoms this much: There is no matter as such! All matter originates and exists only by virtue of a force which brings the particles of an atom to vibration and holds this most minute solar system of the atom together. . . . We must assume behind this force the existence of a conscious and intelligent Mind. This Mind is the matrix of all matter.

Since everything is made of energy, making corrections on an energetic level will usually yield the fastest and longest-lasting results.

Western medicine often ignores the spiritual and emotional aspects of our lives—the energy that is us. Viewing the body as separate from the mind is no longer possible. We now know that energy, emotions, experiences, and beliefs affect every cell of our bodies.

Our cells are constantly dying and being replaced, and it has been estimated that our bodies have a near complete turnover of cells every seven years. If you continue to hold on to distorted frequencies, or imbalances, you will continue to recreate unhealthy cells. If you have enough unhealthy cells, you may manifest disease that Western medicine cannot fix. In the following story, a man was able to walk and dance again after his doctor told him he would never get better.

Dancing Again

An uncle of a friend of mine had a bad stroke. After being in the hospital, he was in a rehabilitation center. He was not able to stand straight, even with help. The doctors told my friend that her uncle had to leave the rehabilitation center after three weeks because there was no chance of him ever getting better. I did six Body Code sessions with him at a distance in one month. Meanwhile he continued to improve while in the nursing home. After all six sessions, he got up from a chair, stood up, walked, and even danced with a nurse! My friend sent me a video so I could see it for myself. I had tears in my eyes as I watched it. Now he can live in his home again, and only needs a little bit of support.

—Heidi R., Vienna, Austria

I'm sure it's no surprise to you that our mental state affects our physical health. Believe it or not, that was a revolutionary idea to some of the great thinkers that shaped Western society.

Back in the early 1900s, deeply affected by the Industrial Revolution, the Western world was well entrenched in the idea that everything worked like a machine. The body was seen as a machine with separate parts that are unrelated to other parts. It was thought, if you have a toothache, pull out the tooth, but disregard the diet because what you eat doesn't matter. If you're not breathing so well, address the lungs, but disregard the severe grief of losing a loved one.

Today we are still entrenched in that same model of the parts making up the whole, instead of the whole being far more than the sum of its parts. It's no wonder that doctors today specialize in single systems, without much regard to how all the other aspects of people's lives might contribute to their suffering. For example, although the popular adverse childhood experiences (ACE) study of more than seventeen thousand people that was done between 1995 and 1997 clearly correlated adult physical disease with childhood trauma, not enough has changed in the established ways of treating these people since then.

Under the existing mechanistic perspective, remedies that have been used successfully for thousands of years were effectively set aside and essentially ignored by Western medicine. If doctors and scientists couldn't fit those concepts into their frames of reality, then those ideas were seen at best as placebos, and they were discredited and dismissed. Herbs, homeopathy, meditation, ritual, religion, and the wisdom of traditions were ridiculed and eliminated from the Western health-care world long ago, and, for the most part, remain ostracized.

For example, when your grandmother checked into the hospital with COVID-19, were any alternative remedies recommended or tried, or even thought of by Western-trained doctors? Unlikely. Western medicine is at the mercy of the pharmaceutical-industrial complex, which only recommends treatments that benefit the bottom line, even though their costs may outweigh their benefits.

Yet while the "body as a machine" perspective was driving our medical community's view of illness, physicists and mathematicians were discovering quantum physics—a much more comprehensive view of the world—starting with the behavior of the tiny unseen particles that make up everything. Einstein brilliantly taught us that light energy not only behaves as waves, but also as particles. This shift in understanding moved us down the path to discovering laws now used today, opening us to a world of new possibilities.

We can apply this new understanding to the human energy field, leveraging new understandings in quantum mechanics, such as the laws of superposition, the collapsing of the wave function, nonlocality, entanglement, and others, many of which are beyond the scope of this book, yet are true principles that you will take advantage of in using the Body Code. Mind expanding and faith inspiring, these principles are pure delight to those who want to rationalize how it's possible to heal a lifelong ailment in fifteen minutes through work with the Body Code, an ailment that "modern" medicine could not cure.

Of course, not all issues are as quickly remedied. Some can take many weeks, even months, to address. Imbalances are often layered and may require a specific sequence of issues to be addressed over time, much like peeling an onion one layer after another. The point is that quantum physics helps us to understand how and why the Body Code works. It does successfully alleviate suffering and brings healing and wholeness to those open enough to believe and do the work.

While the scientific community continues to validate and leverage the laws of quantum physics, the Western medical approach continues to focus on a limited set of principles, providing a limited set of outcomes, much to the disadvantage of their patients.

Even so, if I break my leg, I'm deeply grateful I can go to a standard orthopedic doctor to get it reset and stabilized. Especially in emergency situations, we are immeasurably benefited by current understandings of how to help the human body. By all means, stop the bleeding, stabilize the patient, and deal with shock. Standard medicine serves brilliantly in many instances. But when it comes to comprehending all the reasons for pain or discomfort, especially the chronic issues, a wider net is needed to get to the source.

Gratefully, researchers are digging deeper, and thousands of studies already demonstrate the interrelationship of thoughts, emotions, experiences, and disease.

One study showed that having a diagnosis of depression alone carries with it a 65 percent greater likelihood of premature death. Other studies demonstrate that a diagnosis of depression predicts a higher chance of developing a future disease. Depression and anxiety are associated with multiple diseases that affect the heart, gastrointestinal system, and nervous system, as well as a role in autoimmune diseases and chronic pain. And that is just the tip of the iceberg.

Studies exist showing a clear link between childhood trauma and adult physical health. But how to use that information to improve healing methods remains a mystery to those still limited to the old models our mainstream medical world lives in. Prevention of childhood abuse is the primary action from some of these studies, which is great for the next generation, but what of those hurting today from long-ago injustices? While significant emotional trauma may be an obvious source of chronic physical disorders, more pervasive are the effects of far more common experiences. Heartbreak, disappointment, anger, frustration, and the full gamut of normal reactions to life can create trapped energies that affect us physically and mentally years later. In this next story, Helga discusses a man who finally found relief from his fear of heights.

Clearing Childhood Abuse

A client of mine, let's call him S to protect his identity, suffered from fear of heights. When he was four years old, his father put him on top of the fridge and told him to jump, that he would catch him. Well, S jumped, but his father did not catch him, and his words were, "This is to teach you never to trust anyone, not even your father."

I worked on him in person and he visited me at our home, which is on an island. Unbeknownst to me, in the beginning, when crossing the bridge, he had to concentrate and look only straight ahead. One day, after our first session, he said, "Wow, I did not know that bridge was so beautiful and the river was just magic." After four sessions, his fear vanished, and this is what he sent to me:

"Great news! As you know, Hindmarsh Island Bridge is a breeze for me to cross now, but today I was able to stand on an A-frame ladder, with my shoes SIX FEET above the ground. Unbelievable, Wow!! I had no symptoms of fear or nervousness. Normally I am so weak in the legs that I have to get down, as I can't stand. Feeling faint, visions of me falling and hurting myself, the pain of my father's cruel act; it has all gone! And I can't thank you enough, I haven't felt this way all over and all inside for a long, long time. The highest I could go was a meter, and that was bad enough.

"I lost count of how many times I went up that ladder, as I couldn't believe it, and had to keep testing myself out (must have been a lot, my leg muscles are sore). I really felt good up there, like all the baggage is starting to drop off my shoulders, a great feeling! Once again, a big thank you, thank you, thank you!"

—Helga C., Goolwa, South Australia

While contemporary methods exist to effectively address and release the energetic imbalances of the past that are creating the pain and suffering of the present, few mainstream doctors will point their patients to these sources, simply because they do not fit into the current medical paradigm.

Before we attribute this new awareness of how energy affects us, let's give credit where credit is due. This rich understanding of energy started thousands of years ago. The oldest form of energy medicine, I've found, was practiced by the Chinese, who discovered energetic pathways in the body. Acupuncture is practiced by manipulating the flow of energy through the body to improve function and wellness. Since then, tai chi, meditation, yoga, hypnotherapy, acupuncture, massage therapy, Reiki, quantum healing, qigong, emotional freedom technique (EFT), and many other methods have emerged as independent protocols, using the laws of physics to manipulate energy to improve health.

It didn't take an understanding of quantum mechanics for me to use its principles. In wonderment, I watched my patients make remarkable recoveries as I identified and addressed the imbalances that were at the root of their suffering. Once found and released, the body and mind were free to mend, and often, mend immediately. Quantum theory validated what I was experiencing every day.

2. ENERGY BODY OR SPIRIT

Energy makes up both the physical body as well as the other energetic components of our being, such as the biofields, the chakras, the electromagnetic field, etc. But an even more significant aspect of the energy field is something held in reverence by many different cultures now and throughout time. It has been called the prana, the chi or qi, the life force, the spirit, and the energy body. We can differentiate the energy field into distinct components, but for simplicity in this conversation, let's wrap them all into one thing—the blueprint for the physical body—and call it the spirit.

Knowing about your spirit is essential to this work because your body and your spirit must be aligned to be fully happy and healthy. Garri Garripoli, author of *Qigong: Essence of the Healing Dance,* illustrated this point nicely when he stated,

> *Married to a soul and a mind, the body provides us with carnal pleasures and serves to reflect our overall spiritual and mental condition like a polished mirror. . . . To the extent that we can discover our own, unique balance, we are whole . . . and once whole, we can truly dance like the free spirits we are.*

In the following story, Phillip experienced feeling his energy body and what it was like to be whole.

Discovering My True Self

When I ended the longest and most meaningful relationship of my life, I fell into a deep spell of depression. No matter what I tried, from meditation to yoga, I could not pull myself completely out of the throes of despair. I cycled on and off, over and over again, feeling one day like I was finally emerging from the darkness, only then to be thrust back in the following day.

After a couple of months of this, and what seemed like no progress at all, I came across a chance encounter with a family friend. Over lunch, listening to her describe how the Emotion Code works, I figured, "Why not? I might as well give it a shot."

During our session, she discovered that I had two trapped emotions, grief and heartache, that were linked together, and had to do with my previous relationship. With three swipes of the magnet down the back of my spine, they were gone. Within less than five minutes after that, I felt a huge sense of relief, like an incredibly heavy blanket had been pulled from my energetic body. For the first time in months, I could tangibly feel the energy that I know to be what I call my "true self." It wasn't just in my mind; it was real and tangible, and it felt amazing to have found such a profound method of healing that is also incredibly simple and easy to perform.

—Phillip K., North Carolina, United States

I believe that the Creator made everything energetically or spiritually before He created anything physically. Your spirit is a blueprint for your physical body. It is a three-dimensional template that your physical body grows into.

For decades scientists have been trying to regenerate human tissue. Many of them have come to the same conclusion: there is an energy field within living things that actuates the cellular processes, builds, and maintains the body.

Here is an example: Scientists have done many studies on animals like the newt, which has the amazing ability to regenerate its tail if it gets pulled off. The newt uses this defensive mechanism to escape predators. When the tail grows back, it looks exactly like it looked before. How does that happen? The newt's energy field, I believe, provides a three-dimensional template for the tail to grow into, and the physical form simply fills in that invisible blueprint.

Your spirit is ultimately who you really are. It is your sentient intelligence and being, an invisible body of light. If you go to a funeral and look at the person lying in the casket, it's obvious that there is something that has changed. You can feel the absence of the individual, even though the physical body looks familiar. It's like an empty shell without the spirit or life force inside.

A controversial study that dates back to 1907 found that the human body loses, on average, twenty-one grams of weight at the moment of death. Could this be the weight of the human spirit?

One's spirit animates one's physical body, like a hand animates a glove. At death, the spirit or energy body moves on, and the body decays because it no longer has its life force. During one's mortal lifetime, the spirit and body interface in a profound way that we don't yet understand. Because of this interface, when the energy body becomes imbalanced, the physical body is always affected. Imbalances in the energy body must be corrected for a person to be able to be truly well.

Your Truest Identity

Let me go into just a little more detail about what I believe about who you really are—your truest identity. For centuries, human beings have been described as selfish and dominating, with a strong impulse to compete and try to accumulate power and possessions. While this may be true in some instances, particularly for people who have ignored and shut off access to their own heart, humans have a part of them that did not begin with earth life.

Your spirit body has existed long before you came to Earth and will continue to live beyond death. You came from the presence of your maker. So your truest identity is an eternal, spiritual, intelligent child of the Creator. You are a glorious being, journeying through earth life to learn and progress.

Growth requires resistance and new experiences. You may not remember now, but I believe you chose to come to Earth because of all you could do and learn here. Acquiring a physical body with a powerful brain is immensely challenging. The brain is naturally designed to keep you alive and protect you at all costs from what it perceives as threats. Painful past experiences can easily cause the brain to take more control of your life than necessary, interfering with the delicate balance between your spirit and physical body. When you are not fully integrated with your physical body, or when you are out of balance, full vibrant health is significantly hindered. Like a washing machine with an off-balance load inside, when the spin cycle starts and the stress increases, you can find yourself being painfully pounded by life. Addressing your spiritual needs is a powerful aspect of finding physical and emotional wellness.

Your spirit, the real you, is special but often obscured and unrecognized by what you can see and touch. Your body is actually a sacred "temple" for your spirit to inhabit.

Anytime we are working to help the body function better, we are doing a sacred thing. If we are sewing up an injury, if we are helping someone who is disabled, if we are helping someone heal, we are doing something special that deserves sincere respect. Your body and brain do not know these things, because it's your spirit that knows, receives, and recognizes truth from the source of all truth.

Many near-death experiences reveal that people who have "died" and have left their bodies for a time didn't realize that they had died until they looked down and saw their physical body lying there as they hovered above it. People who have been through this understand that they are not their physical body. Instead, their body is more like temporary housing for their spirit-self.

I once had an experience that I will never forget because it taught me the truth of this concept. One day, after asking for help from above, I turned my attention to the patient lying on the table before me. At that moment, I was given a gift of understanding from above. It was as if I had been blind all my life and suddenly could see with a clear, spiritual form of sight. I instantly and clearly perceived that I was standing in the presence of a sacred temple—the temple of the body that belonged to this patient. I was instantly filled with the deepest sense of awe and reverence. This powerful revelation lasted only a few seconds, but it was unforgettable, and it revealed the truth about the body on a much higher level of understanding than I'd ever had before.

Our sense of purpose in life, our desire to grow and learn, and our desire for connection to others, all stem from a deep inner knowing about the truth of who we really are. There is more to life than self-preservation. Our spirits connect us to the truth that life has deep meaning. We innately know that people are more important than things, and relationships with people are more rewarding than ownership of "stuff." The more we grow ourselves and reach out to serve, the more inclined we are to be good to each other.

C. S. Lewis, the atheist turned Christian author, wrote:

> *It is a serious thing to live in a society of possible gods and goddesses, to remember that the dullest most uninteresting person you can talk to may one day be a creature which, if you saw it now, you would be strongly tempted to worship, or else a horror and a corruption such as you now meet, if at all, only in a nightmare. All day long we are, in some degree, helping each other to one or the other of these destinations. It is in the light of these overwhelming possibilities, it is with the awe and the circumspection proper to them, that we should conduct all of our dealings with one another, all friendships, all loves, all play, all politics. There are no* ordinary *people. You have never talked to a mere mortal. Nations, cultures, arts, civilizations—these are mortal, and their life is to ours as the life of a gnat. But it is immortals whom we joke with, work with, marry, snub, and exploit—immortal horrors or everlasting splendours.*

When we know that we are each eternal beings having a mortal experience, we have the motivation to be our best, to seek healing and peace, and to live a life of service and love. We each have a mission and a reason for being here on Earth. And it's no accident that you're learning about the Body Code now. Perhaps it will be a tool for you in becoming who you came here to be. Life is not always as it appears.

These spirit bodies of ours are matter, albeit highly refined matter, which is why most people cannot see them, most of the time. They can go out of balance, which then affects the functioning of the physical body. As real as your spirit is, it does not have a "voice" as obvious as your physical body's vocal chords. So when there are imbalances, trapped emotions, or other issues in the energy body, or even issues in the physical body that the spirit is keenly aware of but you do not know consciously, how do you get to that information?

Fortunately, your subconscious is ready to let you know where the problems lie and what is needed. The Body Code provides the necessary interface between the conscious and the subconscious mind to give you that access and make it simple.

3. SUBCONSCIOUS

Let's discuss the difference between the conscious and the subconscious mind. Your conscious mind is where you spend all your waking hours, where you make your decisions, where you receive and analyze thoughts and ideas and make conclusions and decide which actions to take. It has been said many times that we humans use only a fraction of our brains. Recent studies have found, in fact, that the conscious mind needs almost none of the brain's total resources. In other words, thinking, moving about, making choices, planning, seeing, hearing, tasting, touching, and smelling are all conscious activities that take up a minimal portion of the processing power of the brain. If this is true, what is the vast remainder of the brain doing?

The bulk of your intelligence is subconscious. Most people give the subconscious little recognition, even though it is actually super active. It's archiving and remembering everything. The entire history of every cell in your body, down to the quantum level, is archived and stashed away in that amazing holographic computer system that is the subconscious mind.

This silent intelligence within you is constantly busy storing information and keeping your body's systems running efficiently. It is also important to understand that the subconscious mind exerts an unseen yet profound influence over the things we do and over how we behave and feel.

Most people give little consideration to the existence of their subconscious minds. But imagine for a moment having to take over the functions that your subconscious mind performs. Imagine the difficulty of instructing your digestive system how to digest your lunch, or telling your cells how to create enzymes and proteins. Imagine if you had to worry about keeping your heart beating and keeping air moving in and out of your lungs every moment of every day. And you think you have a full schedule now!

Your subconscious mind is so intelligent, it can take your breakfast and convert it into new cardiac muscle tissue or new red blood cells. It's been said that a single cell compares in complexity to a modern full-size aircraft carrier, with aircraft on the ramp ready for takeoff and thousands of people working at their own often-complex individual jobs. When you realize that the human body has an estimated thirty-seven trillion cells, and when you realize that the subconscious mind is controlling, organizing, and orchestrating all of this to keep you alive from one moment to another, it is quite humbling.

An image of an iceberg can help you visualize these two minds, with the vast bulk of the iceberg (below the waterline) representing the subconscious mind. The smaller part of the iceberg (above the waterline) represents the conscious mind.

In the following story, Lorraine witnessed the subconscious mind's ability to not only remember but to also reveal the underlying causes of things while working on Bronson's night terrors.

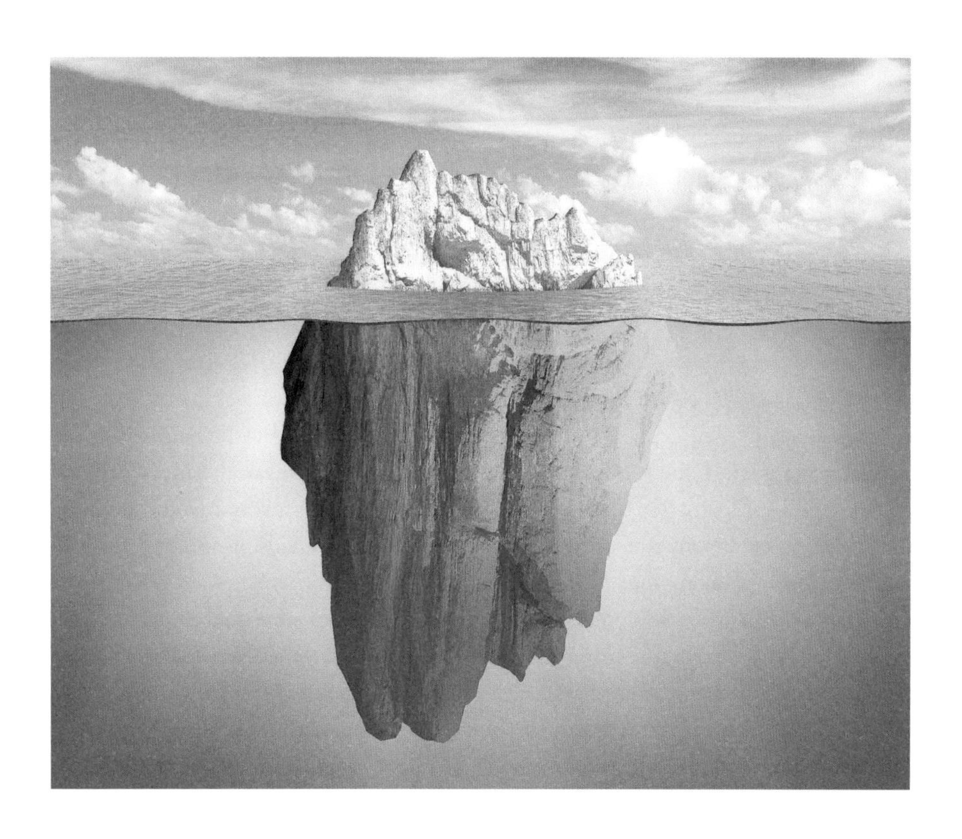

Bronson

Bronson was a seven-year-old suffering from night terrors. He couldn't sleep in his room at night even though he was with his sibling. His mother would lay with him in bed until he fell asleep, and would then go to sleep in her room. She and her husband kept a small mattress on the floor beside their bed, knowing that when he awoke during the night in fear, he would end up sleeping in their room for the rest of the night. They tried everything to help him feel loved and safe, but nothing helped.

I had worked with Bronson and found several trapped emotions. What his subconscious revealed astounded his mother. The trapped emotions identified through muscle testing were shock, terror, horror, and fear. When we asked if we needed to know more about them, the answer was yes. We needed to find an age, and it was around two. His mom recalled a distressing event that took place just prior to Bronson's second birthday, when he ran out of the driveway and onto the highway. It was getting dark and a car was traveling down the road. To avoid hitting the child, the driver swerved around him, and then landed in a ditch. It was a terrifying incident, as she remembered.

One can only imagine how that child felt seeing the headlights of a car coming right at him. Bronson's mind subconsciously trapped all those emotions, which then came out in the form of night terrors or nightmares and fear of going to sleep. Once the trapped emotions were released, he was able to sleep well every night. They felt it was nothing short of a miracle!

—Lorraine L., New Hampshire, United States

Your subconscious mind is aware of any imbalances your body may be harboring, and it also knows exactly what effect these imbalances are having on your physical, emotional, and mental well-being. This information and more is tucked away in the subconscious mind, as Dr. Jill Carnahan, MD, states: "Your subconscious mind controls all the vital processes of your body. It already knows the answers to your problem and it already knows how to heal you."

Your subconscious mind knows what the solution is to your physical, emotional, and mental problems, and it is constantly available to answer your questions. As we learn to access that information, we get the answers we need. As a massive database of information about you, your subconscious is like a computer that knows your exact problem and how to fix it—whether it's recovering from an illness, making more money, or improving your relationships.

Your subconscious mind is heavily influencing your decisions, thoughts, and actions. When you want to get in shape and you think of going to the gym daily but fail to get out of the door all month, which part of your mind do you think is making the choice to stay home? It seems as though your conscious mind has a solution in going to the gym to get in shape, but there is something in the subconscious that may be holding you back from actually doing it.

In sum, your subconscious mind is the part of your intelligence that is not only keeping you alive from moment to moment, it is also quietly directing your steps and running your life.

When we have symptoms, most of the time we aren't sure why. We know that our back hurts. We know that we don't feel well. We know that we can't conceive a child. We know that we are depressed, or that we have anxiety or digestive problems. We know that something might not be right with us, but we usually don't know why.

Do you think it's possible that the subconscious might actually know why symptoms like these exist? It is my premise that healing is all about accessing that internal computer, the subconscious mind, where all the answers are available for the asking.

Subconscious Mind vs. Spirit

You might wonder then what the difference is between the subconscious and the spirit. Now we're getting into deep water, with lots of interesting different opinions. In this model, the subconscious is part of the mind and is therefore information-based and a bit like a computer. The spirit has all the information, and also, as the truest and most eternal aspect of you, has values, emotional intelligence, ethics, critical thinking, and curiosity.

Both the spirit and the subconscious are tracking everything about your experiences, and neither has dominant access to "speak" its truths; but they are as different as your cell phone is from your pet. One is informational and the other is relational. This is why accessing the subconscious is so valuable. It has the answers. It's not judging the answers or feeling anything about the answers. The access to answers is in the form of yes or no. We can work very quickly with the subconscious, averting the complexities of life experiences and getting directly to solutions.

If the subconscious mind is likened to the part of an iceberg that is below the waterline, the ocean of water that the subconscious mind is immersed in represents something often referred to as "universal intelligence." Also called "the database of all that is," or the "morphic field," or "the light of Christ," it is the energy that fills the universe, that is somehow governed by divine intelligence, the intelligent mind that is the "matrix of all matter," to quote Max Planck.

This field of energy fills the interspaces of the universe and connects the subconscious minds of all people into one vast whole. When we work on someone at a distance, we do so through this field of energy that is infinite. Our subconscious minds, therefore, are truly connected into a database of genius. All knowledge exists in this database of energy. So, although your subject has never heard of the Body Code, his or her subconscious mind has complete access to it through this field of intelligence. Because of this, through muscle testing, the subconscious mind can immediately take you to the relevant imbalances.

We can access all the information in this amazing computer system by simply using muscle testing. Not only can we get answers to just about every question about the body, but I believe there is a list in every single person's subconscious mind of all the things that need to be done to bring the body back to 100 percent functioning, or as close to it as is possible.

In other words, every person has the answers to his or her own issues. You have the answers to your own issues. While working to help another person, the person that is using the Body Code and asking questions is a blank slate, with no agenda other than to assist with balancing the body of the other person. By asking simple questions that can be answered by the body with a yes or a no, imbalances can be identified and corrected, addressed or cleared. Most imbalances can be cleared immediately, but some may require additional effort to be corrected. Maybe you need more water, or a specific vitamin or mineral, exercise, or to get out of a toxic relationship. Who knows? The subconscious knows. Most often, we find that clearing or balancing the frequencies or energies is all that is needed to pave the way for the body to restore itself, let go of the symptoms, and be happy.

When you are working on someone, be open to any possibility at all. Remember once again the old saying of the holistic physician: "Anything can cause anything!" In the following story, a grandmother shares her realization about how an unexpected cause was the key to solving a difficulty.

Sore Thumb

You always say that anything can cause anything. Well, in the middle of the night, my thumb, all of a sudden, developed a trigger in it; it was very painful to move. Over the next six months it became stiffer and more inflamed. The joint even became enlarged. . . . It was just stuck, and I could not bend it.

We finally found inherited emotions from two ancestors on both sides. Halfway through releasing the trapped emotions, my thumb started working. My thumb function is improving with no trigger, and the inflammation is subsiding from the joint.

—Bonnie L., California, United States

If you allow yourself to quiet your conscious mind and tune in to your body, you will learn that your subconscious is quite able to communicate with you.

4. HIGHER POWER

Two essential aspects of becoming a healer are (1) to be humble enough to realize that you need help, and (2) to be willing to ask for that help from whatever Higher Power you believe in.

Your ideas and mine about the Higher Power probably differ. I don't think it matters so much that we give the Source or Creator different titles, but that we do acknowledge and lean on it. What I do think matters is the character of this Higher Power. To quote Augustine, "God loves each of us as if there were only one of us."

A connection to the Divine is the one thing that will guide you to truth, to help you get to the underlying causes of disease most rapidly, and to connect with those who are ready to be helped. This work puts you in a position to be an instrument of healing. Always ask for help before working with anyone, and be open to the subtle thoughts, ideas, and impressions that will come. You will be amazed at the good that will unfold through you, as Patty was in the following story.

Getting Help

I had a client in her early thirties who had struggled for many years with infertility. She and her husband finally saved enough money to start infertility treatments, but they were very disappointed because her body was not responding to hormone therapy and she could not begin in vitro fertilization (IVF) treatments.

Using the Body Code, I identified that she had misalignments of her reproductive organs and several trapped emotions. She began treatment but was still unable to conceive.

During her next session, after my prayer to ask for help with this client, it occurred to me to ask specific questions about how she felt about becoming pregnant. Questions kept coming to my mind to ask, like: Is she okay with being pregnant, okay with being a mother? What is blocking her from conceiving? What can I clear that will allow her to conceive a child? With help from above, deep layers started to be revealed. The beauty of this modality is that she didn't have to reveal the situations and she didn't have to relive any traumas.

We did six sessions in total, until I got no to all my questions regarding any imbalances or "blocks," and yes to my questions regarding whether each organ/structure was balanced. Her body was able to heal itself. After about four months, I received an email from her and her husband that she was pregnant and that they *did not* need IVF treatments! Now they have a beautiful, healthy baby boy.

—Patty C., Florida, United States

FOUR ACTIVATING PRINCIPLES

To utilize the Body Code fully, and to become the most effective healer you can be, there are four principles that you need to be aware of and to practice. When you use the Body Code, be conscious of your "state of mind," because being present as you use these principles will "turn on" the power of this work. They are:

1. Love
2. Intention
3. Prayer
4. Gratitude

Your growing understanding of these ideas will be foundational to your success using the Body Code.

1. LOVE

Love is central to this work. Why? Because love is the energy by which transformation and healing occur. As Deepak Chopra once said, "The use of love is to heal. When it flows without effort from the depth of the self, love creates health." When you feel love for the person you're serving, gratitude for the opportunity to serve, and love for the source that makes this all possible, you become a conduit of light for the Divine.

None of us are perfectly qualified to do this work. You're not perfect, but you are enough. Love yourself in spite of your faults, and your work with the Body Code will be easier and more fruitful.

One of the fascinating things I have noticed about the experiences of people who "die and live to tell about it" are the questions they are asked when they have temporarily passed over to the other side. They are never asked, "How big of a house did you live in?" Or, "How much money did you make while you were alive?" Instead, they are asked, "How much did you love others?" Or, "How much did you learn?"

I think this should be a clue as to the importance of these things and should help us to understand what the purpose of life really is. It's all about love and learning.

In the Book of Corinthians, the apostle Paul wrote that without love, we are nothing.

When we die, no matter how much money we have made, no matter how much success we have attained in this world, we only take with us the knowledge that we have gained and our ability to love others.

To successfully use the Body Code to help another person, allow your heart to fill with love for that person. That love is instantly communicated from your heart to theirs. It's disarming on a subconscious level. Barriers and protections are lowered in the face of unconditional love. True healers always come from the heart. You can't lie to the subconscious mind of another person. If all you're really interested in is their money, or in feeding your own ego, they will feel and know the truth about you. If you have any other agenda besides truly wanting to help from your heart, they will know it, at least subconsciously.

If you want to work on yourself using the Body Code, the same principle applies. Choose to fill your heart with love for yourself. If you find it hard to love yourself because you feel that you are not good enough or worthy enough or smart enough or whatever enough, realize that these feelings do not come from the light. Our love makes us able to connect with divine love, which is perfect. So you are enough to do this work, since divine love will fill in what you feel is missing. As you accept this, you will grow into that very love. Like everyone, you have healing to do. Love yourself in spite of your faults, and you will feel yourself begin to heal from the inside out, and your work with the Body Code will be easier and more successful.

Sometimes we need to do some work for ourselves to clear out what might be in the way of our ability to both give and receive love. In this story, Reham did just that.

Feeling Love

Life is not easy. I became so disconnected and numb that I couldn't feel any emotions anymore. But once I found and cleared my Heart-Wall, that all changed. Now I can feel my emotions! More importantly, I can feel my two boys' love! I will keep clearing to fully experience love.

—Reham M., Ontario, Canada

One way to begin to feel more love for yourself is to personify things that are bothering you. For example, if your thumb has arthritis and is throbbing and aching, simply think of your thumb as an innocent small child that is crying and needing tenderness. How would you talk to a hurting three-year-old? Love it, say kind things to it, even thank it for all the great work it has done for all these years. Let it know you're sorry it is in pain and that you're here to help. That might feel awkward at first, but if that mental image helps generate love for whatever is painful in your life, then it's worth the effort. It will pay off.

Another way to feel love for what's not working well is to see it as a gift. The pain may be the only opportunity for you to notice and identify an imbalance that could create something much worse later if it's not dealt with now. It's a metaphorical hand in the air, waving, saying, "Over here! I have some important information for you. Focus on me, so I can lead you to something we need to address that's down this path. Let me lead you to it, so you can fix it." Appreciating the discomfort for what it can show you is the first step to loving it. Once you appreciate it, choose to love it, and that love will create a vibration of trust and an ability to get to the bottom of the problem.

To quote Dr. Wayne Dyer:

There is no greater power in heaven or on earth than pure, unconditional love. The nature of the God force, the unseen intelligence in all things, which causes the material world and is the center of both the spiritual and physical plane, is best described as pure, unconditional love.

A wonderful side effect of having a heart full of love is that doubt and fear are driven out by love. John of Patmos said that "Perfect love casts out fear." Fear and doubt cannot coexist in a heart that is filled with love. So if you are feeling doubtful about your ability to help and heal yourself or others, add more love to the mix and watch the fear and doubt depart! In addition, you may want to do a Body Code session to find and release any blocks to your ability to love yourself and others.

2. INTENTION

Intention is having an aim or plan to do something and setting your mind firmly to do it. Intention energy is simply a vibrational frequency that you create by focusing your expectation for a specific result. When you are holding an intention to do something or to help someone, you don't always understand ahead of time how it will happen. But if you set that intention, and feel that it is successful, that intention is the fuel that will drive the end result, as Sofia found in the following story.

Intention Works!

When I heard about the allergies webinar for premium members, I immediately made the intention not only to attend, but to be chosen as a volunteer. Somehow Dr. Nelson heard my desire and picked me.

Eating my favorite dairy, cheese, and milk has been a problem for about twenty years, and I had to avoid it or substitute it all the time, in addition to avoiding certain fruits, like apricots and citruses.

Using the Body Code, Dr. Nelson made the most incredible connections to my subconscious mind and was able to point out the root of the problem and release the imbalances.

A couple of days later, my husband and I were taking a walk in the park when we heard the sound of an ice cream truck. He knows not to offer ice cream to me, as I would have a reaction. And here something changed. He asked me if I wanted to try my favorite kind, and I said yes. Lo and behold, I ate it and absolutely nothing happened. No reaction. The same thing happened when I ate an apricot yesterday.

I am building my student portfolio to become a certified Body Code practitioner. I am so grateful to Dr. Nelson for the session, for the method, and for the entire new life opportunity. *Namaste!*

—Sofia I., California, United States

Feeling love or compassion for the person you're working with and gratitude that your effort is going to be successful are essential elements for generating the intention energy that will facilitate changes in yourself or the person you're serving. Interestingly, I've found that when you are serving others with the Body Code, you may eventually become more balanced and experience healing effects you had not expected for yourself. This is a nice bonus and side effect of your service. It doesn't always happen, but when it does, I believe it's because light and love are flowing through you as a vessel of healing.

We are very fortunate to be living in this time because the world is transforming. There is increasing turmoil and many are oppressed, but we are also growing as beings of light ourselves; we are not stagnant. We are either gathering more light, or we are diminishing in light. What we will eventually see, with divine help, is a better and greater world. With this transition, you may notice that answers come more easily, the power to do good is more readily available, and intentions manifest more immediately. As the intensity of darkness increases in the world, so the brightness of the light increases as well. Now, more than at any other time in the world, we can expect miracles. Just remember, one of the things about faith and intention is that you have to keep having it. If what you intended didn't arrive today, be confident it will tomorrow.

How is it possible for intention to create change? Let's return to the idea of everything being energy. When a person has an imbalance of any sort, at the core of that imbalance is a frequency that either needs to be added to the body, or a frequency that simply needs to be released or neutralized. Your clear intention along with the power God gives you to serve make this possible.

It really is that simple. But for those of you who appreciate a more technical answer, there is plenty to discuss here. Whether you are doing the Body Code work in person with a subject or over the phone or on yourself, your intention energy is one element that fosters the vibrational changes that create healing.

One of the ways the Body Code can be applied by one person to another person in any location around the world to relieve pain or improve health or happiness is due to a principle of quantum physics known as "entanglement." Albert Einstein described entanglement as "spooky action at a distance," because contrary to logical thought, two energy particles or waves can unite into one and be in two places at once even at distances larger than Earth's diameter. Think about this for a moment. Because of the property of entanglement, it is possible to help a parent, child, or pet remotely from work, on vacation, or in the military on duty.

Although in the physical world distance is a great barrier, in the energetic world, entanglement of energy allows immediate connection and communication between energetic particles without any distance limitation at all. Therefore, through desire and intention, two people can become entangled, allowing one person to act as a proxy for the other, to correct energetic imbalances that may be the underlying causes of physical, mental, and emotional dis-ease. Shoko experienced this as she acted as proxy for her father to help ease his pain.

Her Father's Pain

My father is eighty-three years old, living in Asia. I live in the United States. One day on our phone conversation, I found that he was enduring pain in the area where his gallbladder was removed. He said the pain might be caused by the stones in the bile duct, which doctors could not remove during the operation that took place about four years earlier. Since then, he'd been taking medication daily.

I asked him if I could use the Body Code on him. He may not have understood what the Body Code was exactly, but I got his permission anyway. I found and removed entities, Heart-Wall emotions, and his Heart-Wall itself.

I called him the next day. I asked him, "So how do you feel? Do you still have pain?"

He answered, "Which pain?"

"Well, the pain you had yesterday . . ."

"Oh, it is gone. Your magic worked."

I laughed and felt the magic and beauty of the Body Code.

—Shoko S. W., California, United States

Energy, by nature, is defined either as a particle or a wave. Without getting too technical, this thought can be simply understood by thinking of grains of sand on the seashore. If one is standing on the beach looking at the sand, one can bend over, touch a single grain of sand, and instantly see that it is separate from the others. However, if one looks at the shore from a distance, one might have difficulty seeing one grain of sand, but instead see sand laying in wave patterns created by the ebb and flow of the waves of the ocean. Therefore, one can comprehend sand as a single particle or a wave of possibilities of single particles.

Energy is similar. Let's apply this analogy. The energy of a moment often represents all the possibilities of that moment. Let's say you are lying in bed and your alarm goes off.

You can choose to do one of these things:

1. Get up.
2. Lay there and sleep for a few minutes longer.
3. Check your text messages.

These options are like the seashore of possibilities. Let's say you decide to check your text messages. Once that choice is made, it is as if you had bent over and selected that single grain of sand out of the waves of sand. By choosing to check text messages, you have forfeited the other choices for that moment, and no other choice exists.

This means that all the potential waves of potential choices disappear or collapse into one reality—your choice to check text messages. In this way, the human consciousness can consider all possibilities until one makes a choice. The good news is that each moment in our life comes with another set of waves to choose from, and so one can choose to roll over to sleep a bit more or get up, once again creating a new reality in that moment. Thus, we are moving from one collapsed energy wave of possibilities into a single reality, to another, until the end of our lives. These choices become our reality and together make up the whole of a lifetime.

Two intentions can unite to form one, through the property of entanglement. Since choice and intention can cause the wave of possibilities to collapse into a reality, two people united can also create an even stronger reality together. This is how the actual work using the Body Code occurs. The act of uniting intention for the purpose of changing reality is powerful and magnifies—times two—individual wills as the movement of energy responds to the desires of both the practitioner and the client.

The unified intention and the action of the practitioner and the client decide what is to be observed. Therefore, as the practitioner finds negative energies in the client and removes them with permission, in that moment, a new reality and outcome is created. The Body Code allows negative energies of emotions, traumas, allergies, misalignments, beliefs, toxins, and a vast array of specific imbalances to be removed from the energy fields of the body, collapsing all the possibilities of that moment to create a new, more positive, and healing future.

Intention energy is essential for creating change. But it is not enough on its own. The foundation the Body Code rests on is seeking and receiving power from above.

3. PRAYER

I recommend starting each session with a short prayer in which you ask the Higher Power for help. This is how I have found success.

Prayer is a communication from your heart to the source of all creation. It can be offered silently or out loud. It can be offered independently or in a group. Asking for help works. The mind that is the "matrix of all matter" knows all truth and can direct your thoughts and enlighten your mind.

When you ask for help, you are enabled to receive it. Conversely, when we are too proud to ask for help, we are left to ourselves. Then this work becomes just one more of many alternative methods that rely on human wisdom alone.

Measles

My personal experience with healing began in a miraculous way when I was seven years old. I was severely ill with measles accompanied by a high fever, nausea, and weakness. My parents had made a makeshift bed for me on the living-room couch upstairs so that I could be near their bedroom. From their whispered conversations about me when they thought I wasn't listening, I knew about their plan for me, that they were taking me to the hospital the following morning, where I would be put into something called an "oxygen tent." To my seven-year-old mind, the "tent" part of this plan sounded interesting, but I was really too sick to even think about camping.

That night after my other siblings had gone to bed, my parents quietly came into the living room. My mother said to my father, "Bruce, will you kneel down with me and say a prayer for our boy, so that he might be able to get well?" They knelt down by the side of the couch where I was lying, and my father began to pray for me.

In the midst of my father's short, heartfelt request, I suddenly felt a change take place in my body. This change began at the top of my head and rushed through my body to the soles of my feet in the space of about one single second. In the space of that one miraculous second, I was made completely well! I held my tongue until my father was done praying, which didn't take long. When he finished, I exclaimed, "I'm better! I'm better! Heavenly Father fixed me!" My parents didn't realize what had happened. Their reply was, "That's fine, honey. Go back to sleep now." But the next day proved that I was indeed healed, completely. I was back to my seven-year-old self, full of exuberant energy.

This incredible transformation was unforgettable! The experience is etched indelibly into my mind, and if I live to be a thousand years old, I will not forget it. More than fifty years have passed since that evening, and to me the memory is as fresh as if it had happened yesterday. The inescapable conclusion that I came to was that there must be a Higher Power, or some unseen source of assistance that we can draw upon in times of need, and that prayer is a way to elicit that help.

Now, after a lifetime of evidence-based practice, it's impossible for me to separate prayer from the art of healing. Of course, people's experiences with prayer are as different as they can possibly be. Some people believe in a Higher Power and some don't. Some were taught to use memorized, rote prayers, while others were taught simply to pray from the heart.

Paradigm-changing studies on the efficacy of prayer remain ignored by the mainstream press, but the results speak for themselves. In one study from South Korea, 219 infertile women between the ages of twenty-six and forty-six were treated with in vitro fertilization. The women were organized into two groups. One group was prayed for by volunteers in the United States, Canada, and Australia. Neither the women nor their doctors were informed about the research study. The researchers and statisticians did not know how the women had been organized into the two separate groups until all of the data had been collected and the research study was finished. Thus, it was a randomized, triple-blind, controlled, and prospective study.

When the data was analyzed, it became apparent that the women who had been prayed for were much more successful with their in vitro fertilization procedures. In fact, the women that had been prayed for were twice as likely to have a successful procedure than those in the control group.

In another fascinating study from Israel, patients suffering from blood infections had been admitted to hospitals during the years between 1990 and 1996. Volunteers in July of 2000 prayed for the recovery of half of these patients, chosen by a random-number generator. When the data was analyzed, the group that had been prayed for had experienced significantly shorter hospital stays and had recovered faster than the control group.

The fascinating thing about this study is that the patients who were prayed for had been hospitalized for their illnesses between four and ten years before the study even took place. It seems that prayer not only works, it may actually be able to transcend time! Of course, quantum physics explains how this is possible, since time is another dimension that is actually nonlinear, which is hard for us to wrap our minds around.

I've seen many cases of instantaneous healing since I became a physician. And in over thirty years of working with people from all over the world, with all kinds of conditions, I've learned some important principles.

Because I was asking the Higher Power for help with my patients, I expected that He would help me, and I did receive that help, although I learned that His help comes to us in ways that we might not always anticipate.

In all those years of practice, there were times when, in answer to my silent appeal for help, knowledge and understanding would flood into my being about how to look at things in a new way to help my patients better.

When we ask for help it usually comes in the form of a thought or an impression or an idea. These answers can be so subtle that we often miss them.

We may think that the idea is our own and dismiss it. We may not recognize the impression that comes or the feeling that we have as being answers from above, even when they are. We may even receive the right question to ask, as Rachael found in the following story.

The Right Questions

I wanted to share some recent success using the Body Code with some of my pregnant clients. These three women wanted to be physically, mentally, emotionally, and spiritually ready to have the best birth experiences possible.

One of the women I worked with was in her thirty-ninth week of pregnancy. She had been experiencing terrible groin pain for weeks. We did some work to clear that, and then took a few minutes to check if anything could be done to help with a safe and healthy delivery. One of the things that came up was actually an allergy to the idea of giving birth. This was her fourth delivery. We cleared the idea allergy and the underlying associations. She gave birth that night and reported back to me that she had a wonderful experience—her best birth yet.

Another client also asked if we could do Body Code work to prepare her for birthing. The question that I started with was, "Is it safe for me to give birth?" This was her third pregnancy. We released the energy of an image of her own birth experience, which had the emotions of helplessness and heartache associated with it. We also released a memory of her second child's birth, which had been a very stressful experience. We cleared several other imbalances. Then I felt impressed to ask about the baby: Did she have any priority imbalances that needed to be addressed? Indeed, she did. We released those things and also used the question "Is it safe for me to be born?" and cleared the underlying imbalances.

I have learned that asking for help from up above is so important, and the correct questions to ask will often come into my mind. All three of these women were so excited by their wonderful birth experiences. I also love that this work can be done from a distance. All of these sessions occurred with people that lived great distances from me. We were able to complete our sessions over the phone. I am thankful to Dr. Brad for sharing this modality and also for a loving Creator that has enabled this healing process here on the earth.

—Rachael H., Oklahoma, United States

Sometimes our pleas for help are answered by other people. You might be looking for an answer and have someone contact you about something seemingly unrelated, yet they ultimately help you find the answer. Have you ever inadvertently been the answer to someone else's prayers? If so, you know how good that can feel. Next, my wife, Jean, shares an experience of being an answer for a young woman in need.

The Spare Car

In the summer of 2004, we were getting ready to move from California to Utah. We had scheduled a semitruck to haul all of our possessions, and it was supposed to arrive in a couple of days. The Sunday before the move, I was sitting in church. Suddenly I heard a clear voice within myself say, "Go home right now!"

I literally jumped to my feet and promptly left to go home, without the rest of my family. I had no idea what I would find but was sure I was supposed to go home immediately. It felt urgent.

I remember wondering if our house was on fire. Brad's mom once had a similar experience years earlier. She suddenly felt prompted to leave work and go home. She found her house on fire. She was able to notify the fire department and save the house from burning to the ground.

As I pulled up to our house, I noticed a young man that had apparently been knocking on our front door. He was walking away from our house. I met him on the driveway and said, "Hi, I live here. Can I help you? " He seemed embarrassed. He said, "Well, you see the woman in that car parked over there?" He was pointing across the street. "That's my sister. She and I have been driving around all over the place this morning, and she insisted that we stop here. I know it sounds strange, but she wanted me to ask you about that car that's in your driveway."

I smiled. Our daughter, who had moved into an apartment with friends, had bought a car a few months earlier. She had left this other little car that sat in our driveway behind, as she no longer had any use for it. It belonged to Brad and me. A couple of days earlier, I realized we didn't have a driver to get that car to Utah when we moved. We didn't need it and didn't know what we were going to do with it. We'd been so busy packing and getting ready for the move that we'd forgotten about selling the car. This man asking about our car seemed as if he might present a welcome solution.

It was a small, black four-door, about eighteen years old. It sat there, looking rather forlorn, with fallen leaves scattered across the top of the hood.

I assured him that it was okay to ask about the car and invited him and his sister to come inside. They were very apologetic. Then her story poured out. She shared that she had just run away from home. Her husband had been physically abusive and she needed to get out of the marriage to save her life. She had escaped and gone to this brother for help, and he had been driving her around. Now she was beginning to think about her immediate needs. She was desperate to find a vehicle so that she could get a job to start working to support herself. She told us that she had been praying, asking God to help her find a car. They had started out about twenty miles away and had been driving around most of the morning and had ended up in our little suburban neighborhood.

I thought, "How beautiful that God knows all of our needs and is able to get her to our spare car." This was a sweet realization for all of us. They had truly been guided, and I had been prompted to "Go home right now." If I had been even a few seconds later, I'd probably have missed them. Interestingly, I had often prayed to be able to do more to help abused women. So I was also heard and felt acknowledged that day.

When Brad and the kids arrived home, and after explaining the situation, we agreed that our car should belong to this woman who needed it. She had escaped home with not much more than the clothes on her back but gave us a check for $200 to pay for the car. It was all she had. We were more than content, though the car's value far exceeded that.

After finding the title and sharing a meal, they drove away. We thought about it and knew she must need the $200 more than we did, so we promptly put the check in the mail and sent it back to her. She and her brother wrote a letter back, a beautiful letter of gratitude. The answer she received to her prayers solved not only her problem but ours as well. Truly, God does answer prayers!

—Jean Nelson

This story demonstrates that we can ask for help and receive it. If we do not ask for help from above, then we are reliant solely upon our own abilities, upon our own intuition and our own power. If it's true that help is available simply by asking, wouldn't it make sense to ask? Just open your heart to the possibility and give it a try. It really does work!

So, how should you ask for that help? What do you say? The words aren't nearly as important as the feeling in your heart when you pray. As Mahatma Gandhi said, "In prayer it is better to have a heart without words than words without a heart." It is enough for you to silently say, "Please help me." This is simple and specific. Just be sincere and trust that the Creator knows what is best.

4. GRATITUDE

Gratitude may just be the most underutilized superpower on Earth. You won't have to look far to find study after study on the benefits of being thankful. Feelings of isolation and depression decrease, blood pressure goes down, and immunity increases for people who choose to feel gratitude.

Michael Craig Miller, MD, says:

Gratitude is strongly and consistently linked to greater happiness. Expressing gratitude helps people feel more positive emotions, relish good experiences, improve their health, deal with adversity, and build strong relationships.

But all those great outcomes are not why I have placed gratitude as one of the essential elements for turning on the power of the Body Code.

If everything is energy, and it is, and we're using energy to change our experiences, to heal, transform relationships, unblock, be more creative, gain courage—whatever it is—then we need our energy level to be as high as it can be.

The well-known "Map of Consciousness" by Dr. David Hawkins ranks the vibrations of states of consciousness and emotions on a scale of 0 to 1,000. The lowest-ranked emotion is shame at 20, while the highest is enlightenment at 700–1,000. I believe that full-on, sustained gratitude is between love and joy on Dr. Hawkins's scale, a very high vibrational state indeed. American author, coach, speaker, and philanthropist Tony Robbins said, "When you are grateful, fear disappears and abundance appears."

Holding love for the person you're working with, and gratitude that you get to do this work and that it is working, puts you in a state where your intention can change lower vibrations, which all the negative energies are. The negative emotions range from 20–175 on the Hawkins scale, whereas love, gratitude, peace, and joy all resonate at 500 or more.

Here is a story from a practitioner named Joan, who shares her gratitude.

Itching Ears

I've had terribly itchy ears lately. My body was suggesting that it wasn't due to a pathogen. So, out of curiosity, I asked if I could find the answer in the Body Code. And the answer was yes! Using the Body Code, my subconscious mind took me to an imbalance called "memory field," energy trapped in my body from memories of hard things I have been through—similar memories throughout my life. With this hint, I was able to identify something that has been with me since before I was born, and even better, I was able to clear it all the way back to its very beginning. If that alone wasn't amazing enough, my ears immediately stopped itching!

Anybody who uses the Body Code will know that my story is only one of perhaps millions of shifts and improvements that have been accomplished through this system. Speaking for myself, I know that I have been saved from what would have been a highly challenging existence if I hadn't had the Body Code to help me identify the underlying causes for my challenges and clear them. I have been freed to enjoy a life of huge emotional and spiritual growth. For this, I feel profoundly blessed to have had it come into my life!

—Joan H., Ontario, Canada

I had a dream once that taught me that if you hold a belief that you can do this work, and you combine that belief with gratitude to God that you are actually doing it, you will see the results you are looking for. The equation looks like this:

Your belief that you can do it

+

Your gratitude to God or Higher Power that you are doing it

=

The results you want to obtain

Would we ever begin anything if we did not believe we could do it? No. Belief is essential to all we do and is the necessary first step.

I can't overemphasize the importance of the word "doing" in the equation just given. In other words, your gratitude to the Higher Power that you are actually doing the work is significant, because it is to that Higher Power that we owe everything that we have and are, and every opportunity that lies in our path. If you have a goal that you want to achieve, imagine how grateful you would feel if you had already achieved it. If you can feel that achievement before it happens and expect that it will be, it will be, if you are also willing to put forth the necessary effort.

As you learn to cultivate gratitude to God for what you already have, your faith and belief will increase, for you will draw yourself closer to that very source of power from which all things flow.

You will soon find yourself doing the very thing that was once only a dream.

To be a healer, you must not entertain thoughts of doubt; you must leave your fears behind. Your heart must be filled with love and gratitude. If this seems unnatural at first, it will be easier and easier with practice. Try it!

CHOOSE LIGHT OVER DARKNESS

These four aspects of being present are all about choosing the light instead of the dark. We work to clear negative energies of darkness, which are always destructive and sometimes deceiving. We are all being constantly influenced by negative and positive energies. When we choose to love, have gratitude, intend healing, and ask for help from the source of all light, then we eventually become light bearers to the world and servants to those around us.

Love, intention, prayer, and gratitude call forth the power of light. Believe there is light available to you. Believe that the light is flowing through you as you serve. Choose to be filled with love for yourself and for the one you are serving. Choose gratitude that it's working, and always expect a miracle.

PART II

USING THE BODY CODE

Concerning matter, we have been all wrong. What we have called matter is energy, whose vibration has been so lowered as to be perceptible to the senses. There is no matter.

—ALBERT EINSTEIN

4

GETTING ANSWERS

The beautiful thing about learning is that nobody can take it away from you.

—B. B. KING

Now that we have discussed the principles that the Body Code is based on, let's turn our attention to the more practical aspects of what you have to do to not only get answers but correct imbalances as well.

Depending on the imbalance that you have discovered, the Body Code will supply you with specific directions that explain what needs to be done. For example, a nutritional deficiency may need a specific supplement to be resolved.

Dehydration will likely require the subject to drink more water. If the subconscious indicates a need for an essential oil, that oil will need to be obtained. If an infection or a parasitic infestation is discovered, the Body Code System will guide you to anything from a natural remedy to seeking medical intervention. A toxin may need a cleanse of some sort, and so on. Energetic imbalances are the most common sort of imbalances that we suffer from, and I have found that the easiest and most effective means of correcting and releasing energetic imbalances is with the use of magnetic energy.

MAGNETS

Magnets are a pure source of energy. When used the right way, a magnet can act as an amplifier and carrier for your intention. This is similar to how a magnifying glass will visually amplify whatever is behind it, making it appear larger.

You can use any magnet, from powerful magnets to the weak business-card magnet that your plumber left you, or even the magnetic energy of your body. You may not know it, but your body is continually emitting magnetic energy, so if you don't have a magnet with you, your hand will do just fine.

In the following story, Avelino saw dramatic changes with every pass of a magnet while releasing trapped emotions from a toddler.

The Nightmare Girl

A three-year-old was brought to me by her mother, a patient of mine, because she was suffering from nightmares and was very afraid of men. She had urged in her words, "Mom, I want you to take me to the guy who has been helping you with your emotions." She is one of those little girls that impresses at first contact, but she was not herself. I began working on her using the Body Code and found several childhood traumas caused by her father. As we progressed, her reactions were incredible. With every passing stroke of the magnet, trapped emotions and imbalances were released. Her contagious laughter filled the room. She was calmer as she concentrated on feeling the healing. She left the room very happy and gave me a hug.

After a week, her mom contacted the clinic to let me know that her little girl was healed completely. Her nightmares and fears were gone. She's very happy now.

—Avelino L., Florida, United States

DIRECTING YOUR INTENTION

Chinese physicians discovered around three thousand years ago that restoring balance to the flows of energy in the body improved their patients' health. They mapped out energetic "rivers," called *meridians,* which flow throughout the body and connect with each other. These maps of the meridians in the acupuncture system are essentially the same maps that are used by acupuncturists today.

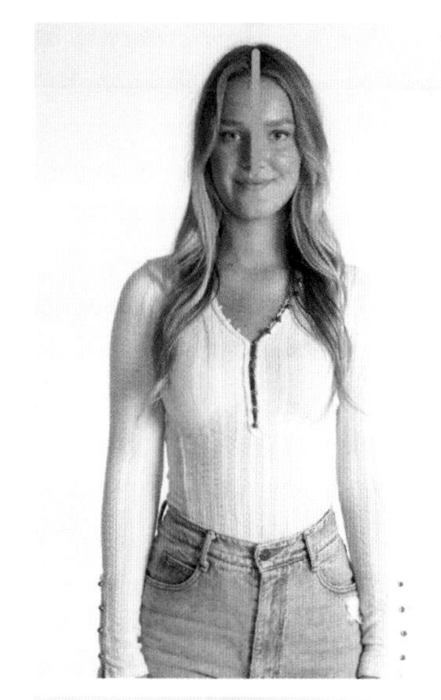

Energy flows through the meridians to maintain balance and function in all the parts of your body. One meridian is particularly important to your use of the Body Code. The governing meridian is an energy reservoir, a primary river in the river system of the meridians. It is the perfect channel into which you can direct your intention energy as you use the Body Code. It connects to all the other meridians, so when intention energy is put into the governing meridian, it flows directly into the other meridians and throughout the entire energy body. The governing meridian starts at the tailbone and travels up the spine, over the head, and down the midline of the face, where it ends inside the upper lip.

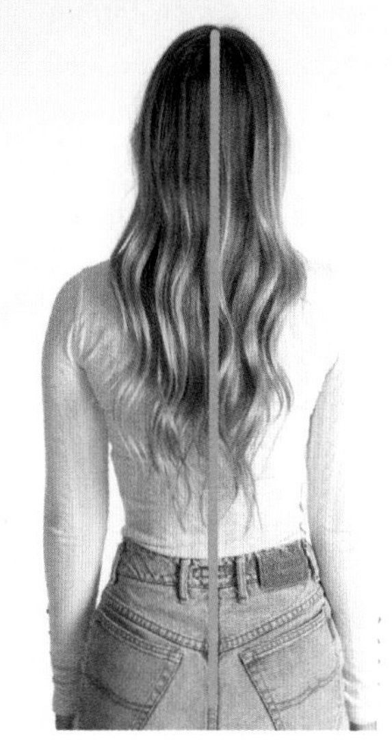

Once you have identified an energetic imbalance and are ready to correct it, swiping a magnet over the governing meridian allows your intention energy to flow into the body, easily releasing or correcting energetic imbalances. Using any portion of the governing meridian works. For example, if you are working on yourself, passing a magnet up the middle of your forehead, over the top of your head, and down the back of your neck is enough. When working on another person, it works fine to pass the magnet from the base of their neck and down their back to the waist.

Most energetic imbalances only require three swipes of a magnet down the governing meridian, but a few require ten, as is needed with inherited trapped emotions, for example. When you follow this procedure, your intention energy flows into the body and does not allow the negative energy or imbalance to remain.

I have personally never seen an energetic imbalance leave the body with my own eyes. However, the changes that occur, such as improvements in the way people feel, their decrease in pain, and so on, are frequent and unmistakable. Occasionally I meet individuals who report that they have seen orblike balls of energy leave the body upon the release of trapped emotions and other energetic imbalances.

When a negative energy such as a trapped emotion is released, it is neutralized—changed into a positive or neutral vibration. If you are having trouble imagining how this works, think of what happens when a magnet is swiped over the magnetic strip on the back of a credit card and the information is erased or changed, rendering the card useless. It's a similar process.

Energetic imbalances, however, are more easily neutralized when there is love and gratitude being focused on the subject.

When you use your intention to release or correct the imbalance, coupled with a few swipes of a magnet or your hand over the governing meridian, any energetic imbalance that is ready to be released can be cleared from the body. That is all it takes. It's simple and incredibly fast.

Now let's discuss the easiest way to find imbalances.

GETTING ANSWERS WITH MUSCLE TESTING

An easy way to get information from the subconscious mind is through muscle testing. This is also known as kinesthetic testing, or simply kinesiology. It is a form of biofeedback that requires no high-tech equipment but is a powerful way to connect with the subconscious to decode vital information. Although some people have never heard of it, muscle testing is not new. Doctors have been using it since the 1940s for various purposes, including to evaluate muscle strength and assess the extent of an injury. Today, physicians and others who specialize in the mechanics of body movement know that muscle testing has many more applications than doctors first understood.

People are sometimes skeptical about whether it will work, but once they've seen the results for themselves, they can't help but be amazed, just as this nine-year-old boy was when his mom helped relieve his sore throat and earache.

Now a Believer

My son is nine years old and one of the biggest skeptics that I have ever met! One night my son was complaining of a sore throat and earache. I panicked at the thought that he might have another infection. Once a year, somehow, he gets incredibly sick and ends up on antibiotics for weeks. I started calling it our annual trip to the ER, because it would happen at the same time every year.

My son sat up in bed complaining to me that his ear hurt and his throat hurt, so I asked him if it would be okay if I tried the Body Code. My son said, "Sure, Mom, but I know it's not going to work." He has always been a little skeptical of my energy-healing work. So I responded with, "Okay, but if it helps, then you have to be open to the possibility that it actually works." He said, "Fine! You have twenty-four hours . . . and I have to feel ninety percent better." I laughed and said, "Okay, deal!"

We worked on clearing emotion after emotion. Honestly, I wasn't sure if it was going to stop. . . . I actually thought I was doing my muscle testing incorrectly. By the time we were done, he said he felt a little better but not 90 percent yet. I told him that he should sleep on it and see how he feels in the morning. So, he did. And in the morning, he came trotting down the stairs like nothing was wrong, and he didn't even mention feeling sick. He had completely forgotten that he was sick the night before. When I mentioned to him that he looked better and I asked him if he was a believer yet, he stopped in his tracks and was a little shocked that he was feeling so good. He said, "Wow, Mom! It did work!" Now, when he gets sick, he will ask me to clear trapped emotions. He will even call me from the nurses' station at school and ask me to work on him over the phone if he is feeling sick at school. He is now a believer!

—Melissa K., Georgia, United States

Muscle testing can tell us about the overall health and balance of our bodies. It can help us identify vulnerable areas before sickness and disease take hold. It can help us find out what's at the root of our various physical, emotional, and mental struggles. It gives us a direct way to ask the body what's bothering it, and, once we've treated the problem, it can tell us whether we've made a change. It can tell us if imbalances are present in the body and let us know the moment they've been released.

The subconscious mind can be compared to a binary computer, so we can ask yes-or-no questions and get yes-or-no answers from the body. Not only can we get answers to just about every question about the body, but I believe there is a sort of list in every person's subconscious mind. This list contains all the things that need to be done to bring the body back to 100 percent function, or as close to it as possible.

Muscle testing helps us to get answers from the subconscious mind because the body gives a physical response when we tell the truth or a lie. The muscles of the body are instantly weakened when we lie. They stay strong when we tell the truth. There are many methods of muscle testing that can be learned. In *The Emotion Code* book, I explain more methods than the following few, but these should be enough to get you started.

SELF-TESTING

The various methods of self–muscle testing that we present here can be used to work on yourself and get answers from your own body, or they can be used as a way for you to get answers about what another person needs when you are standing in as a surrogate or proxy for them.

The easiest self-testing method is called the sway test. Your body will respond by swaying forward when you are holding thoughts of truth, positivity, or congruency. Your body will sway backward when holding thoughts of negativity, falsehood, or incongruency. This works because the human body is an organism like any other. All organisms, no matter how primitive, will respond to positive or negative stimuli. For example, plants grow toward sunlight and away from darkness. A fish in an aquarium will move toward clean water and away from a source of pollution.

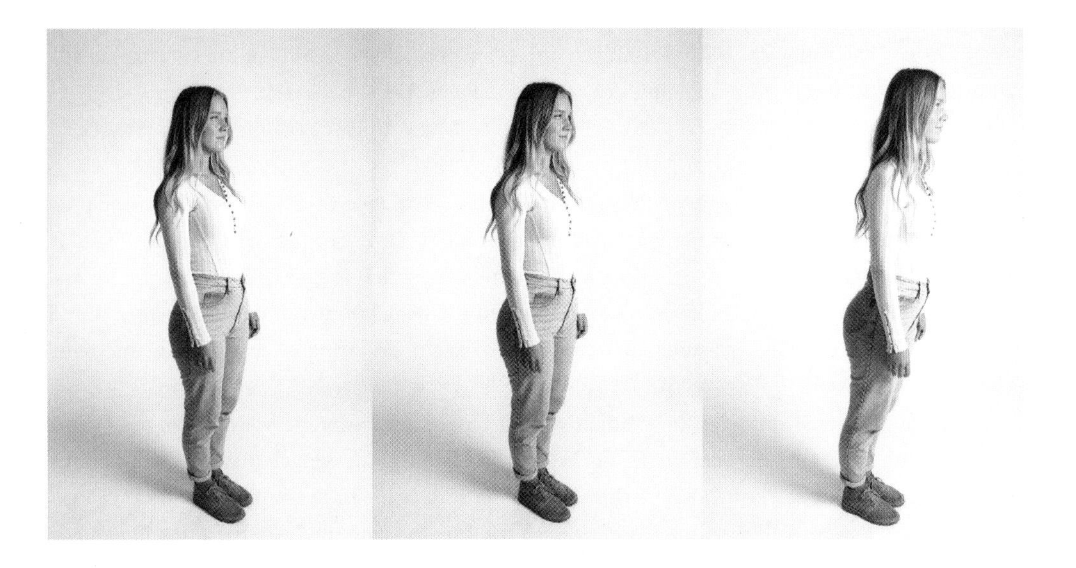

THE SWAY TEST

To perform the sway test, simply stand in a very relaxed way. It's a good idea to turn off any music or TV, just in case they may interfere with the testing. Drop your arms to your sides and completely relax. The first thing you'll notice while you're standing there is that there is a little bit of movement going on all the time. Your body may lean forward just a little or backward a little, or it may lean a little to the side, left or right. These slight movements are simply the oscillation that takes place as your postural muscles continuously work to keep your body standing upright.

Let's see if you notice yourself swaying backward or forward when you hold some specific thoughts.

Let's start with something that is very negative. Think about the word "war" for a moment.

Hold that thought in your mind while you're standing there in a very relaxed way. Think about all the people who have died, all the families that have been torn apart, all the tragedy, all the people who have been crippled and maimed, and all the destruction of property and lives lost. Think about all the sorrow and anguish that's been happening on this earth since the beginning. If you continue to hold these thoughts in your mind, within ten seconds or less, you should notice that your body begins to sway backward, trying to move you away from the sheer negativity of the idea of war.

Now let's try another thought. Think about the feeling of unconditional love. Imagine that you are a being of unconditional love, that the feeling of love in your heart is so big that your heart cannot contain it, and that feeling of love for all people and all of creation expands out from your core and fills the universe. Think about what it would be like to be loved and accepted unconditionally by others in return. As you hold that thought of unconditional love in your mind, within ten seconds or less, you will find your body swaying forward, moving you toward the positivity and the beauty of that potential future.

The sway test can be used for any of the questions that you want to ask the body. It's a useful method of testing and works for just about anyone. It's simple and doesn't usually require much practice. And like most things, the more you do it, the better it works.

There are some other methods of self-testing that are faster than the sway test. These other methods are convenient to use, but they do take some practice to master.

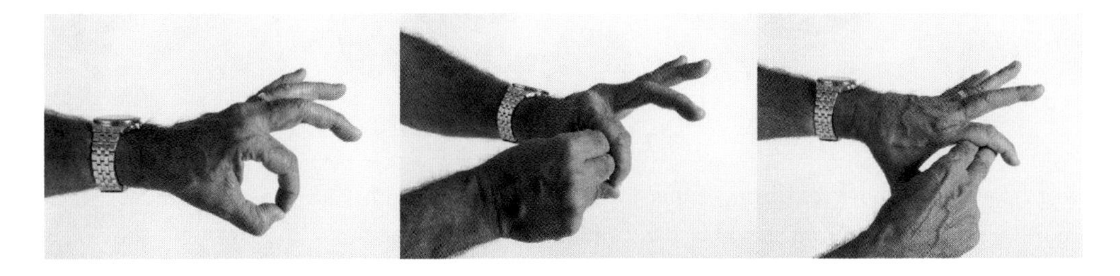

HOLE-IN-ONE METHOD

To perform the Hole-in-One method, you simply make a ring with your thumb and first finger, as pictured. Then insert the thumb and the first two fingers of your other hand into the ring. When performing a muscle test, try to open the ring by pulling apart your other thumb and two fingers. For yes, or a congruent statement, the ring should stay closed. For no, or an incongruent statement, the ring should open because the muscle will weaken a bit temporarily. You can also use other fingers to perform this test if you want to.

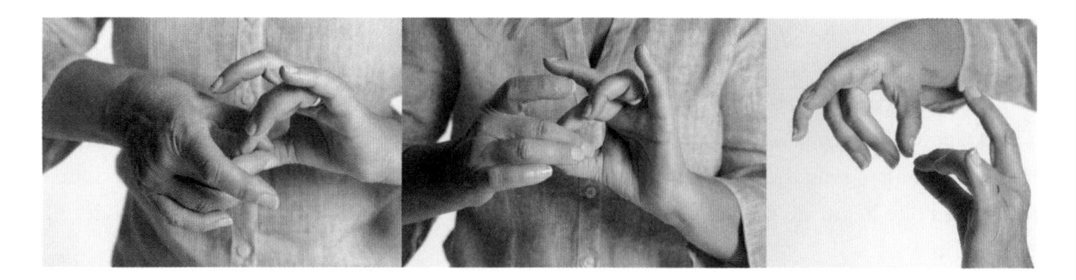

RING-IN-RING METHOD

For the Ring-in-Ring method, use one hand to make a ring with your thumb and index finger. Then make another ring with your other hand, making two links in a chain. To test, make your statement or ask a question, then try to pull the rings apart. For yes answers or in response to statements of truth, congruency, or positivity, the ring (or both rings) should stay closed. For no answers, or if you make a statement that is untrue, the rings will weaken and you will be able to pull your hands apart easily.

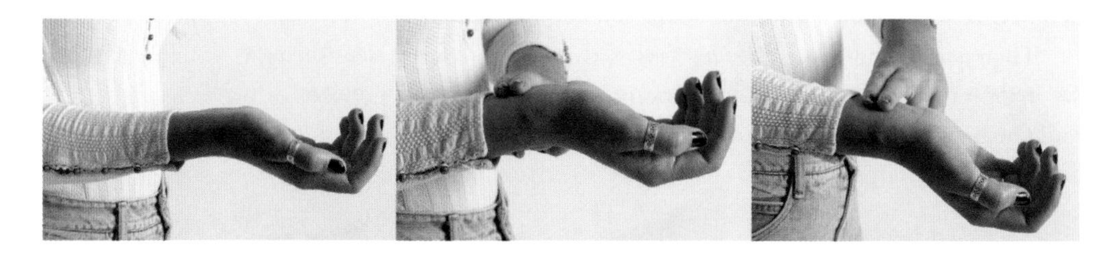

ELBOW TEST

To perform the elbow test, bring either elbow to your side, with your forearm parallel to the floor. Use two fingers from the other hand and place them on the top of the arm right above the wrist bone. Then simply press down. On yes answers, the forearm will stay parallel to the floor, and on no answers, your arm will weaken and drop.

There are a few things that you should note about this method:

- Another variation of the elbow test is to bend your arm at a sharper angle, about 45 degrees or so.
- The amount of resistance force used in this test is simply the amount of muscle strength it takes to keep the forearm parallel to the floor, no more. The amount of resistance used in all of the methods should be minimal. You are simply trying to discern a slight change, not prove your strength.

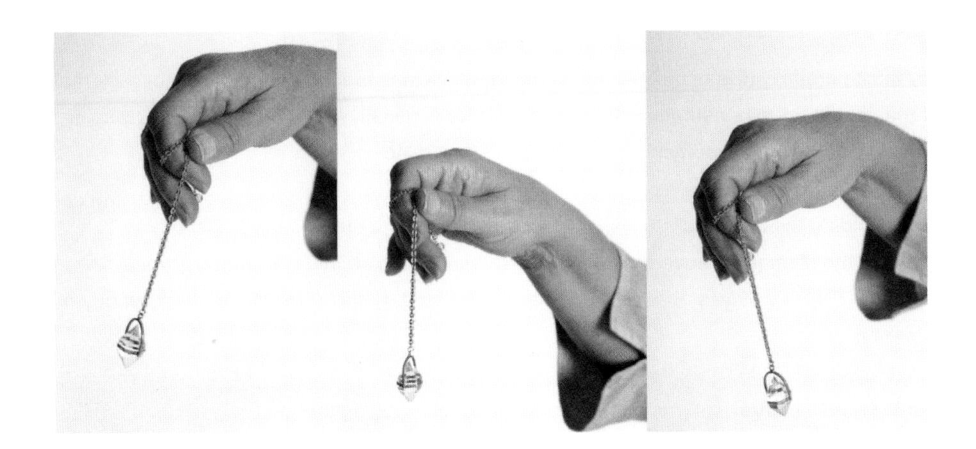

PENDULUM

Pendulums can be incredibly useful tools, especially for those who doubt their muscle-testing abilities. Pendulums and other dowsing devices simply amplify the muscular and nervous-system changes taking place in the most sensitive detecting instrument in existence—the human body.

If you decide to use a pendulum, I suggest you choose one that feels good in your hand. Hold the string or chain with your fingers pointing down. Any small weight or pendant on a chain could be used as a pendulum, but I suggest you purchase an actual pendulum if you want to learn this skill. Intention is key when one is using a pendulum. It's important to note that the pendulum itself is not the source of information. The answers come from the subconscious mind. The pendulum is simply a tool that shows the response in the body when you ask a question.

STEP 1.

Make sure you're comfortable and relaxed.

STEP 2.

Hold the chain so that both chain and pendant are free of interference. Grasp the chain or string between your thumb and forefinger. The ideal length of the chain hanging between your fingertips and the pendulum should be about the width of your palm.

STEP 3.

Brace your upper arm against your body, but do not brace your hand. It will be impossible to stay perfectly still, and this is fine.

STEP 4.

Swing the pendulum back and forth very gently on a diagonal in front of your body to create a bit of momentum. This is your neutral, neither yes or no.

STEP 5.

For most people, yes is usually either a circular clockwise motion or a forward-to-back motion of the pendulum, synonymous with a head nod. No is usually either a counterclockwise or side-to-side motion, synonymous with a head shaking no.

STEP 6.

While holding the diagonally moving pendulum, which is neutral, focus and say "yes." Observe the change of movement of the pendulum, which should take place within a few seconds. This is your yes answer. Return to neutral and try this several times until your yes answer is clear.

STEP 7.

Come back to neutral, returning to a gentle diagonal swinging motion.

STEP 8.

A no answer should be the opposite of what your yes answer looks like. So if your yes was a clockwise motion, your no will be counterclockwise. Say "no" and see what the movement looks like, expecting it to be the opposite of your yes answer. Return to neutral after you get your answer, and repeat several times until the answer is clear each time.

STEP 9.

Now try using different true statements and false statements to test your yes and no responses. Once you have clear and consistent answers, you can begin to use your pendulum to get answers from the subconscious mind.

ALWAYS ASK FOR PERMISSION

Getting permission from others before working on them is critically important, because working on them without their knowledge or permission or against their wishes is a true invasion of privacy and is unethical. Always explain what you are going to do before you do it. If you are going to be pressing down on other people's arms to test them, explain the procedure beforehand and get their permission.

It is technically possible to test other people through self-testing, proxy, or surrogate testing without their knowing it, and this is wrong. Not only that, but because you don't have their permission, it may be harder for you to make a good connection, and you may get incorrect answers. So don't do it even if you're curious, and if asked, tell others that it's against your principles or ethics to do so.

Always ask permission of the person you are going to test, and always honor that person's wishes. Never test or work on minors without the permission of their parents or guardians. If it's an adult child of your own, you must get permission even though it is your child. If you're going to work on someone who is comatose or unconscious, permission must be acquired from his or her next of kin. In the case of domestic animals or pets, you must get permission from the owner.

I have been asked multiple times if getting permission from the subconscious mind of a person is enough. It is not enough. Always get either spoken or written permission from people before working on them, their children, or their animals. Asking permission only from their subconscious mind is unethical and should not be done, unless it is accompanied by conscious permission.

RESISTANCE VS. PRESSURE

Your brain controls how strong or weak a muscle is or how hard it resists. Experiment with any of the testing methods by using more or less resistance. One of the common mistakes that most people make, especially in self-testing, is to use too much force and resistance.

Keep the pressure light and resist only as much as you absolutely need to. Remember that the harder you resist, the harder you're going to have to press down to overcome that resistance, so you're really working against yourself. You'll also probably experience discomfort sooner or later if you are using too much strength. I find that using about 1 percent or less of the strength available is all that is needed to pick up the subtle changes that happen in muscle strength when you are asking questions. The more you practice using very light resistance, the more you will find that muscle testing is not a strength contest. Self-testing, in particular, does take practice, but it's definitely worth mastering. And remember to confirm your testing with a yes-or-no test each time you start testing yourself or someone else to make sure the subject is testable, whether the subject is you or someone else.

If any muscle testing method hurts, it means you're using too much pressure. The goal is not to wear yourself out or hurt yourself, but to find your perfect strength and resistance settings to make it easy.

DON'T FOCUS ON YOUR FINGERS!

A common mistake that people make when learning self-muscle testing is focusing on their fingers. Anyone who can type forty words a minute or more knows very well that they shouldn't think too much about what their fingers are doing or it will slow them down and they'll make more mistakes. Every typing teacher will instruct you not to look at your fingers for this reason.

Self-muscle testing also works best if you don't focus on your fingers when you are attempting to get an answer. Instead, focus on the question or on the person you are testing, and allow the muscle test to take place slightly disconnected from your focus, just like a typist looking at a manuscript and allowing his or her fingers to do what they already know how to do.

PRACTICE! PRACTICE! PRACTICE!

Not all methods are for everyone. Find one or two methods you like and practice them until you are proficient. I recommend that most people practice using their favorite method about one hundred times a day for about two weeks or so to get the hang of self-testing. That's simply saying yes and no one hundred times and testing the muscle response every day for two weeks. That should only be a few minutes of practice per day and is well worth the effort, as Natalya found in this next story.

Do It Yourself

After spending thousands of dollars on doctors, prescriptions, and health supplements, I knew I needed to do something different. After being worked on by a Body Code practitioner, I realized how much money I could save by doing this method on myself and my family. I found the Discover Healing online muscle-testing method, and I started practicing self-testing right away. It took me a few days to get used to reading my own body messages and to train my fingers (I use the Ring-in-Ring method, mainly). And it works, and works always!!!

—Natalya B., Russia

MUSCLE-TESTING OTHERS

One way to find out what is going on in someone else's body is by muscle-testing the person directly, using his or her muscle strength.

Before you use this method of testing, always ask people you wish to muscle-test if they have pain in either shoulder. If they do, don't use the sore arm, as it may aggravate their condition. If they have trouble in both shoulders or if they are too young, too weak, or too ill to be tested, you should try a different way to test, such as either surrogate or proxy testing. You could be the surrogate or the proxy yourself if the other person is unable to be tested. These will be explained later in this chapter.

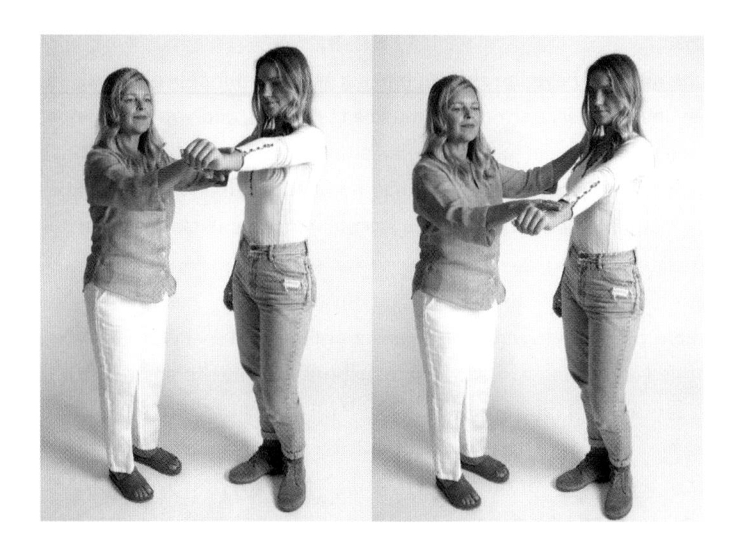

STEP 1.

Ask the subject to stand up and hold one arm out directly in front, horizontal to the floor. The person should not make a tight fist, but let the hand remain relaxed.

STEP 2.

Place the first two fingers of your hand lightly on the other's arm, just above the bump on the wrist. (See the image.)

STEP 3.

Place your free hand on the person's opposite shoulder for support.

STEP 4.

Tell the subject, "I'm going to have you make a statement, and then I'm going to press down on your arm gently. I want you to resist me by holding your arm right where it is. Try to prevent me from pushing your arm down."

STEP 5.

Have the subject state his or her name. If the subject's name is Kim, for example, he or she would say, "My name is Kim."

STEP 6.

Perform the muscle test by smoothly and steadily increasing the pressure downward on the subject's arm, going from no pressure to a gentle-but-firm pressure within about three seconds.

STEP 7.

The arm should stay "locked" against your firm downward pressure and should not give way.

STEP 8.

Now repeat the test, but have the subject make a statement that is obviously false by using a wrong name. Immediately perform the muscle test again, and you should notice the arm is weaker, since the statement just made was untrue. We refer to this as a "baseline test." It is done to see if the subject is testable at that moment, and it should always be performed before a Body Code session is done, if you are planning to muscle-test your subject directly.

Correct finger placement is important when muscle-testing. You'll notice that everyone has a bony bump on the wrist, which is part of the ulna bone. Notice in the photo that the tester's two fingers are positioned *above* the wrist (toward the elbow), not *on* the wrist. With the tester's fingers placed as shown, pressure is being applied on the long bones of the arm. If the fingers are placed directly over the bones of the wrist, it is difficult to get a proper muscle test, because pressure applied to the wrist bones will automatically weaken the arm muscles and make accurate testing difficult. This is because the brain does not want the wrist bones to be injured, which can happen if too much pressure is placed on them. This is a protective mechanism that is built in to prevent injury. You do want to be applying your pressure as far out on the long bones of the forearm as you can be for maximum leverage, but not past the wrist bump.

TIPS FOR TESTING OTHERS IN PERSON

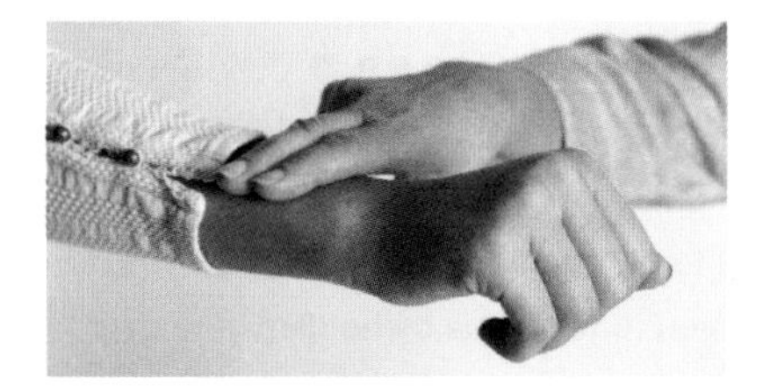

There are a few important things to keep in mind when muscle-testing others in person.

- Use a smoothly increasing downward pressure that starts from no pressure at all, increasing to firm pressure over about three seconds.
- Don't bounce, instead be smooth and gentle, allowing the muscles time to adapt to your pressure instead of confusing them.
- As soon as you have your answer and it's clear to you that the person's arm is either staying locked or feeling mushy, you should let go. Don't wear your subject out!
- If you are muscle-testing a person who is much stronger than yourself, have your subject sit in a chair while you stand, so you are at a mechanical advantage.

- Ask your subject to "resist me gently."
- Use only the minimum amount of pressure needed. Think finesse, not force.
- Muscle testing is about "sensing" the answer.
- Keep an open mind. You should never project what you want the answer to be, as that can skew the result.
- If any muscle-testing method hurts, stop and try another method.
- Keep your fingers in the correct position; don't go past the wrist bump toward the hand.
- You can experiment with various arm positions to see what works best for you and whomever you are working on. Some other options are for the subject to hold his or her arm out to the side rather than straight out in front, or with the elbow bent at a 90-degree angle, with the forearm parallel to the floor (as discussed in the elbow test method).

During my years in practice, I would occasionally have a pregnant woman come to me to see what the sex of her baby was going to be. I found that during the first three months of the pregnancy the answers were difficult to obtain and seemed to be unclear. However, during the second and third trimesters it was usually easy to get an accurate answer. In fact, I was about 98 percent accurate in my predictions through muscle testing, which I felt were at least as accurate as ultrasound. This was entertaining and fun, and I didn't charge for this simple service. However, I eventually learned how important it is to remove any bias in order to avoid getting wrong answers.

Biased Muscle Testing

At one point during my years in practice, our twin boys were born, and the number of our children suddenly doubled. By the time they were three years old, my wife, Jean, was feeling worn out, and was making a decision to not have any more children. As she was having these thoughts one day, suddenly in her mind's eye there was a darling little girl who was saying, "What! You mean you're not going to have me?!" My wife's heart instantly melted, and she realized that there was another child meant to come to our family.

When she got pregnant later, we were excited that our little girl was on her way. We wanted her to come, we would make room for her, and it was all going to be fine.

Once the first trimester was over, I would periodically test Jean to see if this baby was a girl. Every time, the answer received through muscle testing was yes.

We decided to have the baby at home with a midwife. But the baby was a boy! I thought, "What happened?"

As I thought about this, I realized what had gone wrong. You see, the subconscious mind is a bit like a puppy. Puppies want to please you, and so might the subconscious mind. Jean and I wanted the little girl who we were sure was coming to our home. We had done everything except paint her room pink. Because we had this desire, both of our subconscious minds interfered with getting to the true answer. Our little girl finally did come, but it was not until after two more boys had been born that she decided to make her appearance, right on time.

I hope that you will remember this story. Muscle testing, like anything else in this world, is not 100 percent accurate. It can be swayed away from the truth if either you or your subject has a desire for the answer to come out a certain way. Beware of this in your testing, and have an open mind, free of bias.

SURROGATE TESTING

Like a light in a dark room, a person's (or animal's) biomagnetic field is powerful up close but becomes dimmer the farther away from it you get. I have found that our energy field extends out from our bodies powerfully for six feet in all directions. When information surfaces from the subconscious mind, it results in readable changes in our immediate energy field, which can be measured and shown by muscle testing. But what if someone isn't able to be muscle tested directly for some reason? This is where surrogate testing comes in. A surrogate is another person who steps in and, in this case, allows themself to be muscle tested as an extension of the subject. Surrogate testing is the answer in any situation where a person or animal is present physically but is not testable.

Reasons that someone might be temporarily unable to be muscle tested on their own body include the following:

- Age—it may be difficult or impossible to test an infant, a small child, or an elderly person using their own muscles.
- Physical limitation, such as injury, illness, pain, weakness, dehydration, or neck misalignment.
- Loss of consciousness, such as being asleep or in a comatose state.
- Inability to reason due to intellectual disability.
- Being an animal.

In order to use surrogate testing, the subject must be within six feet of the surrogate. When a subject is not testable for any reason, we can still get answers from the subconscious mind using a surrogate. To get those answers, we use either of these two approaches:

- Self-testing, which is when the tester acts as both surrogate and tester.
- Having a third person act as the surrogate.

In either situation, the surrogate doesn't have to touch the subject. We have found that being within six feet of the subject is close enough to receive a strong reading in energy changes when the intention to get answers from the subject is clear.

Suppose you would like to test an infant. Anyone who is testable can act as a surrogate for the infant. In the case of a child, the surrogate could be the child's mother or father or anyone the child is comfortable with.

Anyone who is testable can act as a surrogate for anyone else. I've come to regard surrogate testing as an indispensable application of muscle testing. If you are getting an inconsistent or unclear muscle-testing response while testing your subject, my recommendation is to use surrogate testing, either by asking questions and receiving answers on your own body via self-testing or by adding a third person as the surrogate. In any case, you are still directing your questions to the subconscious mind of the subject, but you are muscle-testing the surrogate, (either yourself or a third person). The answers will be the same. In fact, you will often find that using surrogate testing will help make the answers easier to discern.

HOW TO DO SURROGATE TESTING

Following are two procedures for using surrogate testing: one for using self-testing and acting as surrogate yourself, and the other for when you are using a third person as the surrogate.

When you are acting as both tester and surrogate, using self-testing, follow these steps:

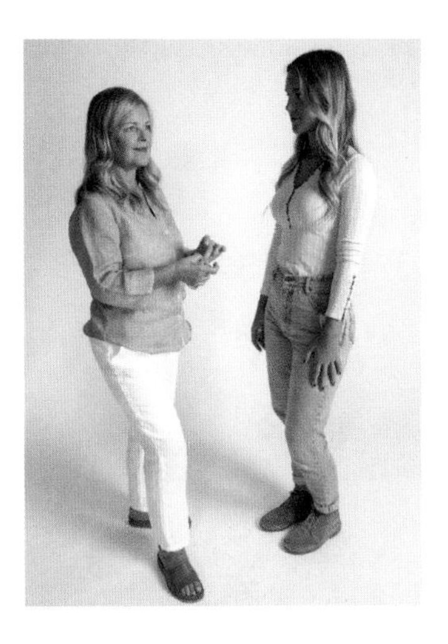

STEP 1.

Feel love for your subject, gratitude that this will help the person, and offer a silent prayer for divine assistance.

STEP 2.

Make sure that you are testable by getting a good baseline test. Do this as previously discussed, by making sure you get a clear and correct answer to each yes-no question.

STEP 3.

Make sure you are within six feet of the subject. Physically touching is not necessary but is fine if desired.

STEP 4.

To confirm that you are reading the energy of the subject, have the subject state his or her name: "My name is ____." If the person is unable to speak, you can state, "Your name is ____," filling in the blank with the name. Then perform a self-muscle test, and the response should be strong.

STEP 5.

To double-check, have the subject make an incongruent statement by saying, "My name is ____," using any name that is false. You can also make the statement for the subject such as, "Your name is ____." Your response here should be weak or incongruent when it is untrue.

STEP 6.

If your answers are not clear, repeat steps 4 and 5 until the answers are clear. At this point, you may continue with the Body Code process.

When you are using a third person as the surrogate and testing on their body, follow these steps:

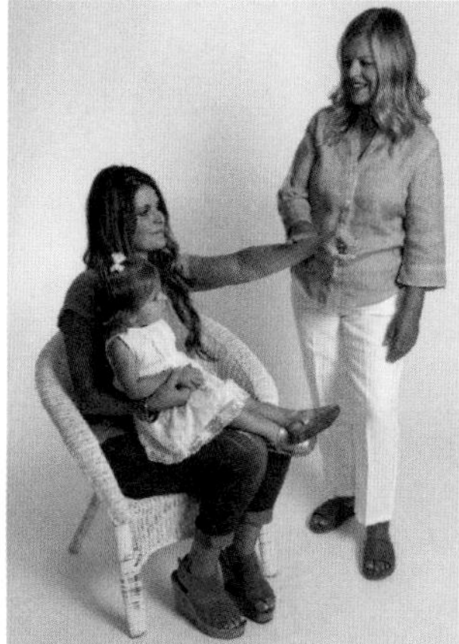

STEP 1.

Feel love for your subject, gratitude that this will help them, and offer a silent prayer for divine assistance.

STEP 2.

Make sure that the surrogate is testable. Get a good baseline test on the surrogate, as previously discussed, by making sure you get a clear answer to each yes-no question.

STEP 3.

The surrogate simply needs to be near the subject, within six feet. They can hold hands if desired, but it is not necessary.

STEP 4.

To confirm that the surrogate person is able to pick up the energetic changes in the subject, have the subject state his or her name: "My name is ____," filling in the blank with the subject's name. If the subject is unable to speak, you can state, "Your name is ____," filling in the blank with the subject's name. Then perform a muscle test on the surrogate, and the response should be strong.

STEP 5.

Then, have the subject make an incongruent statement by saying, "My name is ____," using any false name. You can also make the statement for the person, such as, "Your name is ____," filling in the blank with any name that is incorrect. The muscle-testing response on the surrogate should be weak.

STEP 6.

If your answers are not clear, repeat steps 4 and 5 until the answers are clear. At this point, you may continue with the Body Code session.

Remember that during this process, you will ask questions of the subject or have the subject make the appropriate statements, but the muscle testing will be done on the surrogate's body, not the subject's body.

SURROGATE TESTING CHILDREN

Young children are not usually able to be muscle tested reliably. Surrogate testing provides a simple and efficient way to get the answers you need to help them.

You can help children by using a surrogate for testing. The Body Code works the same way for children as it does for adults. Any child can have trapped emotions and other imbalances, no matter how much love the child receives or how favorable the home environment may be.

SURROGATE TESTING ANIMALS

When I test animals, I always talk to the animal as if it were a human being. Animals may not understand our spoken words, but they do understand the intention that our thoughts convey. Animals have subconscious minds just as we do, and they implicitly understand what we're trying to do for them. When working on an animal, direct your questions to the animal and test the surrogate (either another person or yourself) to get the responses.

Surrogate testing works with cats, dogs, horses, and all kinds of animals. There are so many remarkable stories about using the Body Code on animals that I've devoted an entire chapter to the topic toward the end of the book.

SURROGATE TESTING FOR PEOPLE WHO ARE UNCONSCIOUS

Surrogate testing also makes it possible to test someone who is asleep, unconscious, or in a coma. Even if a person is unresponsive or unable to make verbal contact, the subconscious mind is still at work; it never sleeps. Unconscious people's bodily functions are still working. They are still breathing. Their hearts are still beating. Their subconscious minds are still alert to the environment and working to keep things on track. When you ask the subconscious mind a question, it will know the answer, but if the person is unconscious, he or she will not be able to actively participate in the test. So testing through a surrogate is the perfect solution.

However, muscle testing should never be used in an emergency situation, when CPR would be a more appropriate response.

A number of years ago, my father suffered a massive brain aneurysm and fell into a coma. I was deeply concerned and eager to help him in any way I could. When Jean and I went to the hospital to see him, we found it impossible to get close enough to work on him directly, due to all the tubes and wires that surrounded him.

I asked Jean to act as surrogate for my father. Even though he was in a coma, we were immediately able to tap into his subconscious mind and determine what we could do to help him the most, in addition to all that was already being done by the hospital staff. He did wake up, and we had one more precious year with him before he finally passed. Being able to work on him in that comatose state was an unforgettable experience that made me grateful indeed for the gift of surrogate testing.

Remember that in surrogate testing, questions are directed toward the subject, but testing is actually done on the surrogate person. Imbalances are found by testing the surrogate, but corrections are made on the subject. However, you can also make corrections on the surrogate if that is a better option at the moment.

One of the great things about surrogate testing is that the answers you get will often be amplified through the surrogate. It's almost as if by using a surrogate the signal coming out of the subject is boosted, so your answers will often be clearer than they would have been otherwise. In this next story, Wendy used surrogate testing to help her son's allergies.

High Confidence

My first experience using EC was with my eleven-year-old son. We took a vacation to Colorado for fall break and stayed in an Airbnb that has cats. I completely forgot he was very allergic to cats. I had brought the Emotion Code book with me on the trip to read. After reading it and seeing all the amazing stories in the book, and watching my son being so miserable with three days of cat allergies, I decided to try it. I really didn't know what I was doing, but I was good with a pendulum. I followed the flow chart and found six trapped emotions specific to cat allergies. After releasing them with the magnet, within minutes he stopped scratching his face and sneezing. I was amazed! I asked him how he felt twenty minutes later and he took a deep sigh, rolled his eyes like a good preteen would, and said, "Mom, I was just thinking, your necklace [pendulum] thing really works." It was so fun, and I got home and started practicing muscle testing and practicing on my friends. They all have seen results at various levels. I love it.

—Wendy H., Utah, United States

It's important to note that it is not necessary to physically touch the subject. If the surrogate is within six feet of the subject, you should have no problem testing accurately. Your body will detect the energetic changes that take place in the subject's body in response to yes-or-no questions, and these changes will show up in your muscle testing as strength or weakness in the surrogate.

If you're working alone with a subject who isn't testable, and you don't have a surrogate person nearby, you can act as surrogate yourself and use self-testing. Just direct your questions to the subject and test on yourself using any self-testing method, and then release or correct whatever comes up on the subject's body, or on your own body, if needed.

PROXY TESTING

When someone has been given authority to act for someone else, we commonly refer to the authorized person as a proxy. A proxy is someone who acts as a substitute. In proxy testing, the proxy temporarily "becomes" the person being tested. By voluntarily putting themselves into the position of standing in for someone else, a proxy person can be tested and worked on with the Body Code as if they were the subject.

Proxy testing is used when the person or animal that you want to test is farther than six feet away from you. Let's say you want to work on your friend who is several states away, or who lives on the other side of the planet. You can make a perfect energetic connection with them using proxy testing, no matter how far away they are. We have found this ability to be absolutely indispensable. It enables you to test someone and release or correct any imbalances the person has, no matter how far away he or she may be. It is similar to surrogate testing except that the subject is not physically present. The person who stands in for the subject is called the proxy, and, in effect, that person's body will set aside its own needs temporarily to help the subject. Once the connection is made, the proxy person *is* the subject for all practical purposes.

This image illustrates a proxy-testing scenario with three people. Note that the tester and proxy are in the same place working together, while the subject is somewhere else.

SUBJECT
PROXY
TESTER
PROXY SCENARIO
Muscle testing a 3rd person (proxy) for the subject

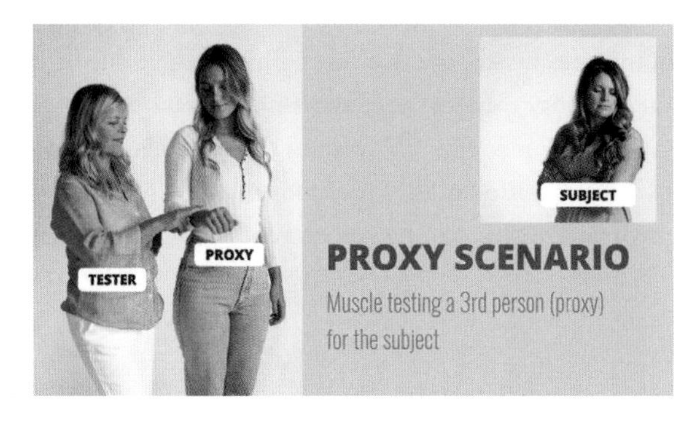

This picture shows the subject on the far right, who happens to be my daughter Sara, and on the left are the proxy, my daughter Lizzy, and the tester, my wife, Jean. Imagine that Sara is in Paris and Lizzy and Jean, pictured on the left, are in the United States. Sara has telephoned Lizzy and Jean asking for help with a headache. What follows is how Lizzy and Jean can connect with Sara to help her with her headache.

ESTABLISHING A CONNECTION

To establish a connection with the subject, have the person who will act as the proxy repeat the following: "My name is [subject's name]." In this particular case, Lizzy, acting as proxy for Sara, would say, "My name is Sara." At first this will probably test weak because, of course, her name is not Sara. But if she continues to repeat this statement, it will eventually test strong, as soon as an energetic connection is made. In other words, when she connects with Sara she will test strong if she says, "My name is Sara." If at that point she says, "My name is Lizzy," she will actually test weak. Why? Because her body will have set aside its own needs to stand in and act as proxy for Sara, so Jean can figure out what is going on with her and help her with her headache. At that point, everything that Jean finds on Lizzy will really be for Sara's benefit. Any corrections that are made, anything that's released or corrected on Lizzy's body, will actually end up being corrected or released in Sara's body. So here, Jean is actually working on Sara through Lizzy's body. This is a perfect example of the principle of quantum entanglement, allowing you to make any corrections to the subject on the proxy's body.

BREAKING THE CONNECTION

You always want to remember to break the connection when you're done. To break the connection, have the proxy repeat, "My name is ____," stating her own name, until a strong test is obtained. In this particular example, Lizzy would simply say, "My name is Lizzy." She would continue to repeat this statement until she tests strong once again. Initially, the first time she says it she will probably test weak because she is still acting as proxy for Sara. But if she continues to repeat the statement "My name is Lizzy," the connection will be broken and this statement will test strong.

In proxy testing, although muscle testing and releasing or correcting imbalances is performed on the proxy person, the person who is receiving the benefit is the subject. It's really quite amazing, as Alison found out in this next story.

Allergies at a Distance

My father was visiting, and he suffers from severe sinus problems and pain. He wasn't enjoying his visit or his granddaughter much. I shared with my mom and dad that I knew the Body Code and wanted to help. By proxy, I was able to clear trauma and anger and allergies from him. The next morning when he awoke, he had more energy and cheer than I've seen in him in a very long time. He wanted to go out and see the town.

I have also been able to use muscle testing by proxy to test foods for my daughter for nuts and eggs that she was allergic to. It worked wonderfully. Over time I was able to clear the energies that were causing these allergies in her, and she is no longer allergic to anything. I am working on the same for myself; I have cleared an almond allergy that I have had since I was ten.

—Alison S., British Columbia, Canada

PROXY TESTING WHILE ALONE

Just as you can work without a third person in surrogate testing, you can also act as the proxy yourself, using self-testing, allowing you to "stand in" for another person, no matter how far away he or she might be, without any limit. Anything you test, correct, or release will be done on your body, but for the benefit of the subject. You may not always have another person that can act as proxy, and if you are able to get answers on your own body using any form of self-testing, you don't need anyone else. You can act as both the tester and the proxy yourself.

Here is my method for establishing a proxy connection with a subject who has given permission for me to work on them, when I am working alone, acting as both tester and proxy:

SUBJECT
TESTER
PROXY
PROXY SCENARIO
You use self-testing (you are proxy)
for the subject

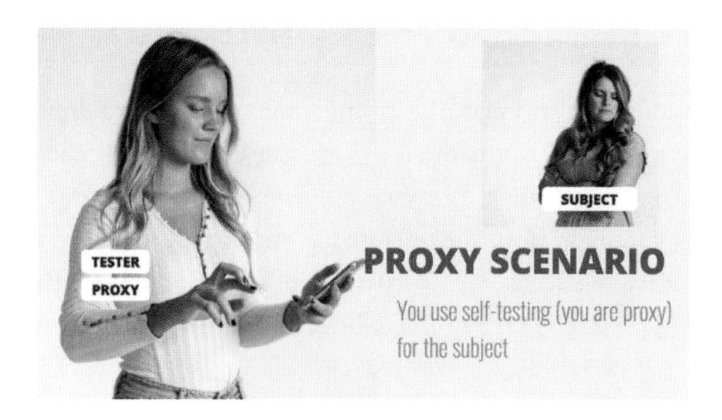

STEP 1.

I start out by saying a silent prayer for divine help.

STEP 2.

To establish a connection with the subject, I repeat, "My name is [subject's name]" until this statement tests strong, indicating an energetic connection has been achieved. For example, if I were attempting to connect with a person named Kim, I would repeat "My name is Kim" until I got a strong muscle test.

STEP 3.

Once the connection is made, I would use the Body Code to find imbalances and correct them on myself. Most of the time, correcting imbalances will consist of simply swiping a magnet or your hand from your forehead, over the top of your head, to the back of your neck a few times as indicated.

STEP 4.

When I'm done, I would break the connection by repeating "My name is Brad" (inserting your own name here, of course) until the statement tests strong, indicating the energetic connection has been broken.

TIPS FOR MUSCLE TESTING

SURROGATE VS. PROXY

The basic rules for using surrogate testing or proxy testing are as follows: If you're within six feet of the subject and he or she is untestable, use surrogate testing. If you're further away from the subject than six feet, use proxy testing. Either method can be done when you are working with a partner or alone.

KEEP YOUR THOUGHTS IN CHECK

Clear thoughts are the key to getting accurate answers. Keep it simple, focus on the statement or question, and keep other thoughts out of your mind. Instruct the person you are testing to do the same.

Thoughts that you might be holding in your mind can affect the outcome of muscle testing, so it is important not to have expectations that might influence your answers. Do your best to stay focused.

Distracting or negative thoughts can override the answers you're seeking. If you are holding negative thoughts about the person you're testing—even if that person is you—your body might respond accordingly by returning a weak muscle response, even if the answer to your question was yes. Try to have a heart full of love for yourself or the person you are testing, and be open to whatever answer you might receive. Remember, "Anything can cause anything!"

SENSING THE ANSWER

All of our sensory organs are best able to do their jobs when they are not overwhelmed. For example, you get the best sense of a sweater's softness by running your fingers delicately over the fibers. If you were to run your hand over the sweater in a fast and rough manner, you might not get a good idea of its softness.

In the same way, muscle testing is best performed lightly and delicately. It is not at all about sheer physical force. What you will eventually learn to detect is a slight change in muscle strength, the difference between the muscle being "locked" and being "mushy." Learning to sense this change is part of the skill you will develop with muscle testing, and it applies to testing other people as well as yourself.

ESTABLISH A BASELINE

It's crucial to establish a baseline every single time you want to use muscle testing. You need to make sure that you are testable if you are working on yourself, and if you're using muscle testing directly on another person, you need to make sure they are testable. This will help you make sure you've determined the proper resistance and pressure settings and also that you know what yes and no answers look and feel like when you are testing another person's muscles.

CAUSES OF UNTESTABILITY

You may find that some people are temporarily untestable. In this case, their arm will usually test strong no matter what statement they make, true or false.

There are a few reasons why a person may not be testable at any given time. If your subject is dehydrated, you'll want to stop and have him or her drink a glass of purified water, then try again in a few minutes. If you're the person doing the testing and you're dehydrated, you may have a hard time doing the testing, so drinking some water yourself may help.

If you're working on someone who has a neck misalignment, that will make it difficult to test as well. The person may need to see a chiropractor, but you can also try rolling a magnet down the spine with the intention of realigning whatever bone is misaligned in the neck. I will be explaining how to find and remove the underlying causes of structural misalignments in detail in a later chapter, but this simple method can often make an untestable person testable, at least temporarily.

Trapped emotions may also make a person temporarily untestable. If you're working on someone and a trapped emotion is suddenly welling up and coming to the surface to be released, you may temporarily be unable to get a clear muscle test. This is just one reason why knowing a method of self-testing will come in handy, because you can always test an untestable person via proxy or surrogate testing.

CAUTIONS ABOUT MAGNETS

Don't use a magnet directly on anyone who is pregnant, has an older pacemaker or medical device, is sensitive to magnets, or is under a doctor's care for a serious illness. Anyone who fits any of these descriptions can still be worked on using the Body Code, but you should use the magnetic energy from your hand instead, or you can use surrogate or proxy testing to work on them without touching them directly. By the way, magnets do not hold on to the energies they release. They do not need to be "cleansed" or anything of the sort.

IT'S A GIFT!

Muscle testing is a gift from the Divine, to allow us to help ourselves and each other. It is not to be used to test for the winning lotto numbers, nor is it to be used to ask who you should marry, etc. Asking about anything unrelated to health probably won't work anyway, in my experience. Muscle testing to ask about present and past imbalances works very well, but it seems that there is too much variability in the future to get good answers about it.

DO NOT USE MUSCLE TESTING TO MAKE BIG DECISIONS!

You will have to trust me on this one. Muscle testing is a God-given tool for restoring light and truth (healing) by serving the "injured." It's not to be used to predict the future, win the lottery, or make big decisions. "Service" is the key word here. Use it only to serve others and help them to heal. Why? We are all on a journey of growth and progression. Our Higher Power has entrusted us with this gift to be used in a specific way. If we steal the tool to use it for our own purposes, we are misusing God's trust, and missing a great opportunity to grow in light and love. Speaking from experience, it has become clear to me that muscle testing is a gift that has a specific purpose, but that purpose is limited. You can muscle-test every decision you make, but you won't get anything but neurotic, in my opinion. Use muscle testing to find imbalances in the body and to help yourself and others to get and stay physically well and successful, and leave it at that.

Miracles come when we get out of our own way and allow that Higher Power to work through us.

DON'T GIVE UP!

While some people seem to pick up these self-testing methods easily, most people take more time and have to practice. Find a self-testing method that works for you. If one of these testing methods is more comfortable or feels more natural to you, practice it every day, and like riding a bike, it will become second nature to you before long.

Learning self-testing is optional to using the Body Code, but mastery of any self-testing method can make things easier and more efficient for you. When I became proficient at self-testing, I saw the advantages immediately. I no longer needed another person to help me test patients who were far away or temporarily untestable. I could test them on myself and receive answers more rapidly and effectively. I could also check them for imbalances and correct them on myself. It works to find out what your body needs, as Shannon H. discovered and said, "I have had tremendous success using self–muscle testing for food and supplements!"

If you persevere, it will become easy for you, and it will open a whole world of healing to you.

There is nothing better than the feeling you get when you have really helped someone. And it doesn't happen every time you work on someone, but it will definitely happen if you just have it in your heart to help as many people as you can. The first time someone looks into your eyes and tearfully thanks you for what you have done for them, you will understand what I mean.

For additional help, be sure to visit discoverhealing.com/muscle-testing for training videos on even more methods of muscle testing.

USING YOUR INTUITION

Everyone who uses the Body Code or the Emotion Code for very long eventually notices something peculiar. They inevitably find occasions where a split second before they obtain an answer through muscle testing or using a pendulum, the answer appears in their minds. Somehow, they know what the answer is going to be. This is their intuition speaking to them, and it will speak to you, as well.

I know people who have cultivated that little inner intuitive voice to the point that they don't need to use muscle testing at all. Instead, they rely solely on their intuition, on their inner knowing of what the answer is going to be. I think that's powerful, and a great thing to strive for. I believe that that little inner voice of your own intuition, if you pay attention to it, will guide you to more and more truth.

If for some reason you feel that you just cannot get the hang of muscle testing, don't give up. Keep practicing. Experiment with your intuition. After asking a question, relax and listen for a moment, and the answer may suddenly appear in your mind.

There are different ways that intuition can be experienced. Whether you just feel it or know it or see it in your mind's eye or hear a subtle voice in your head or feel a sensation in your body, you can allow your intuition to give you the answer you are looking for. For me, the first answer that pops into my head is usually the actual answer from the subconscious mind.

Even if you consider yourself the least intuitive person in the world, you have the gift of intuition, because it's built into you. The more you use that intuition, the stronger it will become.

During my years in practice, I was always trying to find simpler, faster, and more efficient ways to identify my patients' imbalances. Ultimately, I was able to organize all the imbalances from which we suffer into six main areas.

I have dedicated a section of the book to each of these categories. Under each category you will find a description and exercise that enables the subconscious mind to guide and direct you to the underlying imbalances and then instruct you on how to decode and address them.

It even works when you have no symptoms at all. When I came across a patient who had no symptoms of any kind, the person's imbalances could still be detected and corrected using the Body Code to help prevent problems from developing in the future. This is true preventive medicine, to find and correct the imbalances that might ultimately cause illness before they have a chance to do so!

For more information about muscle testing and to watch videos showing how it is done, visit discoverhealing.com/muscle-testing.

5

THE MECHANICS OF THE BODY CODE

By banishing doubt and trusting your intuitive feelings, you clear
a space for the power of intention to flow through.

—DR. WAYNE DYER

IDENTIFYING AND RELEASING AN IMBALANCE

Using any of the testing methods outlined previously, you can use the Body Code Map in part III (page 101) to find imbalances.

Since there are always underlying reasons for symptoms or for the issues that we struggle with, the answer to the question "Is there an underlying reason for this symptom?" should nearly always be yes. If the answer is no, refocus, pray for assistance, and try again.

When the answer is yes, what the subconscious is telling you is that it has an imbalance in mind. In other words, out of all the thousands of possibilities within the Body Code, your subconscious mind has chosen just one that you can now decode or figure out.

Since the subconscious has an imbalance in mind already, and while looking at the Body

Code Map at the beginning of part III that shows the six major categories of imbalances, you might simply ask, "Is the imbalance in the left side of this chart?" In other words, you would be asking if the imbalance is in the "Energy" area, in the "Pathogens" area, or in the "Circuits and Systems" area.

If the answer is no, then the imbalance must be in one of the categories on the right side of the chart, in "Misalignment" or "Toxins" or "Nutrition and Lifestyle."

At this point, you should have identified that this first imbalance is in one of the categories on the left or one of the categories on the right. If you've gotten this far, congratulations! You're well on your way to finding your first imbalance.

Now that you have identified which side of the Body Code Map this imbalance is in, the next step is to find out which *category* the imbalance is in, using the same process as discussed earlier.

While asking questions in this way and getting answers from the subconscious mind may seem laborious at first, with practice, this process becomes second nature and quite rapid.

It's important to understand that the subconscious mind wants to help you find the imbalances. After all, it's these imbalances that have been creating whatever symptom it is you are trying to correct right now. If you can find the correct imbalances and release them, the symptoms can resolve.

Once you drill down to the imbalance that the subconscious has in mind, you will find easy step-by-step instructions that are specific to that imbalance, as follows:

- **EXPLANATION:** Every imbalance includes a descriptive section that explains what the imbalance actually is. You are likely to find imbalances that you know very little about, especially when there are so many possibilities. Fortunately, the explanation sections fully describe the imbalances, common symptoms that are likely to arise from those imbalances, and how they affect other parts of the body. To understand the imbalances fully, in this book you will also find either my personal stories or testimonials from others as examples.
- **DECODING:** In most cases, simply determining what the imbalance is will be enough to fulfill this step. However, sometimes further questioning might be required. On occasion, the subconscious mind will want more information brought to conscious awareness about a particular imbalance before it will allow that imbalance to be released. I refer to this process as decoding. For example, you may be directed to ask, "Do we need to identify more about this trapped emotion, or this pathogen, etc.?" If the answer is no, you have finished the decoding step, and you can move to the next step. If the answer to this question is yes, you will follow the directions to uncover more about the imbalance you have discovered.

- **ASSOCIATION:** This is where we find out if this particular imbalance is related to (or is being caused by) yet another imbalance. If you receive a yes answer when you ask, "Is there an associated imbalance that needs to be decoded?" then you will find and clear that associated imbalance first. Then you will come back to the original imbalance and ask if there are any other associated imbalances and repeat until you receive a no answer. For example, a misaligned bone will often have an associated imbalance that is causing the misalignment, usually a trapped emotion. In this way, we can find the root causes and eliminate them, obtaining the best possible results in the shortest time frame.
- **INTENTION:** Once an imbalance has been decoded, including resolving all associated imbalances, then it is ready to be released or corrected. This is the last step in the process of correcting an imbalance. Most of the time this step will involve simply swiping a magnet or your hand a few times over the governing meridian, with an intention to correct the imbalance.

SIMPLY FOLLOW THE INSTRUCTIONS

The beautiful thing about the Body Code is that you can safely follow the instructions and never be at a loss for what to do next.

As you use the Body Code and find things to correct, you will often be instructed to ask, "Is it necessary to identify more about this imbalance?" The reason it's important to ask this question is because sometimes the subconscious mind will not allow an imbalance to be released without bringing a little more information about that imbalance to conscious awareness. If the answer to this question is yes, you may need to identify when this imbalance occurred. In other words, you might need to determine your subject's age when this particular imbalance originated.

For example, if you are working on yourself and find that a particular imbalance needs more information, you might begin by dividing your current age by two. In other words, if you're forty years old, you might ask, "Did this occur prior to age twenty?" If the answer is yes, you might ask, "Did this occur prior to age ten?" and so on, until you arrive at the age of occurrence. Most of the time if you need to identify more information about any particular imbalance, identifying the age will be enough.

Sometimes you might need to dig deeper and find out if there was some life event, such as an injury or an illness or an emotionally charged event that was the driving force behind an imbalance. However, most of the time the answer to the question "Is it necessary to identify more about this energy?" will be no.

The next question is important to ask. "Is there an associated imbalance that needs to be decoded?" If the answer to this question is yes, it means that there is another imbalance that needs to be uncovered, an imbalance that is either causing the current imbalance or that the current imbalance is connected to in some other way.

This may seem complex at first but let me explain.

Let's say you're driving down the highway and your check engine light comes on. You pull into a car repair business and ask them to take a look. Fifteen minutes later the mechanic emerges from the shop and says, "We found the problem. Your car was completely out of oil. We've added oil to your car, so you should be good to go."

You may be wondering why your car ran out of oil in the first place. You recall hitting a curb pretty hard earlier in the week and wonder if that might have something to do with it. You tell the mechanic about this, and he agrees to take a look again to make sure you don't have anything else going on. A few minutes later he returns and says, "It's a good thing we looked. You knocked a hole in your crankcase when you hit that curb. We'll have to fix that hole in the crankcase or your oil is simply going to drain out again."

Looking for an associated imbalance is looking just a bit deeper to see if there is anything else you can address. Finding associated imbalances is simply a way to make sure that whatever you correct stays corrected.

If the answer to the question "Is there an associated imbalance that needs to be decoded?" is yes, you would simply return to the Body Code Map in part III (page 101) and ask which category this particular imbalance is in. Remember that anything can cause anything, so keep an open mind.

If the answer is no, you can continue on to the next step and release the energetic imbalance. I've broken this entire process into five easy steps.

THE PROCESS

STEP 1.

Ask: "Is there an underlying reason for this symptom?"

If there is no symptom present, ask, "Do I [or you] have an imbalance that can be released now?"

STEP 2.

Muscle-test to receive the answer. Let's say it is a strong response or forward sway, a yes answer.

STEP 3.

Using the Body Code Map in part III (page 101) as a reference, you will ask the subconscious mind through muscle testing where the imbalance is located on the chart.

Ask: "Is the imbalance on the right side of this chart?"

If you get a yes answer, you know the imbalance is in one of the categories on the right. If you get a no answer, the imbalance is in one of the categories on the left. The next step is to find out precisely which category the imbalance is in.

Let's say that you have found that the imbalance is in one of the categories on the left. Start at the top and ask, "Is the imbalance in the energies section?"

If yes, at this point you will turn to that section in this book (you will find the page number to turn to under the category icon on the chart), or if you have downloaded the Body Code System app, you will tap the energy icon on the home page. If you receive a weak response or sway backward, it is a no answer. Keep asking: "Is the imbalance in the ____ category?" until you receive a yes answer.

This is the beautiful simplicity of the Body Code. By asking simple questions we can receive simple answers, and be guided deeper and deeper by the subconscious mind until we arrive at a specific imbalance. You will know that you have found the imbalance when you can go no farther.

STEP 4.

When an imbalance has been found and nothing more about it needs to be identified, it is ready to be released. You will hold a clear intention to release or balance the disruptive energies, then swipe anywhere along the governing meridian with the magnet or your hand, following the instructions on where to guide your intention.

Remember, the governing meridian starts at the tailbone, goes up the midline of the back and neck, over the top of the head, and down the midline of the face to the inside of the upper lip. You do not have to pass a magnet over the entire meridian. Most people will swipe from their foreheads over the top of their heads to the back of their necks when working on themselves. If you are working on someone else, you will probably swipe from the base of their neck down to their waist, but swiping a magnet (or your hand) on any length of the governing meridian will work.

Being thorough with the imbalances you find by following the instructions carefully helps ensure that you get to the root of the issue as much as possible and prevents imbalances from recurring.

STEP 5.

After releasing or correcting an imbalance, you can start the process again to find and release another one, if you wish.

The more you practice the Body Code, the more intuitive you will become. The most important aspect of your sessions is your intuition. Pay attention to it, do what you feel is needed, and more ideas will be revealed to you as you get more confident with the process.

SUBJECT PREPARATION

Be sure you and your subject are hydrated, comfortable, and have a basic understanding of what you're about to do with them. Here is a simple introduction you might recite to your subject:

> *The Body Code is how we "decode" the imbalances that are blocking you from being healthy or successful. Let's help your body return to a more balanced state. We will look for the imbalances that are in your way and correct those imbalances. The Body Code works for both physical and emotional issues as well as any desires you may have to be your best self. I'll ask basic, specific questions, and we'll do this together.*

ASK FOR HELP

Perhaps the most important thing you can do to ensure that this work is effective and life changing is to ask for help from the Divine. Draw upon your own faith and belief system. You can do this privately if you wish. Or you could create a moment of silence with your subject, requesting help in the way you each feel most comfortable. By doing this together, you are uniting in purpose and entangling your energy through the laws of quantum physics, allowing divine power to flow through you.

I recommend that you do this with each subject, each time you work with the person. Do it for each session, even if you're working with several people in a row. It only takes a moment, after all. I always start by asking for help from above, because I want to take advantage of the immense power and intelligence that is available to me. I want the angels to be with me as I work, so they can whisper to my mind the things that I might otherwise miss.

To give you a clearer picture of what it looks like to work on another person, let's imagine that you are about to work on your friend Sarah, using surrogate testing by muscle-testing yourself, and that she is sitting with you in your room. Note that the Body Code can be used at any distance, but for this example I will explain how it can be used live and in person.

Make sure that you are seated within six feet of each other, and the answers to any question you ask of your subject's subconscious mind will manifest in your body through self-testing. The easiest way to confirm this if you are using self-testing is to have your subject state his or her name. If your subject's name is Sarah, have her say, "My name is Sarah," and muscle-test yourself to see if you get a yes answer. Then have Sarah say, "My name is Bob," or any other name that is not her own, and see if you get a no answer on self-testing.

PRIORITIZE THE ISSUES

Ask your subject if there is a particular issue to be addressed in the session. A subject's issue or "complaint" is just a way to refer to any concern they are dealing with, from physical pain, to emotional distress, to being unable to make a change, to blocks to achieving one's dreams. Your subject may want help with back pain, depression, painful memories, stage fright, or something else. Ask the person to choose one issue for now, whichever issue is most bothersome, and rate it on a scale of 0–10, 10 being the worst, and 0 being no concern at all. This measurement is widely used in research and is known as the "analog discomfort scale."

Let's say your friend Sarah is suffering from a migraine headache. You might ask Sarah, "On a zero to ten scale, with zero being no pain and ten being the most you can imagine, how would you rate the pain right now?" Let's say that Sarah replies, "I would say right now it's an eight." When possible, establishing the severity of a complaint like this is very useful as it will allow you to more easily see the effect your session will have on your subject's current symptoms.

If the person that you are working with does not have an issue that comes to mind, that's okay. Because the subconscious mind is a search engine, you can use it to find imbalances even though no symptoms are present.

If you are working with someone who has no physical, mental, or emotional issues that they can identify, you can simply ask, "What is the most important imbalance we can identify today?" or, "Is there an imbalance we can address that will help your body function better?" Questions like these will lead you to imbalances that matter but that may not be causing any symptoms, at least not yet. This next story illustrates the power of asking the right questions and using the analog pain scale.

Frozen Shoulder from a 10 to a 0

I had a client who suffered with a painful frozen shoulder for three years. Her traditional medical treatments included uncomfortable injections, and she also tried many different holistic therapies and treatments with little or no relief. When she contacted me we started Body Code sessions. I asked what her level of intensity was on a scale of 0–10, 10 being the worst. She said it was a 10++++.

It was so interesting what kept coming up in most of her sessions as causing all this discomfort. She had found out her boyfriend of seven years had been cheating on her. She was absolutely devastated and had manifested all this horrible pain, which was causing her frozen shoulder. She started to feel a reduction in discomfort from our sessions right away, and it continually reduced with each session down to 0. Tracking her pain level on the 0–10 scale helped us quantify the progress and kept us motivated to keep working on it over the weeks.

Today her shoulder is pain free. As a bonus, her ongoing migraine headaches disappeared, even though we didn't work on that issue directly. I often find overlapping benefits when doing this work. Sometimes we'll be working on one issue and another gets taken care of. She now plays sports with ease of movement and has been pain free for the last seven years. She told me her gratitude in one word—"*amazing*." As a practitioner, this technique never ceases to amaze me. I love it!

—Carmen D., Ontario, Canada

SAMPLE BODY CODE SESSION

Using the Body Code is a bit like playing a game with the subconscious mind. It knows what the imbalances are, and your challenge is to find them. By asking questions, you use the Body Code to find imbalances, one at a time.

When you first start working with someone, it's not unusual to release a lot of trapped emotions before getting to the other types of imbalances.

For example, I once worked with a woman who had fallen off a balcony and had broken her back. Years later doctors were still unable to resolve her pain. We worked together for weeks without any lessening of her symptoms. She was becoming discouraged because she didn't seem to be getting better. However, I knew that every session was getting us closer to success. I had to clear a lot of trapped emotions first before we could discover the low-grade infection at the core of her pain and lack of healing. Once we handled that, her pain was gone, but it took time and effort to get there.

Working to uncover the deeper causes of a person's problems is sometimes like being an archaeologist. You just keep asking questions, uncovering imbalances, and resolving each one, layer by layer, until you either get to the core issue or find nothing left to correct. That may happen in the first session, or it might take many sessions. Not surprisingly, children are much faster to work with than adults. Often, adults have been through more distressing experiences, and they have had more time to accumulate imbalances of all sorts.

AN EXAMPLE

Let's assume that Sarah's migraine is being caused by a misalignment of a bone in her skull, which is in turn being caused by a "physical trauma" energy that became lodged there from a car accident when she was sixteen years old.

There are any number of ways to ask questions through muscle testing and get to the underlying imbalances.

You might ask, "Is there an underlying reason for your migraine symptoms?" Since symptoms always have underlying reasons, the answer to this question should be yes. Once you have a yes answer to this question, it's important to realize that the subconscious mind knows the first imbalance you need to find, and your job is to decode it. So, using this book, you would turn to the beginning of part III (page 101) to view the Body Code Map. To find the answer, you might begin by asking, "Is this imbalance on the left side of the Body Code Map?" Let's say the answer is no. That would mean the imbalance must be on the right side of the map.

The right side of the Body Code Map lists "Pathogens," "Misalignments," and "Nutrition and Lifestyle."

Remembering that anything can cause anything, you might ask, "Is this a pathogen?" No. "Is it a misalignment?" Yes.

So far so good. You've established that a misalignment is contributing to her migraine symptoms. You then turn to section 4, "Misalignments" (page 231), and see a chart with two different possible choices, skeletal misalignments on the left, and soft tissue misalignments on the right. You would determine which direction to take at this fork in the road by asking, "Is the misalignment on the left side of this chart (skeletal misalignments)?" A no answer would mean that the imbalance must be on the right side of the chart (soft tissue misalignments). Let's say you receive an answer through muscle testing that the misalignment is on the left side of the chart, in skeletal misalignments. Under that icon you see a page number, and you turn to that page, to see a chart composed of four possible areas of skeletal misalignments.

You might ask, "Is the misalignment on the left side of this chart?" In our example, this would result in a no answer, meaning the misalignment has to be on the right side of the chart, which contains two choices, cranial bones and appendicular skeleton.

Accordingly, you might ask, "Is it in cranial bones?" Yes.

You can now turn to the "Cranial Bones" page reference, where you will discover more information about the imbalance you have just uncovered. If you are using the Body Code System app on your mobile device you will see more options to drill deeper to find the precise cranial bone that is out of alignment. If you have not yet installed the app, you will still be able to find and correct the imbalance by following the instructions at the end of any given chapter.

Remember, Sarah's subconscious mind knows exactly why she is having these symptoms. It's trying to take you to the first underlying cause. It's a bit like you are playing charades with her subconscious mind to find out what it knows.

You would then ask, "Is there an associated imbalance that needs to be decoded?" Let's say the answer is yes.

It's important to ask if there is an associated imbalance, because finding and fixing an associated imbalance usually means removing an even deeper underlying cause.

To find an associated imbalance you would return to part III (page 101) to view the Body Code Map once again.

The next question might be, "Is this imbalance on the left side of this chart?" Yes. "Is it in 'Energies'?" Yes.

So you would turn to the "Energies" page. On the energy section page you will see a table with four possibilities including emotional energies, post-traumatic energies, allergies and ideas, and offensive energies. You might start by asking, "Is the imbalance on the left side of this chart? No. "Is it in post-traumatic energies?" Yes. At this point you can turn to the page indicated under the icon. Note that if you are using the Body Code Systems app, you will have more choices, but it functions in this same way.

You then turn to "Post-Traumatic Energies" in the "Energy" section and are presented with an option called "Physical Trauma Energy." You ask, "Is it a physical trauma?" Yes.

Here, you can read about what a physical trauma energy is, follow the exercise instructions, find out if there is anything associated with it, and release it through intention.

Most often, an associated imbalance will turn out to be an underlying cause of the issue you are trying to solve. For example, most misalignments of bone or other tissue are caused by trapped emotions or some sort of post-traumatic energy. Releasing the underlying imbalance(s) will usually correct the misalignment.

This phenomenon, where one imbalance is caused by another imbalance, is what I call the "Domino Effect."

If an associated imbalance is not actually causing the imbalance in question, it will be connected in some other way. The subconscious mind is always trying to give you information about what's going on with the body, so it's important to be open to possibilities and ask yourself, "What is the subconscious trying to show me?"

Not all imbalances have associated imbalances, but when they do, you will want to release them to obtain the best results. And, interestingly, releasing any associated imbalances will quite often automatically correct the original imbalance you are working on.

It's a good idea to keep asking, "Is there an associated imbalance that needs to be decoded?" until all associated imbalances are handled.

One thing can lead to another, and you might find a chain of causes behind the issue you are working to correct.

Being thorough with the imbalances you find by following the instructions carefully helps ensure that you get to the root of the issue as much as possible and prevent imbalances from recurring. You can learn more by watching real-life sessions online, attending my seminars, and becoming a certified practitioner by taking our online courses at DiscoverHealing.com.

Here is a brief overview of the types of things the six categories of imbalances contain:

- "Energy" includes trapped emotions, the most common imbalance we suffer from, which is why I wrote the book *The Emotion Code*. However, this category also includes other common energies, such as allergies, trauma energies, mental energies, offensive energies, and more.
- "Pathogens" includes both the energetic and physical forms of infectious organisms, such as viruses, bacteria, fungi, parasites, and more.
- "Circuits and Systems" includes all the systems of the body, such as cardiovascular, nervous, endocrine, digestive, immune, reproductive, etc. Also found in this category are the organs and glands in the body, meridians, the energy body, chakras, disconnections between spirit and physical body, etc.
- "Misalignments" includes all of the hard and soft tissues of the body, since any tissue can become misaligned and can create malfunction.
- "Toxins" is a broad category including everything from dental toxins, such as mercury, to biological poisons, environmental pollution, food toxins, heavy metals, electromagnetic radiation, and more.
- "Nutrition and Lifestyle" contains information that can help you identify specific changes needed at any given time to support your health and well-being, like a particular mineral, herb, food, type of therapy, color, sleep, etc. You can even find the specific essential oil that would benefit your body the most.

When you use the Body Code Map, you begin with a question that sends you into one of the categories. Each new question you ask allows you to narrow things down until you arrive at a specific answer and find exactly what you need to know. We'll explore the six categories in more depth in the various sections that follow. You might find it instructive to watch a live Body Code session on my website, where you'll see me navigate the Body Code Map just as you can.

PART III

THE BODY CODE MAP

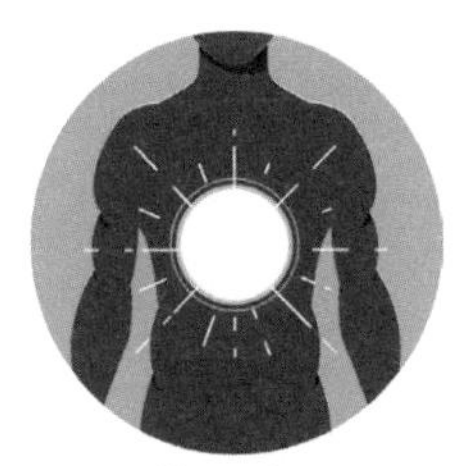

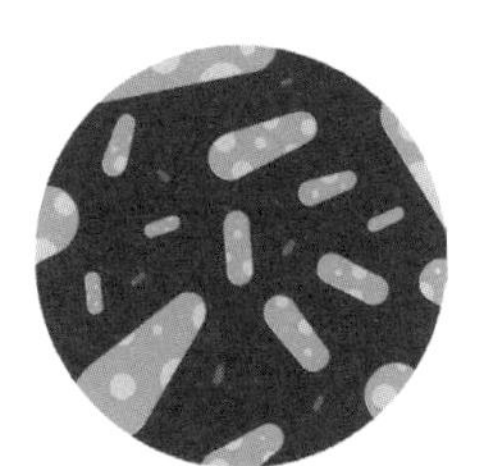

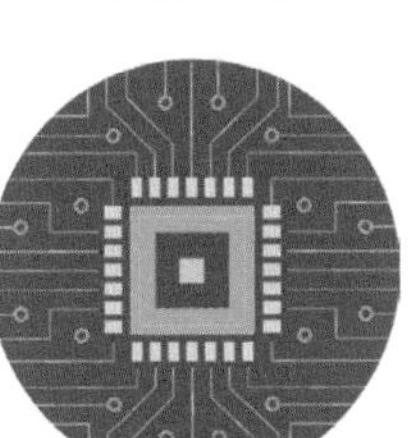

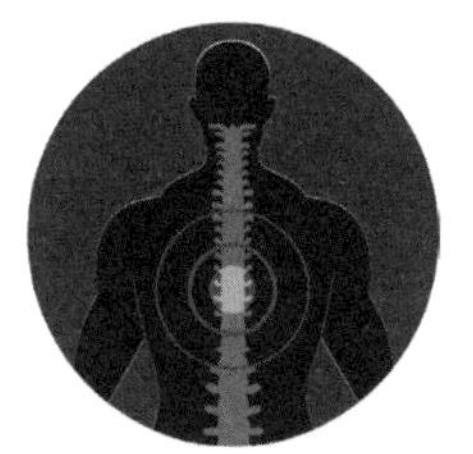

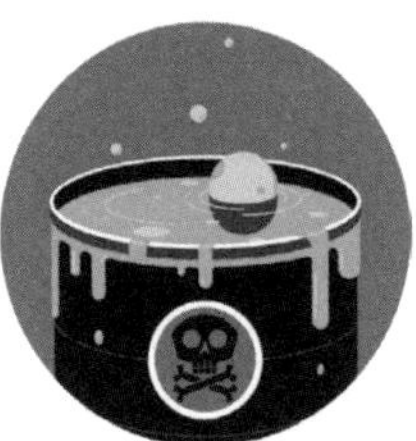

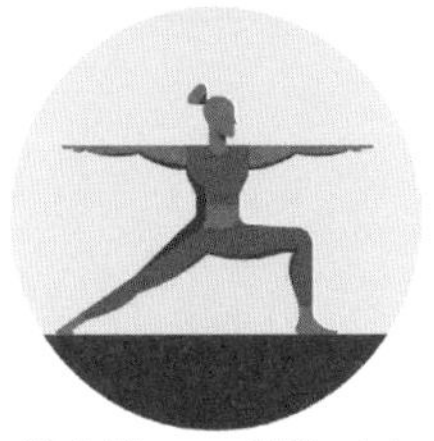

SECTION 1

ENERGIES

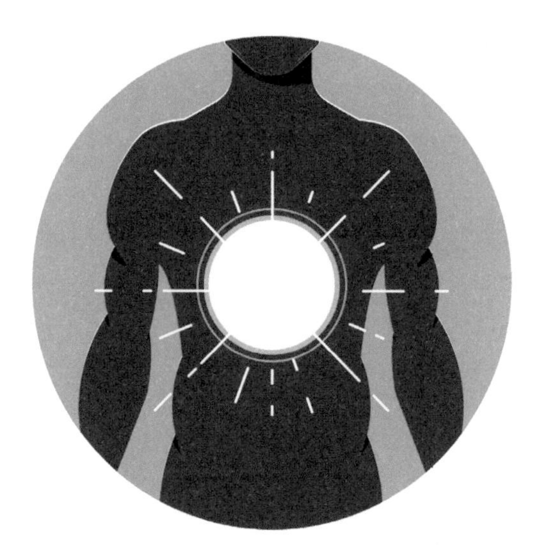

Everything we call real is made of things that cannot be regarded as real. If quantum mechanics hasn't profoundly shocked you, you haven't understood it yet.

—NIELS BOHR

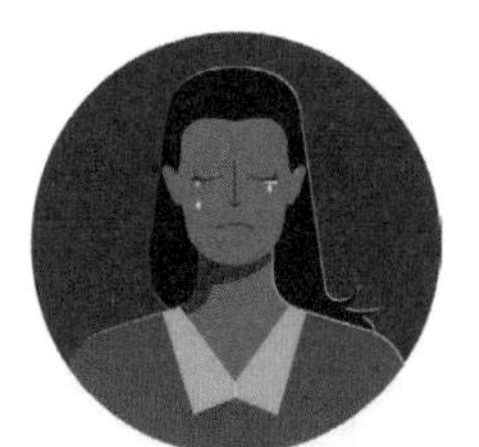

Emotional Energies
(page 105)

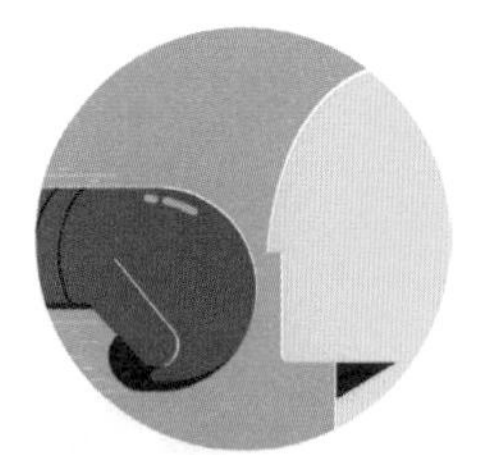

Post-Traumatic Energies
(page 117)

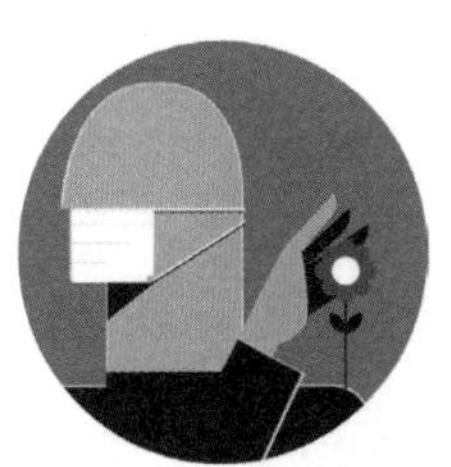

Allergies and Ideas
(page 121)

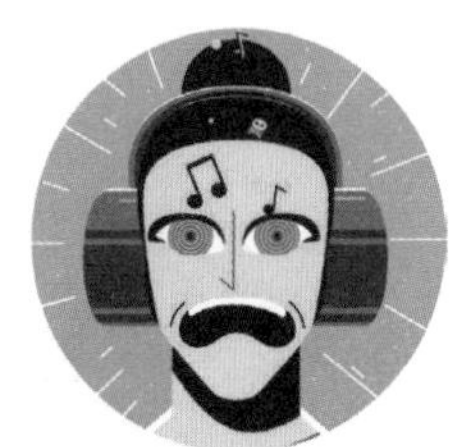

Offensive Energies
(page 130)

Of the six categories of imbalances on the Body Code Map home page, the energy category is the most commonly accessed. In other words, more imbalances are typically found in this category than in any other area. The reason for this is that trapped emotions are found in this category, and they are typically the most common underlying cause of health and mental issues.

There are many different kinds of imbalances in this section. They are grouped into subsets: emotional, post-traumatic, allergies to both physical substances and ideas, and offensive energies. (Note that the Body Code app includes many more than could be included here.)

6

EMOTIONAL ENERGIES

Emotions are energy. Repressed emotions block our energy—exhausting us or making us sick. Whatever is repressed will find a way to be expressed.

—CRYSTAL ANDRUS

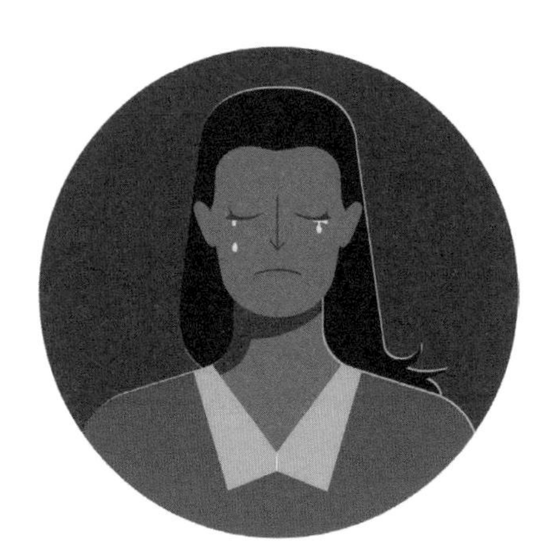

The most accessed subcategory of energy imbalances is referred to as "emotional energies," of which the most common are trapped emotions and the Heart-Wall. In this chapter I will show you how to find and release trapped emotions and start you on your journey in clearing your Heart-Wall.

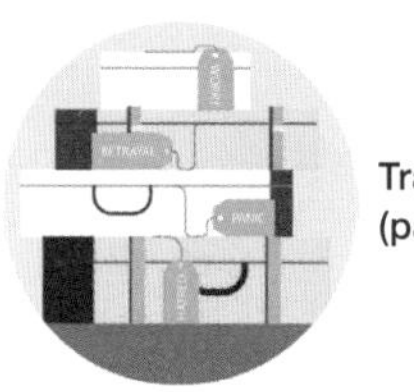

Trapped Emotions
(page 106)

Heart-Wall Emotions
(page 112)

TRAPPED EMOTIONS

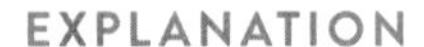

EXPLANATION

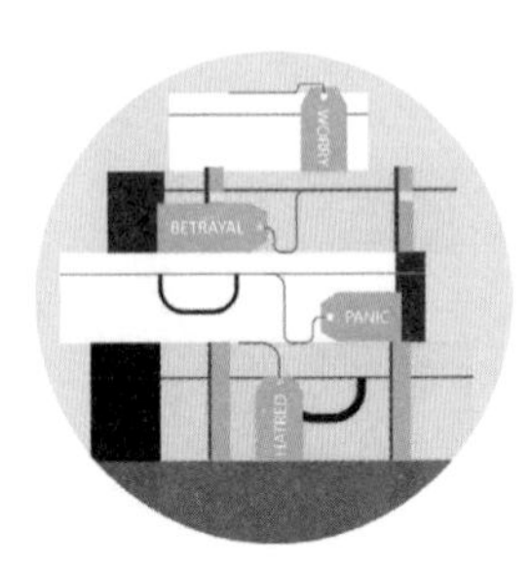

The most common yet unrecognized underlying cause of our physical and emotional pain is trapped emotions. A trapped emotion is a sphere or area of pure emotional energy, ranging in size from a baseball to about the size of a small melon. Trapped emotions may become lodged anywhere in your body, and when they do, they ultimately end up causing emotional, mental, and physical effects. Trapped emotions exert a distorting force on the body's energy field. This distortion affects the tissues of the body, creating physical pain and malfunction. Every biological function taking place within a sphere of trapped emotional energy is going to be affected to some degree, including cellular processes, chemical reactions, blood flow, lymph flow, and the flow of acupuncture meridian energy.

This is the reason trapped emotions cause so much physical pain and discomfort for so many of us. If you're experiencing physical pain right now, there is a high probability that your pain is being caused, in whole or in part, by trapped emotional energy. When trapped emotions are removed, pain often instantly decreases or disappears.

I've personally seen too many cases of instantaneous pain relief to count, pain that was removed by simply releasing trapped emotions. Steve was a remarkable example of this.

STEVE'S ANGER

Steve had been suffering for weeks from severe low-back pain. During the examination, I found that it was difficult for him to bend at the waist in any direction. He was suffering from a great deal of muscle spasm, and rated his pain as a 9 on a 0–10 scale.

As I began using muscle testing to ask his subconscious mind what the underlying reasons for his pain might be, the first thing that came up was that he had a trapped emotion of anger. Further muscle testing revealed that this emotion had become trapped in his body about twenty years before. He thought about it for a moment and then remembered that around that time he had gone through a traumatic work situation that left him outraged.

I released the trapped emotion by passing a magnet a few times down the governing meridian. Suddenly, his excruciating pain was gone. It was entirely and completely nonexistent! He couldn't believe it, and I was only slightly less astonished than he was. He kept bending over and twisting his body this way and that, proving that the difficult and limited range of motion that he had exhibited during his examination was now a thing of the past.

I had experienced wonderful success before this with many patients who were suffering from pain. It was very common that trapped emotions were an aspect of their pain, but this instantaneous and complete improvement was remarkable even to me, and I was grateful that it worked so well.

The story became even more interesting as a few days later, Steve came back to see me and said, "Dr. Nelson, my back pain has not come back. I still can't quite believe it. But I have to tell you something else. When I came in here, I had another problem that I didn't tell you about. For as long as I can remember, I have basically been what you would call a 'rageaholic.' I was always yelling at my wife and my kids. Little things would really tick me off. I've been to anger management several times, and it hasn't really helped me that much. I've had to watch the road rage, and I'm normally wound pretty tight. Since you released that trapped emotion of anger from me, I don't feel the anger anymore. Things that used to really set me off, now don't seem to bother me. I feel kind of peaceful, actually, which for me is unusual. How did you do that?"

When one has a trapped emotion, that part of the body is continually vibrating at the particular frequency of the emotional energy that is lodged there. This makes one much more susceptible to falling into resonance with that frequency and experiencing that emotion more easily and more often.

Steve had become an angrier person than he otherwise would have been because of the trapped emotion of anger lodged in his low back. So, when a situation would arise where he might become angry, he *would* become angry much more easily, because part of his body was already vibrating at the frequency of anger.

Remember that each emotion is ultimately a unique vibrational frequency. Anger is a different frequency than sadness, and so on. When an emotional energy is trapped in the body, it will cause the body's tissues that are within that sphere to vibrate at that emotional frequency. Releasing it then causes an immediate change to take place, relieving the tissues of that negative energetic vibration. Things can then return to a state of balance in that area of the body, something that may have been impossible before. The result is often an immediate improvement or cessation of pain, and possibly the prevention of even more serious problems years or decades down the road.

In the example of Steve and his back pain, you get a glimpse into how trapped emotions can interfere with your life, both physically and emotionally. Trapped emotions can cause you to become erratic and mean, to make wrong assumptions, to jump to inappropriate conclusions, and to sabotage relationships that might otherwise be healthy. Trapped emotions are also a major driving force behind emotional and mental issues such as depression, anxiety, panic attacks, self-sabotage, phobias, PTSD, bipolar disorder, and more.

Trapped emotions comprise the most unrecognized underlying cause of physical pain, as well, they are major contributing factors to diseases such as fibromyalgia, autoimmune disorders, infertility, chronic fatigue syndrome, and even cancer. Every disease process that I have seen has had trapped emotions as part of the underlying reason for its existence. Trapped emotions disrupt the proper function of the body. They disrupt blood, lymph, and energy flow and interfere with proper organ and gland function. They can also create fatigue as well as lower the immune system's ability to fight infection. Even though they can destroy the health of the body, trapped emotions are an unacknowledged factor in illness as far as conventional medicine is concerned, at least for now.

INHERITED TRAPPED EMOTIONS

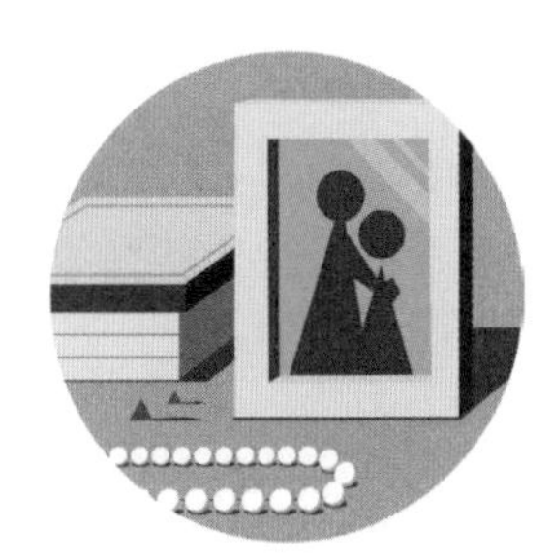

Inherited emotions are trapped emotions just like any other except that an inherited emotion became trapped during an emotional event that occurred in the life of either a parent or another direct-line ancestor. Inherited trapped emotions are passed down the family line similarly to how other genetic traits are passed along. Inherited emotions can be passed down multiple generations, and, like recessive genes, not all descendants will necessarily inherit the same emotion.

Inherited trapped emotions are most commonly uncovered when you are attempting to identify a specific trapped emotion on the Emotion Code Chart and you are unable to do so. The subconscious mind will only take you to the correct column and row that contains the inherited trapped emotion, but no further. So if you are unable to identify the precise emotion you're after because they are all testing either weak or strong, or because you find more than one emotion that tests strong, realize that the subconscious mind has taken you as far as it can. At that point you can simply ask, "Is this an inherited trapped emotion?" Getting a yes answer to this question opens the door to finding the inherited emotion.

It's important to the subconscious mind that you determine the basic genealogy of an inherited trapped emotion. It is easiest to start this identification process working backward from the subject. You might ask, "Did you inherit this emotion from your mother?" or, ". . . from your father?" then ask if it goes back further, that is, "Did your father inherit this emotion from his mother?" or, ". . . from his father?" Continue in this fashion until you identify the ancestor whom the trapped emotion originated with, making note of each generation as you go along. It's amazing what you can find. In this next story, Annelle tracked an inherited emotion back many generations and was able to release it from all those who inherited it.

Twenty-Seven Generations of Hopelessness

One morning, after a light snowfall, I went for a walk through our small town. The trees were feathered with white and were so beautiful! I came home invigorated and hungry. I fixed myself some breakfast, but as I sat down to eat, my stomach started hurting.

Having recently finished the training section for the Body Code Certification process, I decided to do some Body Code on myself to help my stomach before putting food in it. I found my stomach was out of alignment due to some recent trapped emotions of worry and nervousness and one of low self-esteem from age thirteen, all of which I released. Then I found an inherited trapped emotion of hopelessness. It had been passed from father to daughter to son, to daughter, to son, etc., and went back twenty-seven generations! I got excited about releasing this inherited trapped emotion and envisioned all the people I was helping.

As soon as I finished releasing this emotion with ten swipes of the magnet, I felt a wave of feelings come over me—gratitude, relief, letting go of pain, and then joy. The tears began to flow, and I felt as if I were crying a thousand tears for all those people who had carried this hopelessness and were now able to be free of it. What a powerful tool this is! I am so grateful to be able to bless my ancestors' lives in this way.

—Annelle D., Virginia, United States

Since trapped emotions are the most common imbalance from which we suffer, and since they cause so many of our physical, mental, and emotional issues, learning to release them can make a big difference in your life as well as in the lives of your loved ones.

EXERCISE:
FIND AND RELEASE A TRAPPED EMOTION

Using the Emotion Code Chart, I will explain how to identify and release trapped emotions. Use whichever method of muscle testing works best for you and perform a muscle test for each question. Remember that a strong answer or swaying forward is yes, and a weak answer or swaying backward is no.

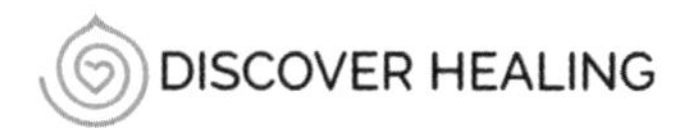

The Emotion Code® Chart

	A	B
1 HEART OR SMALL INTESTINE	Abandonment Betrayal Forlorn Lost Love Unreceived	Effort Unreceived Heartache Insecurity Overjoy Vulnerability
2 SPLEEN OR STOMACH	Anxiety Despair Disgust Nervousness Worry	Failure Helplessness Hopelessness Lack of Control Low Self-Esteem
3 LUNG OR COLON	Crying Discouragement Rejection Sadness Sorrow	Confusion Defensiveness Grief Self-Abuse Stubbornness
4 LIVER OR GALL BLADDER	Anger Bitterness Guilt Hatred Resentment	Depression Frustration Indecisiveness Panic Taken for Granted
5 KIDNEYS OR BLADDER	Blaming Dread Fear Horror Peeved	Conflict Creative Insecurity Terror Unsupported Wishy-Washy
6 GLANDS OR SEXUAL ORGANS	Humiliation Jealousy Longing Lust Overwhelm	Pride Shame Shock Unworthy Worthless

STEP 1.

Start by asking, "Do I [or you] have a trapped emotion that can be released now?"

- If no, you may need to try again later, or there may be a Heart-Wall present, which we will be discussing next.
- If yes, continue to Step 2.

STEP 2.

(Decoding) Ask: "Is the trapped emotion in column A?"

- If no, it is in column B.
- Once you determine the column, you've eliminated half of the list, and have thirty emotions left out of a total of sixty possible emotions. Move to Step 3.

STEP 3.

Ask: "Is the trapped emotion in an odd row?"

- If no, it is in row 2, 4, or 6.
- If yes, it is in row 1, 3, or 5.
- Once you have identified that the emotion is in one of the even or odd rows, you have fifteen emotions left out of sixty. Move to Step 4.

STEP 4.

At this point, you can simply name the rows one by one and muscle-test to identify the correct cell:

- For odd, "Is it in row 1? Row 3? Row 5?"
- For even, "Is it in row 2? Row 4? Row 6?
- Once you identify the correct cell, you have five emotions left out of sixty, and you can move to Step 5.

STEP 5.

With the final five emotions to test for, start at the top of the list, and muscle-test the emotions one at a time.

- Ask: "Is the trapped emotion ____?"
- Test each emotion in that cell, one by one, until one tests strong.

STEP 6.

After identifying the emotion, ask, "Do we need to know more about this emotion?"*

- If no, move to Step 7.
- If yes, ask one or more of the following questions. Return to Step 6 once the answer to any of these questions is determined.
    - Ask: "Do we need to know the age of occurrence?"

*Sometimes the subconscious mind will need more information to be brought to light about a trapped emotion before it will allow it to be released.

- Ask: "Was this emotion absorbed from someone else?"
- Ask: "Is this trapped emotion about a specific event (or person)?"

STEP 7.

(Intention) Swipe three times with a magnet or your hand on any length of the governing meridian, or ten times for an inherited trapped emotion, while holding the intention to release the emotion.

STEP 8.

Ask: "Did we release that trapped emotion?"

- If yes, you can start at the beginning on Step 1 and repeat the process to find and release another trapped emotion.
- If no, refocus, say a prayer for help, allow your heart to feel love and gratitude that this is going to help, and swipe three times once again with intention.

If you are having a hard time identifying the trapped emotion, ask, "Is this an inherited trapped emotion?"

If it was inherited, ask, "Did you inherit this emotion from your mother?" or, "Did you inherit this from your father?" then ask if it goes back further. "Did your father inherit this emotion from his mother?" or, ". . . from his father?" Continue in this fashion until you identify the ancestor with whom it originated, making note of each generation as you go along. Once you have identified how many generations are holding this specific trapped emotion, you can release it by passing a magnet or your hand ten times over the governing meridian, while holding an intention to release that emotional energy.

You can find and watch video explanations of this process by visiting the Discover Healing YouTube channel at youtube.com/c/discoverhealing.

HEART-WALL EMOTIONS

EXPLANATION

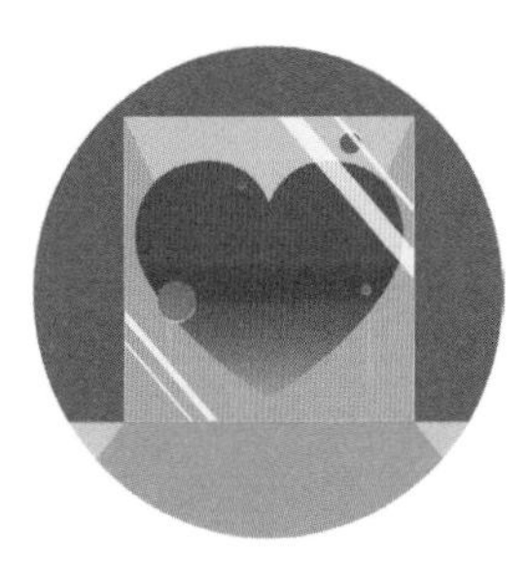

The most important part of the Emotion Code actually has to do with the heart. Ancient societies believed the heart was the source of love and romance, the fount of creativity, the seat of the soul, and the core of our being.

When you've experienced deep grief, hurt, or loss you may have felt that your heart was actually going to break. You may have felt like an elephant was sitting on your chest or that you couldn't breathe. Can you remember a time like this in your life? Perhaps you were going through a breakup or divorce. Maybe you were being abused or bullied as a child. Whatever it was that you were experiencing, in that moment it was all too real.

These feelings of heartbreak can be so uncomfortable, so foreign, and so difficult to deal with that they often result in the formation of an energetic "wall" put up to protect the heart from these profoundly negative emotions. Trapped emotions are moved and arranged by the subconscious mind to surround the heart, layer by layer, like the layers of an onion. This is a protective mechanism to keep the heart from being hurt or broken, which may have been a perfectly appropriate defense mechanism at the time. But there is a price to pay for having a Heart-Wall long-term.

Having a Heart-Wall can make life much more difficult. When your heart is surrounded with layers of negative emotional energies, it makes it harder to feel positive emotions and easier to feel negative emotions. It makes it harder to connect with other people and not only to give love but to receive it as well. Removing that wall of trapped emotions that surrounds your heart can be life changing, as Giacomo found in the following story.

Changed for the Better

After my Heart-Wall was released, my life completely changed. I became far more open to the Divine and I started lucid dreaming. After a few months I entered into my first long-term relationship with an amazing partner, in which I am very happy. At first, I thought I wanted to pursue a completely different profession, but after one month my resolve for my current passion strengthened and I am achieving better results than ever in it. I am so grateful that I discovered the Heart-Wall and had it released!

—Giacomo R., London, United Kingdom

Scientists who have measured the magnetic field of the heart using a device called a magnetocardiogram find that the heart has a magnetic field that can be measured several feet away from the surface of the body. When you're feeling love or affection for another person, you're literally sending energy—from your heart to the other person's. Having a Heart-Wall can impede your ability to love others and to have a happy life, but getting rid of it can make all the difference, as Raluca found in this story.

A New Person After Removing the Heart-Wall

My story is a happy one. I've been married since 2005, but my marriage ran badly for years. In 2013, I sought out a Body Code practitioner who lived in Budapest who was able to remove mine and my husband's Heart-Wall from a distance. I got a "new" husband! I mean a tender, lovely, and cheerful husband, since his Heart-Wall was removed! Also, I feel much more confident with myself, more peaceful inside, since my own Heart-Wall was removed.

—Raluca S., Padua, Italy

Removing the trapped emotions that make up a Heart-Wall is almost entirely the same process that I have outlined earlier for releasing trapped emotions, since a Heart-Wall is made of layers of trapped emotions.

Now let's talk about how you can actually determine if a person has a Heart-Wall and how you can release it.

To find a Heart-Wall, you simply ask. Unless you actually ask the person's subconscious mind if they have a Heart-Wall, it will not be revealed.

The Heart-Wall is made of trapped emotions, but the subconscious mind no longer categorizes them as such. These emotions are now part of a wall and are inaccessible until you ask if there is a Heart-Wall present, or if you can release a trapped emotion from the person's Heart-Wall. Either way, you have to get the subconscious mind to admit that there is a Heart-Wall before you can get to the trapped emotions that are creating it. For simplicity, you can refer to these trapped emotions as Heart-Wall emotions. As you release them, one by one, the wall will come down.

EXERCISE:
FIND AND RELEASE A TRAPPED EMOTION FROM A HEART-WALL

First, you need to find out if you or the person you are trying to help has a Heart-Wall.

You would ask, "Do I [or you] have a Heart-Wall?" Then use the muscle test of your choice to get the answer, and use the step-by-step instructions that follow. Most people can release between one and ten Heart-Wall emotions in one session and can release their entire Heart-Wall in anywhere from one to three sessions. (For this exercise you will once again use the Emotion Code Chart in the exercise section for finding and releasing a trapped emotion.)

If you find that a Heart-Wall is present, decode and release a Heart-Wall emotion as follows. (If you did not find a Heart-Wall, note that roughly 7 percent of people do not have a Heart-Wall.)

STEP 1.

Ask: "Can we release a Heart-Wall emotion now?"

- If no, you may need to try again later when you or the other person is ready to do this work.
- If yes, you can continue on to Step 2.

STEP 2.

(Decoding) Ask: "Is the trapped emotion in column A?"

- If no, it is in column B.
- Once you determine the column, you've eliminated half of the list, and have thirty emotions left out of a total of sixty possible emotions. Move to Step 3.

STEP 3.

Ask: "Is the trapped emotion in an odd row?"

- If no, it is in row 2, 4, or 6.
- If yes, it is in row 1, 3, or 5.
- Once you have identified that the emotion is in one of the even or odd rows, you have fifteen emotions left out of sixty. Move to Step 4.

STEP 4.

At this point, you can simply name the rows one by one and muscle-test to identify the correct cell:

- For odd, "Is it in row 1? Row 3? Row 5?"
- For even, "Is it in row 2? Row 4? Row 6?
- Once you identify the correct cell, you have five emotions left out of sixty, and you can move to Step 5.

STEP 5.

Start at the top of the cell and muscle test the emotions one at a time.

- Ask: "Is the trapped emotion ____?"
- Test each emotion in that cell, one by one, until one tests strong.

STEP 6.

After identifying the emotion, ask, "Do we need to know more about this emotion?"*

- If no, move to Step 7.
- If yes, ask one or more of the following questions. Return to Step 6 once the answer to any of these questions is determined.
    - Ask: "Do we need to know the age of occurrence?"

*Sometimes the subconscious mind will need more information to be brought to light about a trapped emotion before it will allow it to be released.

- Ask: "Was this emotion absorbed from someone else?"
- Ask: "Is this trapped emotion about a specific event (or person)?"

STEP 7.

(Intention) Swipe three times with a magnet or your hand on any length of the governing meridian, or ten times for an inherited trapped emotion, while holding the intention to release the emotion.

STEP 8.

Ask: "Did we release that trapped emotion?"

- If yes, ask, "Did we clear the Heart-Wall?"
  - If no, you can start at the beginning on Step 1 and repeat the process, finding and releasing more trapped emotions until you get a yes.
  - If yes, congratulations, you have cleared a Heart-Wall!
- If no, refocus, say a prayer for help, allow your heart to feel love and gratitude that this is going to help, and swipe three times once again with intention.

HELPFUL TIPS FOR REMOVING THE HEART-WALL

The Heart-Wall is made of different layers of trapped emotions, much like an onion. I find that I can usually release four to ten trapped emotions in a single session, sometimes more, sometimes less. The average person seems to have twelve to twenty-four trapped emotions making up a Heart-Wall, but it may be more or less than this, depending on the person.

I believe that removing your own Heart-Wall and that of your loved ones is one of the most important things you can do. It may change your life—and theirs as well!

7

POST-TRAUMATIC ENERGIES

Each thought you have informs your energy, and your energy manifests into your experiences. Your thoughts and energy create your reality.

—GABRIELLE BERNSTEIN

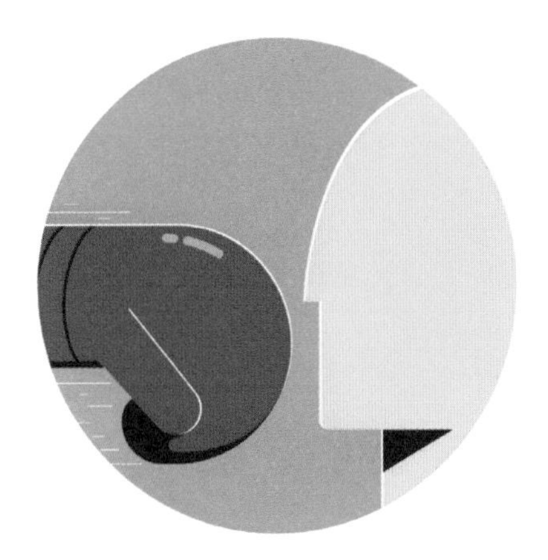

Post-traumatic energies form another category of energy that distorts the energy field of the body. Note that the Body Code System app contains several types, but the most commonly found imbalance in this category is called physical trauma energy.

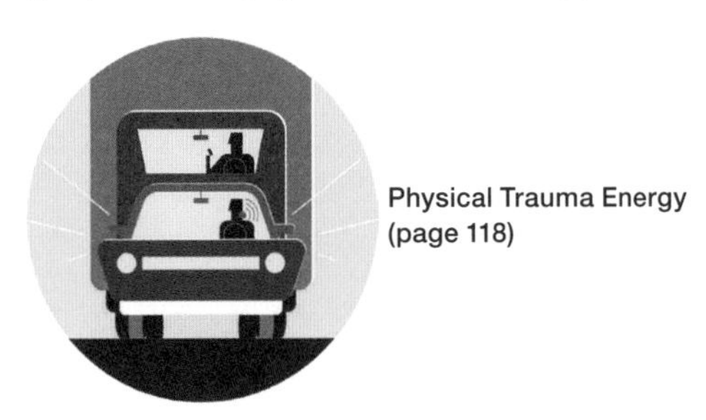

PHYSICAL TRAUMA ENERGY

EXPLANATION

Physical trauma energy occurs when you receive a physical blow or when the body is under extreme physical stress. Usually, this sort of energy will pass through the body, perhaps doing some physical damage to tissues as it does so, but without remaining. Sometimes, however, the energy from a trauma can actually become lodged in the physical body.

I learned about physical trauma energy one day when a young man came into my practice complaining of neck pain. He said, "Dr. Nelson, I was in a car accident in which I was rear-ended by another car. This happened four years ago, and my neck has never stopped hurting since that day. I've been to different doctors, I've been adjusted by different chiropractors, I've been to physical therapy, but my neck pain has never left me. In fact, it currently feels pretty much the same way it felt the day after the accident."

I asked him to describe for me how much pain he was actually in by choosing a number between 0 and 10, with 0 being no pain and 10 being the most he could imagine. He chose the number 9.

I thought about this for a moment. He certainly had tried to get rid of this pain. Nevertheless, it was still very severe. I had treated many auto-accident victims during my years in practice, but this one seemed a bit unusual to me. As was my habit, I sought for help, and in my mind, I prayed, "Father, if there is something unusual going on here that I need to be aware of, will you please help me to understand it?"

The answer to my question flowed instantly into my mind. I suddenly understood that some of the energy that was created in the accident four years ago was still in his neck, disrupting the normal function of his tissues.

Anytime we receive a physical blow, kinetic energy enters our bodies. For example, if you are sitting in your car stopped at a red light and another car hits you from behind, even at a relatively slow speed, tons of kinetic energy can be produced. It's that kinetic energy that crumples the fenders and causes damage to both cars. This same kinetic energy will pass through your body in most cases. However, occasionally, some of that energy may become trapped in the body and essentially become a ball of "physical trauma energy."

Now that I understood the real source of his pain, I used a magnet and swiped a few times over his governing meridian, with an intention to release the energy of this physical trauma. Immediately after doing this I looked at him and said, "Okay, go ahead and move your neck around, look to the left and right, look up and down, and tell me how your pain level is now compared to what it was before."

"Wow! I would say the pain level now is at a two. This is the best my neck has felt since before the accident! What did you just do?"

Physical trauma energy like this is not an uncommon cause of physical pain and malfunction. And it doesn't take something as severe as a car accident to create it. I have found that seemingly minor traumas—if conditions are right—can also become trapped in the body. Any type of surgical procedure will usually leave the body with physical trauma energy. Stepping off a curb wrong and receiving a sudden unexpected jolt to the body can create a physical trauma energy. Hitting your head when you're getting out of your car might do this as well, and so on.

Here is an example of an old injury that resulted in a physical trauma energy and the ultimate outcome once this energy was found and released. Notice that in this next story, there was a list of things that were found and corrected, which is typical when doing a Body Code session.

Giving Back a Builder's Career

John, a seventy-four-year-old builder, was having difficulty raising his arm above shoulder height and had lost strength since having an accident in 1985 when a piece of scaffolding fell from three floors above and hit him on the back of the head, fracturing two vertebrae. Using the Body Code, I released various emotional energies, the physical trauma energy from the accident in 1985, recovery interference, and a physical/spirit disconnection. This resulted in his arm regaining full range of movement as well as strength. He was incredibly grateful.

—Anthea P., London, United Kingdom

Can you see the importance of finding imbalancing energies like these? It's likely that you have some physical trauma energy from your past. This kind of energy is just as invisible as trapped emotions, and unless you know about it, you will not be able to detect it, but the Body Code makes it simple to find and remove.

EXERCISE:
FIND AND RELEASE A PHYSICAL TRAUMA

STEP 1.

Ask: "Do I [or you] have a physical trauma energy that we can release now?"

- **If yes, continue to Step 2.**
- **If no, you may not have a physical trauma energy at all or one that cannot be released now, so you may want to try again on a different day.**

STEP 2.

(Decoding) Ask: "Do we need to know more about this energy?"*

- If no, move to Step 3.
- If yes, ask one or more of the following questions. Return to Step 2 once the answer to any of these questions is determined.
  - Ask: "Do we need to know the age of occurrence?"
  - Ask: "Was this absorbed from someone else?"
  - Ask: "Is this from an injury?"
  - Ask: "Is this from a surgery?"
  - Ask: "Is this from an illness?"
  - Ask: "Do we need to know the location of this energy in the body?"

If yes, using a process of elimination to locate this may be helpful. For example, divide the body in half, and ask if the energy is lodged in the lower half of the body or upper half. Divide the body from left to right and ask if the energy is lodged in the left half of the body or the right half. Continue dividing in this fashion and asking until you've determined the location in your body in which the energy is lodged, then return to Step 2 (Decoding).

STEP 3.

(Association) Ask: "Is there an associated imbalance that needs to be decoded?"

- If no, move to Step 4 (Intention).
- If yes, which is unlikely, return to the Body Code Map to decode and address any associated imbalances, then return here and repeat the question in Step 3 (Association).

STEP 4.

(Intention) Once all associated imbalances are released, and all questions are satisfied, swipe three times with a magnet or your hand on any length of the governing meridian, while holding the intention to release the physical trauma.

- Ask: "Did we release that physical trauma energy?"
  - If yes, you can start at the beginning on Step 1 and repeat the process to find and release any more physical trauma energies.
  - If no, refocus, say a prayer for help, allow your heart to feel love and gratitude that this is going to help, and swipe three times once again with intention.

Releasing the energy of a physical trauma will often result in immediate changes to how a person feels, so watch for those changes to occur and measure them by asking your subject how to rate the discomfort before and after the release.

*Sometimes the subconscious mind will need more information to be brought to light about a physical trauma before it will allow it to be released.

8

ALLERGIES AND IDEAS

It is health that is real wealth, and not pieces of gold and silver.

—MAHATMA GANDHI

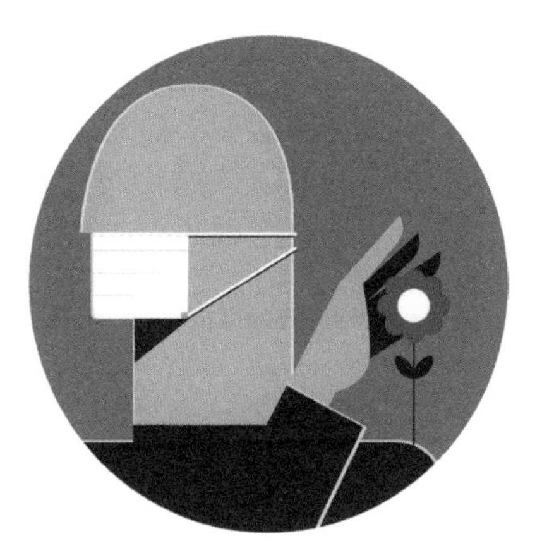

Most people think that if they are allergic to something, they will always be allergic to it. This is not necessarily true, however. Like every other symptom, allergies usually manifest in our bodies when other underlying imbalances exist. If those underlying causes are corrected, allergies can and do disappear.

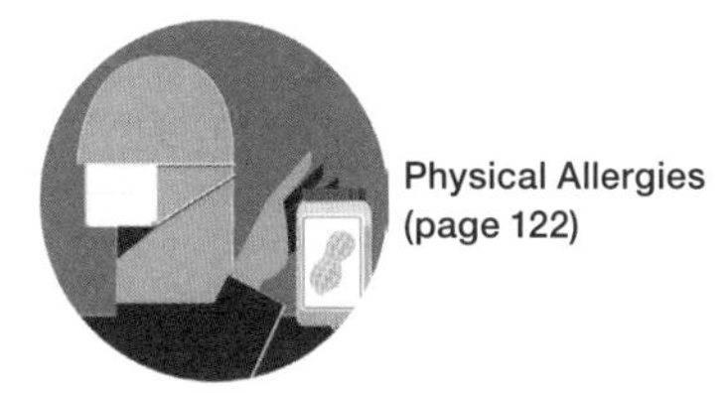

PHYSICAL ALLERGIES

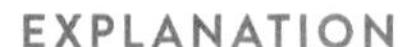

EXPLANATION

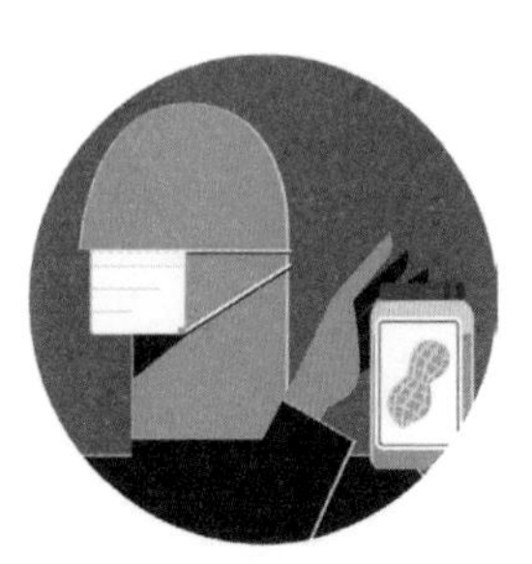

Do you suffer from allergies? While it's possible to be allergic to literally anything, foods such as peanuts, cow's milk, wheat, and eggs are some of the most allergenic foods that exist. In addition, animal dander, pollen, molds, dust mites, certain medications, insect stings, cockroaches, perfumes, and household chemicals round out the list of the top allergens. It's estimated that up to 40 percent of adults and children in America suffer from a form of allergy known as hay fever, a particularly miserable kind of allergy that results from a sensitivity to pollen that fills the air in the spring. If you suffer from seasonal allergies like this, you know how miserable it can be.

One of the fascinating things about allergies is that, in many cases people have not had the allergy their entire lives. People often say things such as, "I never had allergies until about five years ago. Now every spring I'm totally miserable for a couple of months."

Physical allergies are most often the result of multiple imbalances that combine to throw the immune system into a state of malfunction. There are often imbalances in the liver from trapped emotions, heavy metals, or other toxins from food additives, pesticides, and herbicides. However, in some cases an allergy has no underlying cause and can simply be deleted, since the allergy itself can be considered to be an energetic imbalance.

Physical allergies are also created when the subconscious mind makes a faulty connection with a particular substance during either prolonged or sudden emotional and/or physical stress. The immune system then considers the substance to be an allergen, and a negative response or reaction will occur when this allergen is encountered in the future. For example, if you experience something upsetting or traumatic while you are eating or drinking something, you may become allergic to that food or drink. Releasing the trapped emotions around that event will usually result in the disappearance of the allergy.

The subconscious mind may create a physical allergy as a protective measure, in order to defend you from the stress that it has associated with the allergen. For this reason, you can become allergic to literally anything.

Allergy symptoms may include rashes, inflammation, respiratory problems, congestion, sinus irritation, itchy eyes, achy joints, and more.

Fortunately, most allergy symptoms may be relieved using the Body Code and finding the trapped emotions and underlying causes, as Joela found in this story.

Allergy-Free at Last

I had been working on myself trying to clear my hay fever allergies. After clearing several trapped emotions, I am now symptom-free!

—Joela J., Switzerland

The severity of allergies runs the gamut from life-threatening to barely noticeable. And it's important for me to point out that if you have a life-threatening allergy, by all means find and remove the underlying causes using the Body Code, but, just to be on the safe side, don't leave your EpiPen at home.

Do you always know if you have allergies? Allergies always cause symptoms, but the symptoms are often not understood. For example, are there certain foods that make you lose your energy? Are there certain foods that, if eaten late in the day, will keep you awake at night? These are two of the more common symptoms that people complain about that are often the result of an allergic reaction to something that they are eating or drinking.

If you find that you have a physical allergy, you may want to identify what substance you are allergic to. If you can't figure out what the allergen is, don't worry. It is more important to decode and release any associated imbalances than it is to identify the allergen itself. The easiest way to do this is to identify what category of allergen it belongs to, the most common being foods, organic matter, and chemicals. Sometimes it is enough to simply identify the category.

EXERCISE:
FIND AND RELEASE AN ALLERGY

STEP 1.

Ask: "Do I [or you] have a physical allergy that can be released now?"

- **If yes, continue to Step 2.**
- **If no, you may not have a physical allergy at all, or you may have one that cannot be released now, so you may want to try again a different day.**

STEP 2.

(Decoding) Ask: "Do we need to know more about this allergy?"

- **If no, move to Step 3 (Association).**
- **If yes, ask one or more of the following questions. Return to Step 2 (Decoding) once the answer to any of these questions is determined.**
  - **Ask: "Do we need to determine the allergen?"**
  - **If yes, some common allergies you can test are as follows:**

Peanuts	Fish	Dust mites
Cow's milk	Sesame	Medications
Wheat	Eggs	Insect stings or bites
Soy	Animal dander	Cockroaches
Tree nuts	Pollen	Perfumes
Shellfish	Molds	Household chemicals

- Ask: "Do we need to know the age of occurrence?"
- Ask: "Was this absorbed from someone else?"
- Ask: "Is this from a specific event?"

STEP 3.

(Association) Physical allergies nearly always have associated imbalances, such as trapped emotions that must be cleared in order to reset the subconscious response to the allergen.

- Ask: "Is there an associated imbalance that needs to be decoded?"
- If no, move to Step 4 (Intention).
  - If yes, which is likely, return to the Body Code Map and decode and address any associated imbalances, then return here and repeat the Step 3 (Association) question.

STEP 4.

(Intention) Swipe three times with a magnet or your hand on any length of the governing meridian, while holding the intention to release the allergy.

STEP 5.

Ask: "Did we release that physical allergy?"

- If yes, you can start at the beginning on Step 1 and repeat the process to find another allergy, if you wish.
- If no, refocus, say a prayer for help, allow your heart to feel love and gratitude that this is going to help, and swipe three times once again with intention.

HELPFUL TIP FOR RELEASING ALLERGIES

If you are able to figure out what the specific allergen was and treat the underlying causes of it, it's a good idea for the subject to avoid any contact with that particular substance for about twenty-four hours. This allows the body to process the allergy release completely.

IDEA ALLERGIES

EXPLANATION

I've found that it's actually possible to become allergic to an idea! Let me explain. If you are allergic to a strawberry, your subconscious mind, hence your immune system, has a problem with the unique frequency and vibration that makes a strawberry a strawberry. Ultimately, a strawberry is energy. A specific idea is an energy as well, and it has a unique frequency and vibration. As a result, it's possible for you to develop an allergy to a specific idea.

What do you think the results might be if you are allergic to the idea of getting well, for example? What if your partner is allergic to the idea of commitment? Idea allergies like this can play havoc with your ability to create the life that you want. What do you think the results might be if you have an allergy to the idea of money? In Ann's story, you will see just how big an impact an idea allergy can have.

Allergic to Success

Before I started working with the Body Code, I had been self-employed for many years. I had created some success, but I just kept bumping up against an income barrier that I could never seem to get past.

Using the Body Code, I decided to see if it could help me finally "break through" in this area of my life. I was immediately led to an idea allergy, and with a little testing, I was able to figure out that this idea allergy boiled down to a subconscious belief that if I made a lot of money, it would ruin my marriage!

I cleared that idea allergy with three quick swipes. I had no idea how quickly I would see the results of removing that one block. In less than a month, my income more than doubled, and I finally achieved and went over a monthly income goal I had been chasing—and *never* hitting—for years. And what's more, in the six years since then, my monthly income has not once gone down below that goal I had chased for so long.

Meanwhile, I just celebrated my twenty-fifth wedding anniversary, during which my awesome husband and I renewed our vows. It's extraordinary the difference it made in my life using the Body Code on that abundance block!

—Ann H., Rhode Island, United States

Idea allergies are generally created when the subconscious mind makes a faulty or negative connection with a particular idea (any thought, emotion, concept, event, action, person, place, or thing). This usually happens during either prolonged or sudden emotional and/or physical stress. This idea then is considered to be a problem by the subconscious, and a negative response or reaction of some kind will occur when this idea is encountered. An idea allergy can even cause physical pain, as Teresa found in this next story.

The Idea of Loneliness

My friend wrote to me and expressed that she had developed sudden and intense pain in both of her hips. Assuming it may have something to do with a preexisting condition, she did what she could to make herself comfortable, even buying a new mattress topper while she searched for a mattress that could offer more relief.

I offered to check her body for trapped emotions and imbalances. What came up was surprising. Her body indicated that she had an idea allergy that was associated with the hip pain. She had developed an allergy to the idea of loneliness when she was five years old. I released the imbalance and told her I would check in later to see how she was doing.

Within twelve hours, she wrote to say, "Bless you, bless you, and bless you again! My hip pain is so minimal this morning, and it feels like it's going away completely! A side bonus is that I can stop looking at mattresses! But, truly, it's a huge relief because the pain was sudden and quite severe, and now it's just as quickly leaving my body. I'm *so much more comfortable!*" Both of us were extremely grateful to have the Body Code as a quick and efficient tool for resolving this pain. What a blessing!

—Teresa R., Calgary, Canada

The subconscious mind may create an idea allergy as a protective measure, in order to defend you from the stress that it has connected with the idea and to prevent the stressful past from being repeated.

Idea allergy symptoms manifest differently than physical allergy symptoms, of course, and often include self-sabotage, emotional reactivity, avoidance, and even phobias. Sometimes an idea allergy may result in a physical symptom, as in the last story. The subconscious mind is free to generate any kind of symptom in an attempt to avoid proximity to a particular idea, so keep an open mind. Remember, "Anything can cause anything."

Idea allergies nearly always have associated imbalances, such as trapped emotions, that must be cleared in order to reset and neutralize the subconscious mind's response to the idea.

By the way, it's common to have a physical allergy to any kind of substance associated with the idea allergy. (For example, if you have an idea allergy to your marriage, you may develop a physical allergy to your partner's perfume.) Idea allergies influence emotional choices by causing negative feelings about a particular idea.

EXERCISE:
FIND AND RELEASE AN IDEA ALLERGY

STEP 1.

Ask: "Do I [or you] have a physical allergy that can be released now?"

- If yes, continue to Step 2.
- If no, you may not have a physical allergy at all, or you may have one that cannot be released now, so you may want to try again a different day.

STEP 2.

(Decoding) Ask: "Do we need to know more about this allergy?"

- If no, move to Step 3 (Association).
- If yes, ask one or more of the following questions. Return to Step 2 (Decoding) once the answer to any of these questions is determined.
  - Ask: "Do we need to determine the allergen?"

If yes, use the Idea Allergens chart shown to dig deeper. Just like the process I outlined previously for finding a trapped emotion, use muscle testing to ask which column this idea allergy is in, then find the row, and narrow it down to a specific idea allergy. Note that this chart is not all-inclusive, but in most cases it is broad enough to do the job.

IDEA ALLERGENS			
	A	B	C
1	Being burdened Being overwhelmed Being hurt Being traumatized Lack of control Bad things you can't control	Being the victim Being the survivor Being in charge (of ____) Control Change Independence	Being valued/important Being needed or wanted Being respected Being deserving Having a support system Loyalty
2	Your perceived flaws Being/feeling ugly Betraying yourself Having anything feel off Feeling unsafe Feeling trapped	Your own thoughts Your own behavior Your personality Yourself Growing up Life	Love Giving love Receiving love Connection Letting go Going with the flow
3	Being sick Fatigue Feeling drained Pain or discomfort Being doubted/mistrusted Being blamed	Being alive Aging Death Needing someone Drama Being wrong	Being okay Self-reliance Self-care Making positive changes Being motivated Being healthy
4	Being lied to Being deceived Being manipulated Being betrayed Lack of loyalty Being let down	People seeing you as ____ Being noticed People wanting things from you Vulnerability Relationships in general The wrong (or right) person	Having energy Being youthful Being attractive Feeling safe to be yourself Feeling peaceful Being creative
5	Being overpowered Another's suffering Other's negative feelings Being rejected Being judged Being criticized	Setting/maintaining boundaries Having/creating a family Childbirth Marriage Changing unhealthy dynamics Being like your parents	Using/discovering talents Joy or happiness Confidence Fulfillment Progress Passion
6	Being disconnected Loneliness Past repeating itself Fighting Divorce Breakup	Leaving your family Moving forward Money in general Spending money A specific person A specific location	Curiosity Contentment Gratitude Excitement Success Wealth
7	Being invisible Failure Losing money Being poor Trouble achieving Emotion (use Emotion Code Chart)	A specific role A relationship dynamic/role Being visible Goals Work Even exchange of energy	Making money Saving money Receiving money Charging money Receiving rewards Receiving gifts, etc.

Once you have found the specific idea allergen, return to Step 2 (Decoding) and ask if there is more you need to know. If you do not need to know more about the allergen, go to Step 3 (Association), otherwise, you might ask the following questions:

- Ask: "Do we need to know the age of occurrence?"
- Ask: "Was this absorbed from someone else?"
- Ask: "Is this from a specific event?"

STEP 3.

(Association) Idea allergies nearly always have associated imbalances, such as trapped emotions, that must be cleared in order to reset the subconscious response to the idea (allergen).

- Ask: "Is there an associated imbalance that needs to be decoded?"
- If no, move to Step 4 (Intention).
- If yes, which is likely, return to the Body Code Map and decode and address any associated imbalances, then return here and repeat the Step 3 (Association) question.

STEP 4.

(Intention) Swipe three times with a magnet or your hand on any length of the governing meridian, while holding the intention to release the allergy.

STEP 5.

Ask: "Did we release that idea allergy?"

- If yes, you can start at the beginning on Step 1 and repeat the process to find another idea allergy, if you wish.
- If no, refocus, say a prayer for help, allow your heart to feel love and gratitude that this is going to help, and swipe three times once again with intention.

THOUGHTS ON IDEA ALLERGIES

Here is a quote that I have found very pertinent to our discussion of idea allergies:

> *The subconscious mind . . . makes no distinction between constructive and destructive thought impulses. It works with the material we feed it, through our thought impulses. The subconscious mind will translate into reality a thought driven by fear just as readily as it will translate into reality a thought driven by courage or faith.*
>
> —Napoleon Hill

Remember that your focus determines your reality, whether it is conscious or subconscious!

9

OFFENSIVE ENERGIES

I will not let anyone walk through my mind with their dirty feet.

—MAHATMA GANDHI

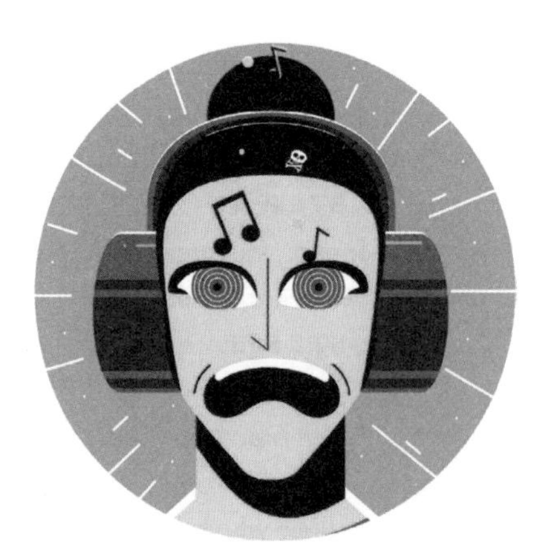

There are several kinds of offensive energies, all of which can create distortions in your energy field and sabotage your life. They can be created by the subconscious minds of other people, by entities, and we sometimes even create them ourselves. This category of imbalances includes saboteurs and entities.

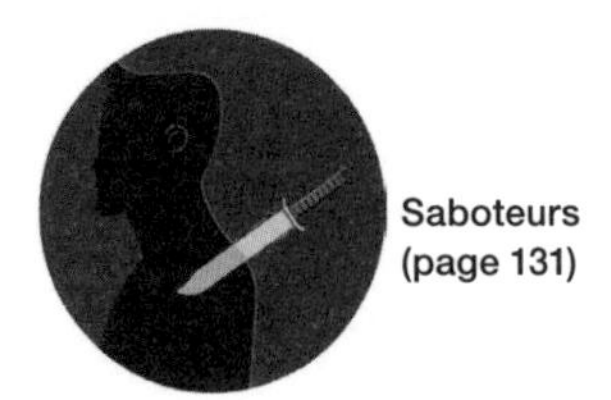

Saboteurs
(page 131)

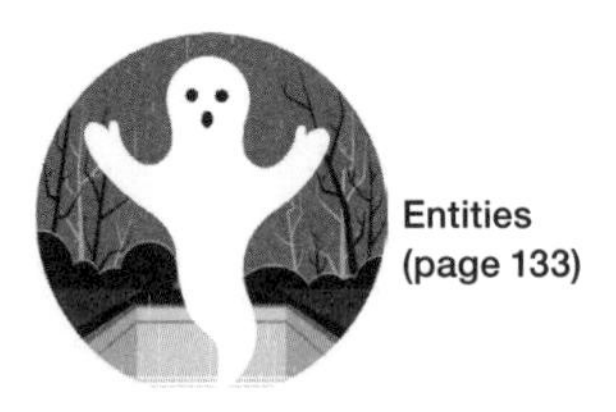

Entities
(page 133)

SABOTEURS

EXPLANATION

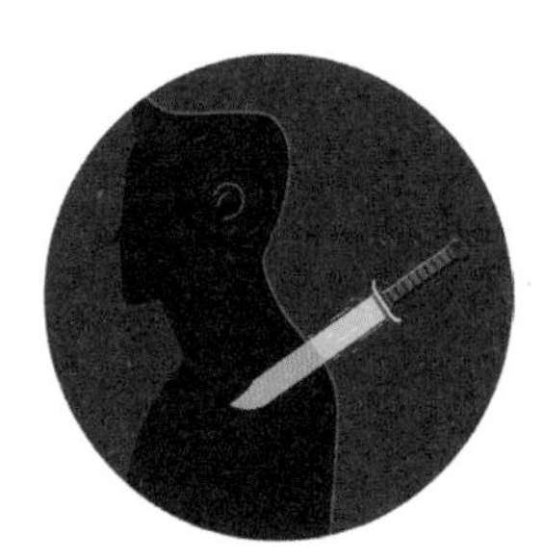

A saboteur is a strong negative energy that is intended to wound and/or sabotage the recipient, usually coming from another person or entity. Saboteurs can be compared to invisible but damaging weapons, wounds, or mechanisms of control.

Most saboteurs are created by the subconscious mind and are expressions of negative feelings toward the recipient. Some sabotage can be self-inflicted, usually if there is ongoing or intense self-abuse. Saboteurs may cause physical discomfort and interfere with the recovery process.

Here is an example of how finding and removing a saboteur helped when nothing else did.

My Favorite Client

I will always remember that wonderful day when Maria, my eighty-one-year-old client, was healed. She barely shuffled into my office for her eighth Body Code session to work on removing chronic sciatica. It was heartbreaking to see the pain on her face and in her body. It was easy to notice that every step she took caused excruciating daggers of pain. About ten minutes into that session, she hollered out, "Oh my gosh, it's GONE!" I said, "What's gone?" She said, "MY PAIN!" That was music to my ears! We both laughed and cried at the same time.

It was discovered that she'd had an energy saboteur. Sadly, someone very close to her had put an energetic "knife" in her lower back ten years previous. Once it was removed, she was smiling and felt like she wanted to do a dance. She has been free of that pain ever since. The client, I have to say, is my favorite, as she is my mother. The healings I have witnessed are incredible! I love being the conduit through which people heal."

—Deborah B., Arizona, United States

It is often not necessary to decode very much information to find and release saboteur energy, however, the type of weapon and the location in the body may have metaphysical significance, which could be interesting or helpful to think about (e.g., a "knife" in the back may signify a betrayal).

EXERCISE:
FIND AND RELEASE A SABOTEUR

STEP 1.

Ask: "Do I [or you] have a saboteur that we can find and eliminate now?"

- If yes, continue to Step 2.
- If no, you may not have a saboteur, or you may need to try again later.

STEP 2.

(Decoding) Ask: "Is it necessary to identify more about this saboteur?"

- If no, move to Step 3 (Association).
- If yes, ask one or more of the following questions. Return to Step 2 (Decoding) once the answer to any of these questions is determined.
    - Ask: "Do we need to know the location of this energy in the body?"
    - Ask: "Is this a weapon?"
    - Ask: "Is this a wound?"
    - Ask: "Is this a control mechanism?"
    - Ask: "Do we need to know the age of occurrence?"
    - Ask: "Was this placed by an entity (or a human being)?"

STEP 3.

(Association) Ask: "Is there an associated imbalance that needs to be decoded?"

- If no, move to Step 4 (Intention).
    - If yes, return to the Body Code Map and decode and address any associated imbalances, then return here and repeat the Step 3 (Association) question.

STEP 4.

(Intention) Swipe three times with a magnet or your hand on any length of the governing meridian while holding the intention to release the saboteur.

STEP 5.

Ask: "Did we release that saboteur energy?"

- If yes, you can start at the beginning on Step 1 and repeat the process to find and release additional saboteur energy you may have.
- If no, refocus, say a prayer for help, allow your heart to feel love and gratitude that this is going to help, and swipe three times once again with intention.

ENTITIES

EXPLANATION

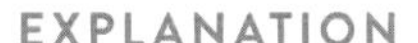

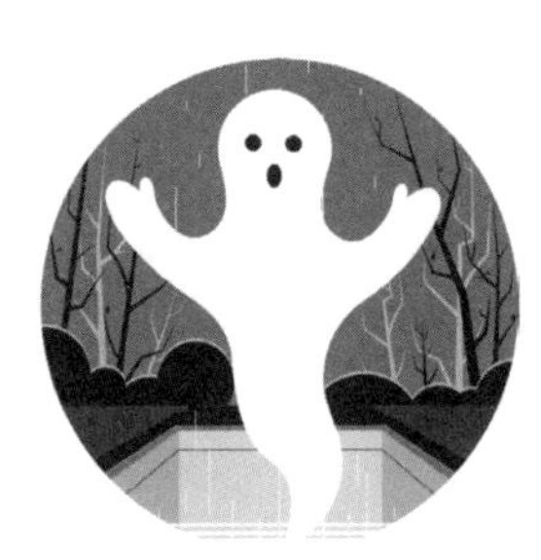

There is an unseen world all around us, a world that we are generally unaware of, yet it has a powerful influence on our lives. But are spirits, ghosts, and other entities real?

Entities or dark spirits are a touchy subject, and I approach it with some hesitation. While every healing method of any great age acknowledges the importance of entities and their effects on physical and mental health, modern Western medicine—a relative newcomer in the world of healing—does not recognize the existence of entities at all.

During his three-year ministry, Jesus seems to have been kept busy getting rid of entities. Seven of his thirty-seven healing miracles included the casting out of dark spirits in order to relieve people of their mental or physical illness.

While Western pharmaceutical-based medicine denies the possibility of the influence of unseen spirits upon us in favor of prescription medications to suppress symptoms, ancient peoples were consciously aware of entities.

Sometimes people are afraid of this topic, of "ghosts" or evil spirits. But you have no reason to be afraid, because they can be dealt with effectively in most cases with the Body Code. If the subject bothers you, or if your mind is closed to the possibility of entities being real, then you can skip to the next chapter. But I hope you will open your heart and mind to realize that there is much about our existence that we do not fully understand.

So who and what are these entities, and how do we most commonly encounter them?

TYPES OF ENTITIES

I've come to believe that there are two kinds of entities in this world: disembodied spirits and unembodied spirits. The disembodied spirits, or "ghosts," are the spirits of people who died but remain "earthbound" because they have not gone to the light and moved on, usually because of the addictions they still cling to from their mortal experience.

For example, a person who is addicted to alcohol may remain earthbound and inhabit places where people are drinking, in an attempt to experience intoxication through a living person's body.

A disembodied spirit who is addicted to pornography may impress thoughts and ideas into a susceptible person to get them to look at pornography, then may attempt to temporarily enter that person's body to feel those sexual feelings again, even if only in a muffled way. Note that disembodied spirits are also often referred to as "unclean spirits."

The other class of entities are often referred to as unembodied spirits, or evil spirits. These spirits have never experienced life in a mortal body of their own but are devoted to misleading people and sowing confusion and chaos.

Entities can be insidious if not identified, removed, and sent away. They enjoy creating unhappiness, taking control, and robbing individuals of their personal freedom. They can cause emotional problems, such as depression and anger, which can be quite severe. They can also cause illness and pain and can interfere with healing and success. Root-cause imbalances can be more difficult to identify when entities are involved.

Entities of either type are drawn or attracted to things on the lower vibrational end of the scale. Violence in all forms, including the portrayal of violence as entertainment, may attract them. Pornography attracts them, and I personally believe that all pornography is a form of spiritual violence. They are attracted to certain kinds of intense or dark music, so be aware of the energy music inspires. If you're experiencing anything with a dark energy about it, then be advised that entities are drawn to darkness in all its forms.

On the other hand, entities may also be attracted to us if we are about to make a breakthrough or bring more light into the world, and they will provide opposition to that. And sometimes they just show up for no apparent reason, as Beth found out in this next story.

A Stubborn Entity

Last week, my sister and I were discussing some spiritual topics, when I suddenly experienced an excruciating and searing pain in my lower back with no explainable physical cause. I could not get up from sitting or support my weight without help. Upon standing, I felt a cold *whoosh* of air blow across my back. We started to look for imbalances using the Emotion Code and found and removed a few trapped emotions, but I became too miserable and had to cut the session short, so my condition remained largely unchanged.

The next day, I had increased and profound distress and was barely able to walk. Nothing helped to alleviate my back discomfort, not even prescription-strength medication. I asked another family member, certified in using the Body Code, for help. He found a saboteur and entities, which he tried to send away. However, my condition did not improve. My discomfort was so overwhelming and relentless for several days following, that out of desperation, I visited a professional masseuse and a Reiki provider, but this also yielded little improvement.

I remembered a previous experience with a stubborn entity that refused to leave without a fight, so I decided to try a second Body Code session to check whether the entities were, in fact, gone. We found that the entities and saboteur were still present. Since I am a Christian, we commanded the entities to leave in the name of Jesus Christ, and to take their weapons with them. We felt a change in the energy of the room, and I experienced *instant* and profound relief in my back. *Wow!* I prayed my thanks to the Lord that night and had the most restful sleep I've had in months. I'm so grateful for the Body Code, which is an amazing tool to help identify negative energies. By calling on the power of Christ, we had the ability to vanquish these negative energies!

—Beth B., Texas, United States

When you are using the Body Code, you are releasing darkness in the lives of those that you are working with. Darkness is dispelled with light and love. Dark energies don't want you to help anyone to get well and be happy. Entities will attempt to thwart your efforts if they can, by influencing you to feel doubt, hopelessness, or some other negative thought or feeling. It's good to be aware of and get rid of them, so you can find the answers that you are seeking. From the experiences that I and others have had, as well as studying other people's experiences, both ancient and modern, it's apparent to me that these entities are not to be feared. They want to create fear in us, it is true. But their tactics are illusions. Their power over us is limited, unless we invite them to have power over us by the choices that we make.

We received a letter from one of our practitioners sharing a beautiful healing story that involved several different kinds of imbalances in the client she brought back to wholeness.

A Weight Lifted

A new client came in that had suffered with PTSD from childhood sexual abuse. She cried through much of the session as we released miasms, entities, and negative emotions. I could see her start to relax and take deep breaths. At the end of the session she burst into laughter because she felt so relieved. This is the email I received from her the following day:

"I feel very relaxed and comfortable. I am trying to find words to best describe what transpired in our emotional clearing. After I left your office, I immediately felt an incredible weight was lifted, like I had lost one hundred pounds. My mind has been silent in a new way. Absence of internal conflict, no nightmares or tremors. Panic and fear are nonexistent. I feel an overwhelming sense of a return to self, completely at ease and comforted by the Divine Light.

"I feel that I was a character in a horror book that was lifted out of that story and a new road was given. I feel incredibly grateful. I feel joy about what my life holds. I feel safe. I have not felt safe and completely comfortable in my own skin in a long time. I am reuniting with the image of me as a child that I told you I saw in your office. I pray with a clear mind and an open heart. I'm actually excited to find out what and where the light will lead me. The best way I can describe it would be, being able to see the world in color for the first time, like in that part of *The Wizard of Oz,* minus the obstacles. I had been stuck in the dark for a long, long time."

—Janet G., Maine, United States

In my experience, I have found that entities have contributed to the following symptoms for my patients:

- Fatigue
- Physical discomfort
- Negativity and mood issues
- Addictions
- Feeling stuck
- Feeling immobilized or overwhelmed
- Self-sabotage
- Anger at self or others
- Self-doubt
- Depression
- Mental illness
- Nightmares

Finding and releasing an entity may help relieve many of these symptoms.

EXERCISE: FIND AND RELEASE AN ENTITY

STEP 1.

Ask: "Do I [or you] have an entity or entities influencing me [or you]?"

- **If yes, continue to step 2.**
- **If no, you may not have an entity influencing you at this time, or you may need to try again later.**

STEP 2.

(Association) Ask: "Is there an associated imbalance that needs to be decoded?"

- **If no, move to Step 3 (Intention).**
- **If yes, return to the Body Code Map to decode and address any associated imbalances, then return here and repeat the Step 2 (Association) question.**

STEP 3.

(Intention)

- Prayer is especially helpful when dealing with entities.
- There are three options for removing an entity.
    - The first option is to simply swipe three times with a magnet or your hand on any length of the governing meridian holding the intention to release the entity.
    - The second option is to acknowledge the presence of the entity, focus the vibrations of compassion and love toward the entity, and swipe three times with a magnet or your hand on any length of the governing meridian to release the entity, intending to send it to the light.
    - The third option is to swipe three times with a magnet or your hand on any length of the governing meridian while saying words to this effect: "Entity (or Entities, if plural) in the name of Jesus Christ (or the Creator, Higher Power, etc.), I command you to depart from this person and never bother him / her again."

STEP 4.

Ask: "Did we release that entity (or entities)?"

- If yes, you can start at the beginning on Step 1 and repeat the process to find and release any remaining entities.
- If no, refocus, say a prayer for help, allow your heart to feel love and gratitude that this is going to help, and swipe three times once again with intention.
- It's a good idea to check for the presence of curses or saboteurs after releasing entities.
- On rare occasions, fasting and prayer may be required to get entities to leave.
- In order to lessen the likelihood of a future entity imbalance, you may want to do some targeted Body Code work focused on raising the vibration and creating wholeness and balance in the energy body and energy field/aura. In addition, it is suggested to avoid anything that interferes with your personal power or the health of your physical and energetic body.

HELPFUL TIPS FOR DEALING WITH ENTITIES

Prayer is especially helpful when dealing with entities. It's a good idea to check for the presence of saboteurs after releasing entities. On rare occasions, fasting and prayer may be required to get entities to leave. In order to lessen the likelihood of a future entity attachment, you may want to do some targeted Body Code work focused on raising the vibration and creating wholeness and balance in the energy body and energy field or aura. In addition, it is suggested to avoid anything that interferes with your personal power or the health of your physical and energetic body.

THE UNSEEN WORLD OF ANGELS AND ENTITIES

Just as there are dark spirits that inhabit this world along with us, there are also spirits of light or angels.

Did you live before you arrived on planet Earth?

We all have different beliefs about where we were before this present life. Some people believe in reincarnation. I believe in a twist on the idea.

If you've read stories about people who have near-death experiences after dying on the operating table or in some sort of accident, for example, it's not unusual for them to suddenly see angels that are observing what is going on. Most often, these angels are connected to the deceased in some familial way. These angels are often ancestors, but sometimes they are the yet-to-be-born descendants of the one that has just passed away.

Many years ago, as I pondered about this and prayed for guidance, I gained an insight into what is going on in our lives.

Before we were born, we visited Earth. I believe that every single one of us has been here before—perhaps multiple times—in the capacity of what might be called a "guardian angel" to someone that is experiencing mortal life. I believe that we accepted these assignments as part of our education, preparing us for our own mortal lives and as part of our progress toward our eternal destiny.

Do angels experience intense emotions? I'm sure they do. Imagine being assigned as an angel to help someone through the mortal life, only to see the person abused, enslaved, or murdered. I don't believe it's necessary to have a physical body in order to trap emotional energy, trauma, or other energetic imbalances.

So these angels develop emotional baggage and are ultimately themselves born into a physical body when they are ready to experience mortality. We sometimes bring into our mortal experience the emotional energies from our assignments as angels.

Trapped emotions that we have brought into mortality from previous experiences as angels are just as real and just as powerful as the trapped emotions we pick up ourselves during our mortal lives.

I believe we have all absolutely had "other lives." I just believe that we experienced those lives as angels on assignment.

I also believe that these angels are usually family members, either those who have already departed mortality or those who have yet to make their appearance in a mortal body. Who would care more about us than our own relatives?

Here is a story of a sweet young mother who received direction from her deceased grandmother because she needed help healing her family.

An Angel's Voice

One warm afternoon I was suddenly visited by a really warm golden light. It had the aroma of rose or something that was very sweet and really, really loving. This energy came and enveloped myself and my two children into its arms. Usually due to my anxiety and my many numerous chronic pains, I have been unable to have any peaceful rest during the day, but because of this mysterious golden light, I was able to take a nap, and so did my superactive children. We all fell into a beautiful nap. That itself was a miracle, but the real miracle started after I woke up from the nap. After a few hours, I woke up, and to my amazement, the years of chronic pain that I had been struggling with, much of it was gone from my back and especially from my neck. A voice came to me from above, or it felt like it came from my heart.

The voice said, "You need to go to your iPad and open the email section. . . ." I had no idea what this was about, but I knew that this voice was coming from heaven and that I needed to follow it. I got up out of my bed and opened my email. There was an email from my beloved meditation teacher whom I have known for a long, long time. The voice said, "You need to open this email." As I did, there was a link, and the link led me to a TV interview by the Gaia TV channel with Dr. Bradley Nelson. The voice said, "You need to watch this."

In those days I was chronically exhausted and so tired. I was not able to do anything beyond my regular chores and looking after my children. Because of the golden light and the warmth of the love that it gave me, I had extra energy, so I was able to watch this. In those days I had a lot of pain in my eyes, too, which made it very difficult to look at the screen, but I don't anymore. I was able to watch this TV series. After watching the show, the voice said, "I want you to study with this man." I knew the voice was coming from my grandmother, who had been in the hospital.

It turned out that the next day I found out that she had passed away.

So that was her voice, and her voice said, "I want you to study with this man, Dr. Bradley Nelson, because during my lifetime, I was not able to heal my relationship with my daughters" (my mother and my aunt). She said, "I did not have the power or the wisdom to heal the disconnection with my daughters. My beloved daughters are suffering and I need you to help me. And this man can help you do that."

I decided to work with the Emotion Code, and ever since then, a lot of my problems have disappeared, which include the eczema problems, hay fever allergies, food intolerances, and the severe pain in my eyes. All those problems that I had have disappeared. I have worked with my husband and our financial problem has disappeared.

> I received an email informing me that Dr. Bradley Nelson was coming to Germany for a Body Code workshop. I told my husband, "Well, he's coming; can we go see him?" My husband said, "Let's book the train ticket." So that's how I came here today to this workshop from the United Kingdom. And it's been a miracle. Thank you.
>
> —Yoriko D., Stourbridge, United Kingdom

Jean and I met Yoriko at an event in Germany and recorded her beautiful story. Visit discoverhealing.com/video/the-voice to watch it.

Sometimes God speaks through our angels to warn us of danger. A friend of mine told me about an experience like this. He was driving slowly on a two-lane road in heavy fog. Suddenly a voice called out, "Get off the road now!"

Without any hesitation, he pulled onto the shoulder, when instantly a car passed him going the other direction at a high rate of speed, in his lane. He told me that he would certainly have been killed if he had not heeded that voice.

When we hear a sudden warning voice, whose voice is it? When we receive a whispered answer to prayer, when we have a sudden stroke of an idea or a solution to a problem, where is it coming from?

I believe that the angels around us are the ones whispering to us, sometimes speaking audibly to us. I believe when we find and remove imbalances, entities, and negative energies in the body, we can more clearly hear our angels' warnings and messages and better feel their love for us.

SECTION 2

PATHOGENS

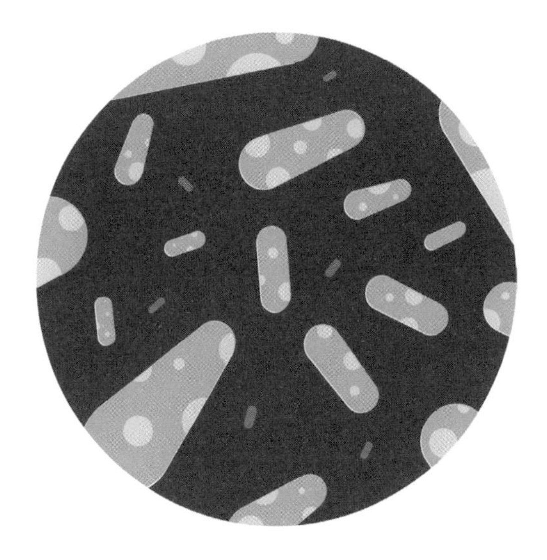

Energy healing is based on the supposition that illness results from disturbances in the body's energies and energy fields and can be addressed via interventions into those energies and energy fields.

—JED DIAMOND

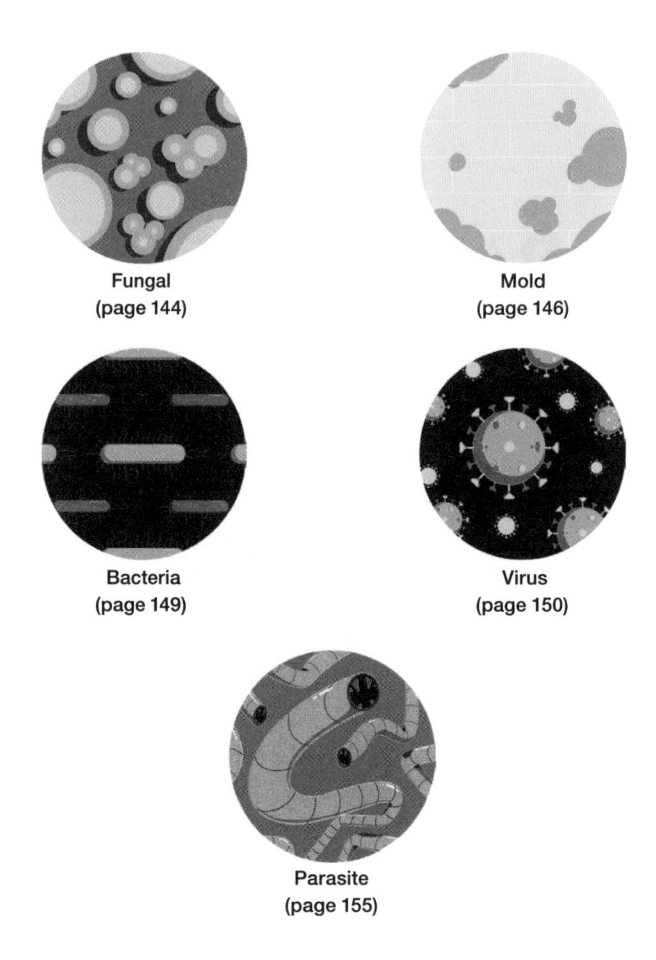

The purpose of this section is to help you to understand the different kinds of pathogens, how to detect them, and what to do to correct them. Pathogens include infections like viruses, bacteria, fungi, molds, and infestations, which refers to parasites.

10

PATHOGENS

Your body has natural healing capacities that nobody in the field of medicine can pretend ultimately to understand.

—DR. WAYNE DYER

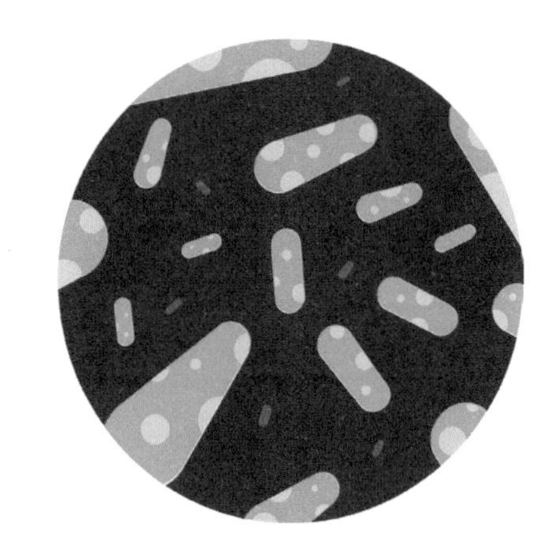

Pathogens are infectious microorganisms, germs, or biological agents that cause infectious diseases or illnesses in the body. The severity of the diseases caused by pathogens varies. Some infections are mild while others may be life-threatening. For example, there is not much comparison between having a common cold and having the Ebola virus.

All a pathogen needs to thrive and survive is a host. Once the pathogen infects the host body, it manages to avoid the body's immune responses and uses the body's resources to replicate before exiting and spreading to a new host.

FUNGAL

Infectious disease is a killer worldwide. Over seventeen million people die from infection every year, making it one of the leading causes of death. Remember that any kind of infection is potentially dangerous, so I would advise you to seek medical assistance if it is available to you. If you are on your own, or if you prefer to try more natural methods first, I outline those in this book.

Historically, infections have been poorly understood. For example, rats in the Middle Ages carried fleas that were infected with bacteria. Due to poor sanitation and filthy living conditions, the abundant fleas would transfer this organism into human beings through their bites. The result was the "Black Death," which resulted in the suffering and death of millions of people in a truly horrific time to be alive. People's symptoms were baffling to the physicians of that era, and the disease was generally thought to be God's revenge on people for their sins, but it was also variously ascribed to things such as bad air, bad water, and even people's bad attitudes.

With the discovery of the microscope and breakthrough use of it by Antoni van Leeuwenhoek, the invisible world of pathogens suddenly became more accessible. Experiments eventually showed that there were actually small organisms at work when food would spoil or when bread left out would grow moldy.

As humankind devoted more attention to improving public health through the use of better sanitation, improved sewage systems, the importance of washing hands, and so on, death by infection fell dramatically.

Most infectious organisms can be considered to be "opportunistic," which means that they will take an opportunity if they are given one. For example, if your immune system becomes depressed, you will be more likely to develop an infection that may ultimately proliferate. In the vast majority of cases, that deadly organism has been living in the body but has been held in check by the efforts of the immune system, which keeps us healthy, most of the time.

FUNGAL INFECTIONS

EXPLANATION

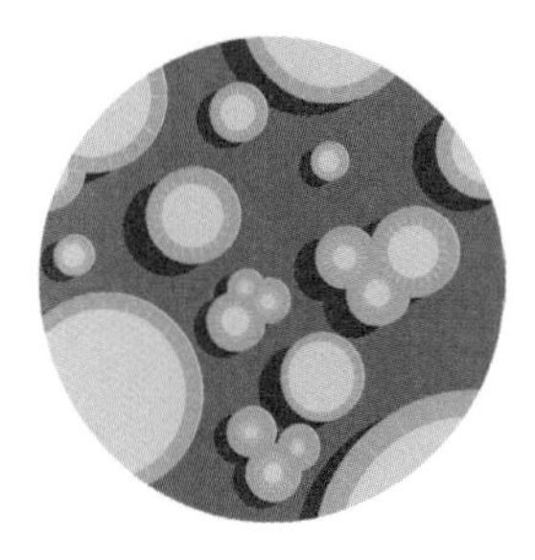

The most common type of fungal infection I have seen in practice is Candidiasis, or Candida. Candida is called "the great mimicker," because it can cause a wide variety of problems, and as a result of this it often is misdiagnosed as something else. Fungi in general are opportunistic organisms, which means that they are everywhere and if given the opportunity to grow, they will. Fungal organisms and fungal spores are in the air that you breathe, and they are in your body, but they're usually kept in check by your immune system. If your immune system becomes imbalanced for any reason, the fungal spores may begin to grow and proliferate.

MOST COMMON SYMPTOMS OF FUNGAL INFECTION

Fungal infections like Candidiasis will tend to create anxiety or panic attacks, abdominal gas or bloating, and brain fog. Fungal infections also tend to create cravings for sugar and starchy foods. This is because fungal organisms feed on simple sugars such as sweets, flour, bread, baked goods, and even alcohol. In fact, this can be one of the underlying reasons behind alcoholism. Alcohol breaks down into sugar in the body, feeding the fungal or mold infection and allowing it to grow even more. This can create a downward spiral unless there is some kind of intervention. Ideally the intake of alcohol should stop and some kind of remedy should be administered to eliminate the fungi (or mold).

Other symptoms of fungal infection include: constipation, diarrhea, depression, eczema, skin infections or skin problems, excessive fatigue, dizziness, headaches, indigestion, irritability, learning difficulties, migraines, headaches, mood swings, poor memory, rectal itching, sensitivity to fragrances and/or chemicals, thrush (where fungus becomes visible on the tongue), and vaginitis (because mold and fungal infections like to live in the dark, moist areas in the body).

COMMON CAUSES OF FUNGAL INFECTIONS

Fungal infections like Candidiasis and mold are common after hormone treatments. For example, going on birth control pills often disrupts the hormonal balance and creates an environment where these opportunistic organisms can start to flourish. Pregnancy also disrupts the balance because of the hormonal fluctuations that occur at this time. Using antibiotics will also create imbalance, allowing fungi and mold to grow. The average person has up to three and a half pounds of healthy flora or bacteria in their intestinal tract. These healthy bacteria form the majority of the immune system, keeping fungal and other pathogenic infections at bay. Antibiotics, particularly broad-spectrum antibiotics, tend to kill off not only the bad bacteria but also the good bacteria that live in your gut, weakening the immune system. Then, when a fungus or a mold is introduced to the body, it tends to flourish without much interference. High sugar intake in the diet will also tend to create an environment where mold and fungal infections can flourish, because the more fuel they have, the more they can proliferate and the stronger they become. Diabetes also creates an environment that is perfect for fungal and mold organisms to prosper because the blood-sugar levels are high.

MOLD VERSUS FUNGUS

Technically, mold is a type of fungus, but they show up differently in the body for some reason. Because of this, mold and fungi are two separate types of infections in the Body Code and they will show up on testing separately, although they are very much related.

The best natural treatments—in my experience—for fungal and mold infections are neem leaf capsules and coconut oil. Neem is a tree from India whose leaves are gentle and cleansing to the body, but tough on fungal infections. It can be easily found at most health food or supplement stores, or online. Pure, virgin, cold-pressed coconut oil can correct and prevent fungal infections, as well as keep your skin, organs, and other tissues healthy. Remember, the subconscious mind knows what a person needs. You can muscle test for whichever one of these remedies your body wants to help it get rid of the infection, and then test for the correct dosage (i.e., how many bottles, how many capsules, drops, teaspoonfuls, etc.).

Be aware that die-off of the fungus or mold may create flu-like symptoms including nausea and vomiting in some cases. People will sometimes muscle test for high doses of neem, but more commonly, people will test for a lower dosage over a longer period of time—for example, ten or twenty neem capsules per day for two or three weeks, or even longer depending on how bad the infection actually is.

Coconut oil can be taken internally by the spoonful, rubbed on the skin, or used in cooking. You can simply ask which method of administration would be the best for the body and for the type and location of the infection. For instance, a skin rash caused by mold could be treated by either rubbing coconut oil on the affected area, by taking it internally, or both.

MOLD

EXPLANATION

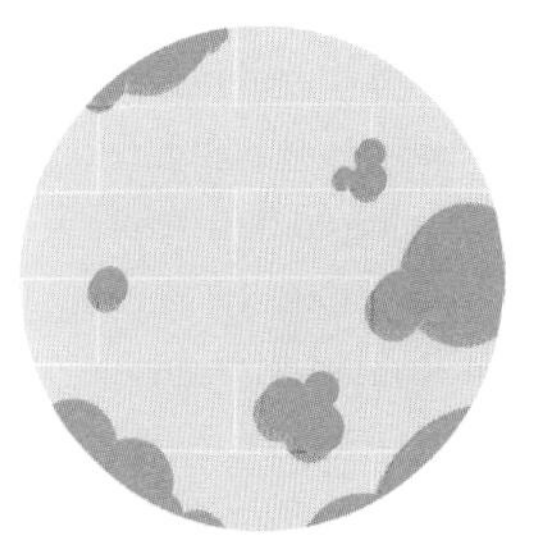

Mold seems to be an increasingly more pervasive problem in the world now. Like any fungus, mold is an opportunistic organism. Mold is everywhere in our environment, no matter where we live, and may take root and grow wherever it is allowed to.

Mold infections can create a wide variety of symptoms and problems, such as joint and muscle pain, fatigue, sinus and respiratory issues, eye and skin irritation, fever, headaches and brain fog, along with cravings for simple sugars. Mold infections can cause all of the same symptoms as other fungal infections that I outlined earlier. Mold can be very dangerous to the body, but it's often difficult to diagnose a mold infection with regular medical testing. For some reason, mold infections seem to be on the increase. The worst mold infections usually arise because of constant and repeated exposure to a mold source, such as mold growing in a house from a water leak or mold in a ventilation system where the spores are breathed in repeatedly.

In the following story, Connie used the Body Code on her infant grandson to identify the true underlying cause of his sickness.

Mold Threatens a Newborn's Life

A couple of weeks ago I wasn't feeling well. I was staying with my son and his wife to assist them with their new baby, so I needed to be a help, not a hindrance. I turned first to prayer to draw upon the powers of heaven to guide me. Then I opened the Body Code app to track down what was causing my extreme fatigue.

In the app, I was taken to pathogens and then to mold, which tested as strong, or yes. That seemed strange because it was a clean, lovely place. No mold was apparent anywhere on walls or plumbing areas. It did seem odd that when I went outside of the apartment, I felt better. When I came back inside, I started sneezing and felt exhausted.

I confirmed with other Body Code practitioners, who also indicated this finding was correct and that it was important that we all get out of there ASAP!

It was not possible for them to pick up and immediately leave at the time. Unfortunately, one week later, their five-week-old baby was in critical condition at a local hospital. The hospital attendants were not able to insert an IV into the baby due to dehydration. He had been unable to nurse due to exhaustion. Muscle testing using the Body Code indicated that he was suffering from a mold infection as well.

He was transferred to a pediatric hospital, where an IV was successfully inserted. When we told them that we suspected mold was the problem, they said that mold testing was not something they were equipped to do at that particular hospital. That was a very frustrating answer after we had requested the test. Instead, the doctors performed a spinal tap that later indicated that no meningitis virus was present.

While we continued to do everything the medical doctors had prescribed, his parents also used the Body Code suggestions. Neem and lavender essential oils were applied. Within several hours, the baby perked up. My daughter-in-law was also using these items in order to get these remedies into her nursing milk.

My son took his own action by purchasing a mold test kit from a local retailer and placing it on the apartment counter for several days. Mold spores grew in the petri dish from being exposed to the air, a sure indicator of a mold infestation.

Once out of the hospital, the baby's systemic mold infection was confirmed by testing at the pediatrician's office. The results indicated very high levels of mold in the baby's system.

The family moved into a hotel until the next living space could be secured. The baby is doing well and is on the mend. Inspectors found the source of the mold in the venting system at the old apartment. They shared that it was the worst mold problem that they had ever seen in many years of doing mold remediation.

Am I grateful for the Body Code? Last week we would have lost the newest member of our family without it. Without the Body Code, my new grandson may have been categorized as "failure to thrive" for some unknown reason. We are so glad we could tune in to the problem in time. Does God answer our prayers? You bet He does. He provides us with the tools to help ourselves. How else can we learn gratitude?

—Connie N. B., Utah, United States

In order to prevent and eliminate infections efficiently, the body's immune system must be functioning properly. Anything that imbalances the body will tend to interfere with the immune system and hamper its natural ability to recognize and eliminate infections. For example, trapped emotions and other energetic imbalances can actually enable infections by distorting and imbalancing the energy field, thence the body tissues, which can allow infection to grow and proliferate. When finding and fixing underlying causes, as Kathy did in the following story, infections can be eliminated, allowing healthy tissue to grow.

A Sick Baby

I had a mother call me one morning concerned about her five-month-old daughter. She had very foul-smelling diapers, diarrhea, and open sores on her bottom that were very painful.

I found out that the baby had a fungal infection. I found an associated imbalance was a misalignment of the large intestine, with another associated imbalance of difficulty absorbing water. This was being caused by a trapped emotion of overwhelm, which the baby had absorbed from someone else, so I released the trapped emotion. I asked if the large intestine was now aligned, and I received a yes answer. I then released the energy of the fungal infection and held the intention for the immune system to eliminate the physical fungal organisms.

The mother called me the next day and said that the sores were almost completely gone, just the deepest ones remained, but they'd significantly improved. Upon checking the baby for water absorption, testing showed that she no longer had a problem. A couple of days later the sores on her bottom were completely gone.

—Kathy H., Utah, United States

BACTERIA

EXPLANATION

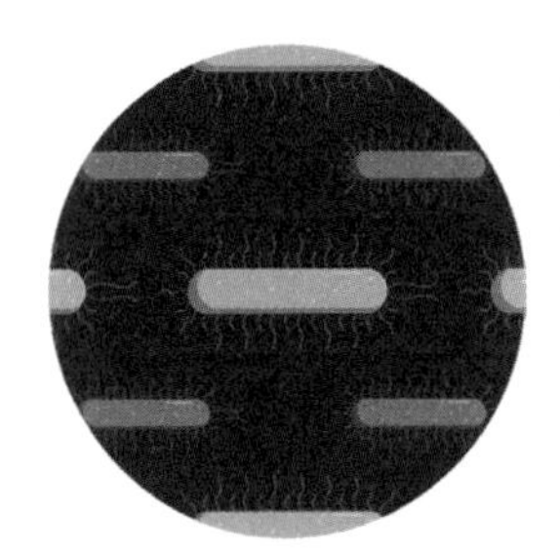

Bacteria are larger, single-celled microorganisms, such as strep, staph, salmonella, E. coli, and H. pylori. Bacterial infections can be deadly, and are responsible for tuberculosis, pneumonia, cholera, syphilis, anthrax, leprosy, stomach ulcers, and bubonic plague, to name a few. In my experience, low-grade infection is by far the most common severity of infection for most people, most of the time. Just like low-grade viral infections, low-grade bacterial infections are typically mild and not life-threatening. They can, however, cause a lot of problems in the body, usually contributing to lack of energy as in chronic fatigue syndrome, muscle pain as in fibromyalgia, stomach ulcers or acid reflux, skin rashes, and other bothersome problems.

On the other hand, low-grade infection is often a hidden contributing factor in grave problems such as cancer. The traditional treatments for infections are primarily based on antibiotics, antiviral, antifungal, and antiparasitic drugs. The problem is that, especially in the case of antibiotics, their widespread use is leading to the creation of superbugs, bacteria that are becoming resistant to every known antibiotic. Another problem with antibiotics is the negative side effects they cause and the damage they do to the physical body. A common saying in the alternative health-care community is that the body needs seven years to recover from taking an antibiotic prescription, but new evidence reveals that the body may never recover fully.

Research has revealed that a variety of diseases may be linked to antibiotic use—especially in the young—including obesity, depression, asthma, type 1 and type 2 diabetes, and inflammatory forms of arthritis. Broad-spectrum antibiotics often wipe out healthy intestinal flora, leading to lifelong problems with digestion. Hippocrates knew what he was talking about when he said, "All disease begins in the gut."

Just as each human being has both a physical and a spiritual side and exists solely as a spirit, or as a spirit coupled to a physical body, pathogens are no different. As a result, it's not unusual to find a pathogen that is only existing in its "spirit," or energetic, form. This most often happens when a physical infection has been eliminated by the immune system, but the "spiritual" energy of the pathogen remains. For example, if you have had a mold infection at some point in your life but were able to rid your body of the mold, you may still have the mold energy, as Sue found in the following story.

Acne Be Gone

I worked with a fourteen-year-old girl who had a severe case of cystic acne and low self-esteem. She had been on toxic medications for a year and was now being put on birth control to try to heal the cystic acne. After one Body Code session, her acne cleared in a few days. I spoke with her three days later and she said 90 percent of the cystic acne was gone! There were many infections such as mold and energies of past pathogens that were released, along with emotional components. This is something the dermatologist could not have found using traditional medicine.

—Sue C., Florida, United States

VIRUS

EXPLANATION

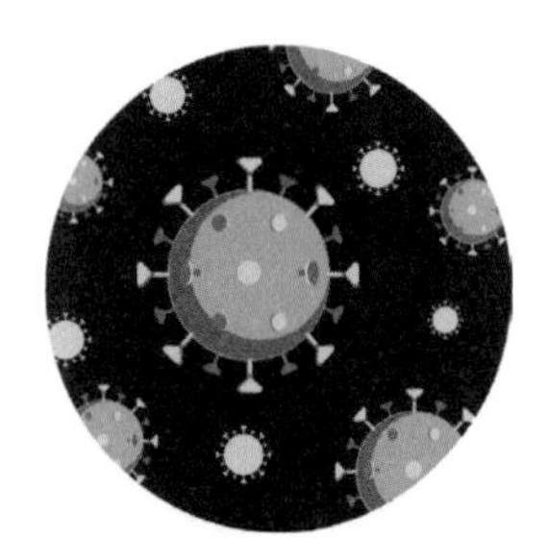

The Latin word "virus" means toxin or poison. This is appropriate considering how destructive viruses can be to the body. Viruses are extremely small, about one one-hundredth the size of the average bacterial cell, and can't be seen with the average microscope. Viruses include the flu, influenza viruses like H1N1 or the swine flu, the common cold, or coronavirus, herpes viruses, various viruses that cause hepatitis, and HIV, or the virus that leads to AIDS. Viruses invade cells, where they induce the cellular machinery to make more viruses, destroying the cells in the process. Viruses are prone to mutate over time, so the medicines and vaccines created to cure them are often ineffective by the time they become available. Many people feel that the new emerging viruses are actually being created in laboratories, either accidentally or on purpose.

Even though a physical organism may not be present, this energy could still be very imbalancing and could potentially create the same symptoms as the pathogen in its physical form.

This was revealed to me one day when an old patient of mine came to my office after I hadn't seen her for a number of years. She explained, "I haven't been feeling well. I had some tests run, and it's been confirmed that I have Epstein-Barr virus." I immediately started thinking about all of the possible natural remedies for her, including things like wild oregano, olive leaf extract, and so on. I thought, "I wish there was a better way to deal with this kind of issue."

I offered a silent prayer: "Father, if there is a better way to approach this problem, will you please help me to know what it is?"

Suddenly, understanding flooded into me.

While it's correct to think of a virus through the prism of traditional Western biology—as a minute mechanical organism—there is another, equally correct way to look at it.

What is a virus? A virus is made of molecules. Those molecules are made of atoms.

Those atoms are made of pure energy. Thus, a virus is made of energy. I was suddenly brought to understand that looking at a viral infection in this way is also valid and true. I realized that a viral infection, in a sense, is no different than the energy of a trapped emotion that can be released.

A viral infection—as well as any other infection—can be viewed as a cloud of energy. It was revealed to me that if I could wrap my mind around this idea and truly accept it, my mind would be free to be able to manipulate a viral infection as a cloud of pure energy.

I started by muscle-testing her and, after establishing a baseline, asking, "Do you have Epstein-Barr virus in your body?" The answer was yes. Holding an intention to release this viral energy from her body, and doing my best to forget everything I had learned in biology about viruses, I swiped a magnet a few times down her governing meridian. I then retested her to see if a change had been made, and it had. I could no longer get the virus to show up on muscle testing. I thought, "Could it possibly be this simple?"

This can be a challenging mental exercise. Most of us, especially those of us with traditional training in biology, are used to thinking of viruses as tiny organisms that cause illness by hijacking the reproductive processes of the cells to produce more viruses. This of course takes time. But one day I had an experience that taught me otherwise.

THE CHRONIC COUGH

One day a patient came in to see me complaining of a chronic cough. She said that this cough had been going on for weeks, and that whenever she took a deep breath she would inevitably start to cough uncontrollably.

Using the Body Code and muscle-testing her body for answers, I found that she had a viral infection. A few more questions determined that this was a common cold virus.

Doing my best to imagine this infection as a cloud of energy, I swiped a magnet down her spine a few times, while holding an intention to release the virus from her body. I said to her, "Okay, why don't you take a deep breath now, and let's see what happens."

She took several deep breaths and turned to me in amazement. "It's gone! How did you do that? What did you do? How is that possible?" I explained to her in simple terms what I had done, and since her treatment was over at that point, I walked with her to the front desk of my office, where my staff and I chatted with her for a few minutes. She left the office with a smile on her face.

I walked back down the hallway, and as I entered my treatment room where I had been working with her, I suddenly felt something enter my chest. I took a deep breath and started coughing uncontrollably! Somehow, I had picked up the energy I had just released from her.

I tested myself and, of course, I had the same virus, the common cold virus that I had released from my patient just a few minutes earlier. When I released it from her, the energy of the virus apparently just hung there in the air, and I walked right into it.

I passed a magnet over my governing meridian a few times, going from my forehead to the back of my neck, with an intention to release this cloud of viral energy from me. As soon as I had done this, I took a deep breath and . . . no more coughing!

This experience helped me to understand that pathogens are really just pure energy, something that regular Western medicine doesn't acknowledge or understand. For a viral infection to immediately start causing a problem like a severe cough just doesn't make any sense if you think about it in terms of traditional microbiology, which would dictate that viruses need time to physically incubate and multiply. Yet it is just as valid to view viruses, and indeed any infection or infestation, as pure energy as well.

Of course, this doesn't just apply to viruses. It applies to pathogens of all types, as a Body Code Certification student found in the following story.

Exhaustion Disappears

While I was taking the Body Code Certification course, I had a volunteer who was exhausted, as if the body's resources were being drained. In the person's first session, I identified and resolved viral, bacterial, and parasitic pathogen energies. Later, the client shared this with me: "I have definitely felt a difference in my energy since my first session! I don't feel exhausted! Before my session, I literally felt like I was dragging my body around. Thank you so much!"

—Jocelyn P., Alberta, Canada

I found that sometimes working with an infection in this way is all that is needed. In other cases, treating a pathogen in this way seems to weaken the organism enough that the immune system can overcome it naturally, and sometimes other physical support, such as herbs or nutritional supplements, may be needed.

It's important to point out that working with pathogens in this way is very belief-dependent. In other words, we know that we affect our reality, depending on what we believe. If you can wrap your mind around this idea, and if whomever you are working with can do the same, with prayer and belief, I think there is no limit to what is possible, no matter what the pathogen might be. This may not make sense in terms of traditional biology, but it makes perfect sense in terms of quantum physics. We are only limited by our own beliefs in this regard, and those beliefs can be powerfully limiting.

Interestingly, it is my observation that having only the spiritual presence of the pathogen may cause symptoms analogous to having an infection with the organism in its physical form.

Knowing that pathogens are energy will help you release them using the exercises in the next chapter.

A quick note before you begin the exercise. To eliminate a pathogen, there are two things that you can do:

- Release the energy of the pathogen.
- Identify and find a remedy to eliminate the pathogen.

To release the energy of a pathogen or parasite infestation, simply focus on the pathogen as being a cloud of energy in the body. You can identify the location of this pathogen cloud if you want to, but it may not be necessary. Then simply swipe a magnet or your hand over the governing meridian three times to release it.

HELPFUL TIPS FOR DEALING WITH PATHOGENS

It's important to point out the necessity of clearing any associated imbalances when you're working with any type of infection. I've personally seen many situations in which low-grade infections would not go away until the trapped emotions or other energies that were blocking them from being released were taken care of.

Physical support may be necessary to complete the process of eliminating pathogens. It is recommended that the subject see a health-care provider, nutritionist, or herbalist. Please understand that any infection is potentially dangerous, so if there is any doubt in your mind at all, seek medical care.

WILD OREGANO

The best natural treatment that I have found for viruses is wild oregano. Wild oregano is a little different from the kind of oregano that you buy in the spice aisle at your grocer. There are a number of different wild oregano products you can find commercially—just muscle test to see which one your body wants. If you have an herb garden, you might want to think about adding wild oregano, but it should be easy to find in most health food or supplement stores as well as online. Note that wild oregano also has antifungal (hence, antimold) properties as well as antiparasitic use.

OLIVE LEAF EXTRACT

Olive leaf extract, which is just made from crushed olive leaves, is another powerful antiviral and antibacterial remedy. This should also be easy to find in stores or online, but if you have an olive tree in your yard you could certainly make your own as well.

COLLOIDAL SILVER

Colloidal silver is another very powerful antiviral, antibacterial, antifungal compound. Colloidal silver is simply silver ions that are in solution, so it doesn't look much different than water to the naked eye. When babies are born, silver nitrate solution is dripped into their eyes to prevent blindness and other complications in case the mother has some kind of infection or sexually transmitted disease. If you get an eye infection, you can put a drop or two of colloidal silver in the affected eye, every few hours for a day or so, and it will usually take care of the problem very rapidly. Colloidal silver is a remedy I've used for many years, and it has always been reliable, whether used orally or topically. It's a good thing to have in your medicine chest as it's multi-purpose and lasts a very long time on the shelf. There are ways to make colloidal silver at home, however it is also very easy to find in stores. I would caution you to be careful with colloidal silver because it is possible to take too much of it, which may turn your skin blue. Make sure to muscle test the body for the correct dosage, not going too far beyond the recommended intake listed on the label. Any natural remedy or herb can be muscle tested for the body, as well as the dosages the body needs. The subconscious will know exactly how many capsules of wild oregano, or olive leaf, or how many drops of colloidal silver it needs.

DETERMINING DOSAGE

Here is how to determine the dosage of any remedy for any kind of infection or infestation.

Ask "Would ______ help the body to eliminate this infection?" When you find a remedy that tests positive, you'll want to find out what dosage the body needs. So you might ask, "Do I [or you] need two capsules per day?" or "Do I [or you] need two drops per day?" If the answer is yes, or strong, this indicates the body needs at least this amount, so you'll want to go higher to test for the maximum dosage, like this: "Do I need three capsules a day?" and so on. If the answer is still strong, test again, "Do I need four capsules? Five capsules? Six capsules?" etc. Eventually, you'll get to the dosage that you need and if you go on beyond that, suddenly you'll get a weak muscle test. For example, if you need five capsules a day and you ask, "Do I need five capsules a day?" you should get a strong muscle test. If you ask, "Do I need six capsules a day?" you will get a weak muscle test. After you determine the daily dosage, you can determine how many days or weeks you need to take the remedy or herb, remembering to retest periodically in case a dosage may have changed. It's always a good idea to see a health-care provider, nutritionist, or herbalist for more information. And once again, keep in mind that any infection is potentially dangerous, so getting professional advice is advisable!

PARASITE

EXPLANATION

It is estimated that 80 percent of the population in the United States has some kind of parasite. Parasites are difficult to identify through traditional methods. In fact, most of the parasites that infest the body don't show up at all on commonly performed tests. The body can become infested with parasites from water, food, insect bites, contact with animals, and even stepping outside on the grass with bare feet.

Parasites can be difficult to find and get rid of. One reason that parasites can be so elusive is that, as they go through their life cycles, they often change their appearance and modes of operation. In addition, parasites have an innate ability to fool or evade the body's natural defenses.

I found for example that even when I suspected a patient of having a parasite, sometimes the answer on muscle testing would be no, that no parasite was present. In those cases, I often found that if I asked that same patient if they needed a particular antiparasitic supplement or herb, I would get a yes answer. At first this seemed illogical to me. But as I thought about it, I realized that part of how parasites survive is by blending in with the scenery.

In other words, I found it wasn't unusual for parasites to be so much a part of a person's body that I could only determine that they actually needed an antiparasitic supplement, which they would test strong for, as odd as that may sound. After a patient like this started taking an antiparasitic supplement, within a few days I would get an affirmative answer from the person's subconscious mind about actually having a parasite.

It's important to realize that parasites are organisms that have a metabolism. They metabolize their food, which they are getting by either feeding on the food that you are consuming, or by actually feeding on your body itself, and their metabolism produces waste matter. Many parasites therefore end up essentially urinating and defecating in your tissues, as awful as that sounds.

I noticed particular patterns as I worked with people who were dealing with parasites. People who complained of pain that was transitory in nature or that seemed to move from one area of the body to another would often have parasites. It was as if the parasites would move into an area of the body, exhaust their food supply, and move on, like a bunch of locusts moving from one ravaged crop to another.

Many parasites produce uric acid, a by-product of protein metabolism. This can elevate the uric acid levels in the body, leading to a condition known as gout. Gout used to be known as the "disease of kings" in medieval times, because only those who were very wealthy could afford to drink wine and eat red meat, which are sources of uric acid. I found that sometimes by putting a patient on antiparasitic herbal supplements, his or her gout would disappear. I believe this was simply because the uric acid production lowered significantly with the death of their unwelcome lodgers. Finding parasites by using the Body Code can be quite accurate, as Angela found in this next story.

Parasites Confirmed

One of my clients in France ran to the hospital to be with her three-year-old granddaughter. For a week now the toddler was experiencing a fever of 40 degrees Celsius (roughly 104 degrees Fahrenheit), and nobody could figure out what was wrong. I asked if she could get permission for me to have a peek. A couple of hours later I got the okay.

Using the Body Code app, I found an imbalance in the hypothalamus (which controls temperature regulation) followed by metabolic waste both in the spleen and the liver caused by parasitic energy. The liver also had inflammation energy. I was curious to see what kind of parasite could cause such a high fever, so I found a list of parasites. I asked if it was in that list and got a yes. It was called the "*Toxoplasma gondii* parasite." One week after I told my client my finding, she received the doctor's diagnosis. It was toxoplasmosis!

—Angela H., Quebec, Canada

There are many different strains of parasites, ranging from microscopic to large organisms. There are three main classes of parasites that could cause problems for humans:

- **PROTOZOA:** Single-celled, microscopic organisms that live inside the host's body
- **HELMINTHS:** Parasitic worms that live inside the host's body, e.g. roundworm, hookworm, pinworm, tapeworm, fluke, etc.
- **ECTOPARASITES:** Those that live *on* rather than inside the host's body, e.g., lice, fleas, bedbugs, etc.

Parasites may create no symptoms at all or they may cause a wide variety of symptoms. Some common problems caused by parasites include intestinal issues, such as constipation, bloating, and diarrhea, as well as muscle pain and weakness, fatigue, anxiety, and frequent skin rashes. Chronic and prolonged parasitic infestation can lead to severe and dangerous diseases, such as ulcerative colitis and Crohn's disease.

The worst case of parasitic infestation I ever saw was also a mystery case that the Body Code helped to solve.

JULIE'S STORY

Julie's parents brought her in to see me when she was twenty-two years old. She was suffering from daily seizures and extreme fatigue and was enduring life in a body racked with constant chronic pain. As if that were not enough, Julie also had memory problems. She had lost most of her long-term memory, making it difficult for her to recall events and friends from the past, and her short-term memory suffered dramatically, essentially making her an invalid in her parents' home.

Four years before, Julie was eighteen years old, fresh out of high school and the picture of health. She wanted to do something to make the world a better place, and when the offer came to serve as a missionary in the Philippines, she jumped at the chance. Conditions in the Philippines were much more primitive than she expected. She ended up working long hours in an orphanage under less-than-sanitary conditions. After a few months, she became very ill and had to return to the United States.

Her symptoms were baffling. Her parents took her from one specialist to another, but no one was able to give her a diagnosis. However, it was obvious to everyone concerned that she was dying. She was losing her life, losing the battle against some unknown assailant that could not be identified. The verdict? She was given four months to live. At the rate she was declining, her doctors could not imagine her living beyond that amount of time.

Somehow, Julie had survived for four years by the time her parents brought her in to see me. She'd managed to hang on, but her quality of life was nonexistent. Her parents explained to me that these are the symptoms she had been dealing with for the last four years, symptoms that had essentially made her a shut-in. They had given up taking her to see more medical specialists and had brought her into my office as a last resort, on the thinnest of hopes that perhaps something might be done to help her.

As I muscle-tested her, looking for imbalances that were causing her illness, I found that she had a parasite. Checking further, the answer that I got was that she didn't have just one parasite, she had a total of nine different varieties of parasites, more than I had ever seen in anyone else. From the various antiparasitic supplements that we used to use in my office, I tested to see which one she needed at that moment, and in what dosage. I told her that she needed to be very consistent about taking the supplements on a regular basis. Her mother spoke up, saying that she would make sure of it. Julie lifted her head and gave me a thin smile and said she would do her best.

The fascinating thing about Julie's case was not that it took an entire year for her to get well, but how that year played out. She suffered through the two-hour-long round trip to my office about eighteen times that year. Each time she would come in, I would test her to see how she was doing with the parasites. One by one, we were able to eliminate the parasites from her body, which often required switching from one antiparasitic supplement to a different one, as one population would die out and yet another population of parasites would hatch.

After about twelve months of care, relying solely on her subconscious mind's direction, Julie was finally well.

At the end of that year, I will always remember her as a young woman once again full of life and happiness, so full of gratitude to be healthy again. She told me that she was trying to get back into her old life again, going shopping, going out to restaurants, and going for walks. She told me that more than once she had run into old friends who'd stopped in astonishment when they saw her, exclaiming, "I thought you were dead!"

Julie went back to college and obtained a degree in advanced sign language.

I don't blame Julie's physicians for not being able to diagnose her problem correctly. I think that would have been more likely had she remained in the Philippines, but in the United States doctors are not used to working with patients whose primary problem is parasitic infestation.

In fact, my experience is that most tests for parasites that are given in the United States often give negative results in cases where people do have parasites. Indeed, in my practice I gave up sending patients out for medical testing of parasites, and came to rely 100 percent on muscle testing to get more accurate answers.

In the next story, Scott used the Body Code System to find and correct the imbalances that had contributed to a woman's blindness, with wonderful results.

Parasitic Energy Wreaks Havoc

A woman was referred to me who had gone blind in just a matter of weeks. Her doctors told her she had parasites that were damaging her eyes and they had no treatment that they thought would help her because this was such a rare condition. She was referred to me for help.

Using the Body Code System, we found numerous misalignments that were creating "fertile ground" for these parasites to flourish. The parasites were identified as amoebas, which were literally consuming the corneas and lenses of both her eyes. Most significantly, it was found that her overall body pH was 6.5, which is very acidic for a human.

We embarked on a three-pronged attack to restore her vision. We found a holistic supplement to clear the amoebas. We created a dietary and energy-balancing protocol to raise her pH to the normal range of 7.3–7.5. And we had eight Body Code sessions where we cleared misalignments, imbalances, and trapped emotions. After three months, the amoebas were gone. Without any further medications, her doctors were then able to give her new corneas and lenses and a year after originally losing all her sight, she now is living a normal, productive life with full vision.

—Scott S., New Hampshire, United States

HELPFUL TIPS FOR DEALING WITH PARASITES

Please understand that parasites can be dangerous, so if there is any doubt in your mind at all, seek medical care.

In my experience, parasites are best killed with herbal remedies that are typically available at health food stores. Remember that you can simply hold or think about a specific herbal preparation, and the subconscious mind will give a strong muscle test, or will sway forward to indicate that this will help.

If there is a possibility that a woman is pregnant or may become pregnant, she should not take any herbal supplement. If there is any doubt, please consult an herbalist or a physician.

Another thing to keep in mind is that parasites can develop a tolerance to the herbs in any formula, so it is important to periodically recheck what is being taken.

Ensuring that food is fully cooked, using insect repellent, and following good hygiene rules can reduce the risk of getting parasites.

EXERCISE: FIND AND ADDRESS A PATHOGEN ENERGETICALLY

STEP 1.

Ask: "Do I [or you] have a pathogen that we can address now?"

- **If yes, continue to step 2.**
- **If no, a physical pathogen may not be present, or it may not be possible to address it now, so you may want to try again later.**
- **Step 2 (Decoding). Ask: "Do we need to know more about this pathogen?"**
- **If no, move to Step 3 (Association).**
- **If yes, ask one or more of the following questions. Return to Step 2 (Decoding) once the answer to any of these questions is determined.**
  - **Sometimes, all that is needed is to identify the pathogen type. Some common pathogens you can test for are in the table at the beginning of this section.**

- Once you have identified a specific pathogen, return to Step 2 (Decoding) and ask if there is more you need to know. If you do not need to know more about the pathogen, go to Step 3 (Association), otherwise, you might ask the following question:
- Ask: "Do we need to know the location of this energy in the body?"

If yes, using a process of elimination to locate this may be helpful. For example, divide the body in half, and ask if the energy is lodged in the lower half of the body or upper half. Divide the body from left to right and ask if the energy is lodged in the left half of the body or the right half. Continue dividing in this fashion and asking until you've determined the location in the body where the pathogen is lodged, then return to Step 2 (Decoding).

STEP 3.

(Association) Ask: "Is there an associated imbalance that needs to be decoded?"

- If no, move to Step 4 (Intention).
- If yes, return to the Body Code Map and decode and address any associated imbalances, then return here and repeat the Step 3 (Association) question.

STEP 4.

(Intention) Swipe three times with a magnet or your hand on any length of the governing meridian, while holding the intention to both release the energy (life force) of the pathogen and to instruct the immune system to seek and eliminate the physical organisms.

- Step 5. Ask: "Did we release the energy of the pathogen?" If yes, you can start at the beginning on Step 1 and repeat the process to find another pathogen.
- If no, refocus, say a prayer for help, allow your heart to feel love and gratitude that this is going to help, and swipe three times once again with intention.
- Note that physical support may be necessary to complete the process of eliminating this pathogen. It is recommended to see a health-care provider, nutritionist, or herbalist for more information.
- Keep in mind that any infection is potentially dangerous. Seek medical advice, especially before taking any remedy.

SECTION 3

CIRCUITS AND SYSTEMS

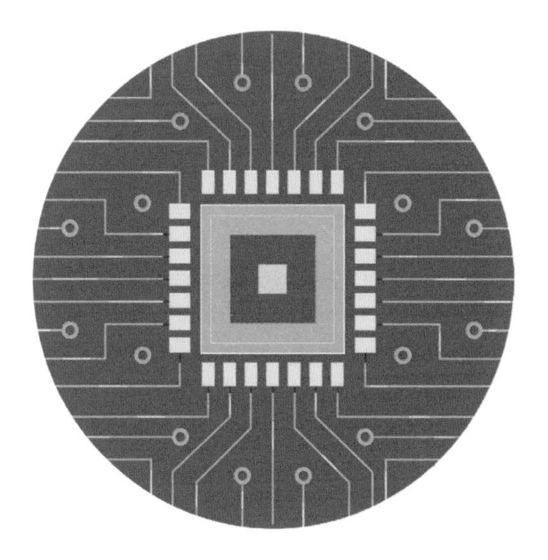

We are slowed-down sound and light waves, a walking bundle of frequencies tuned in to the cosmos. We are souls dressed up in sacred biochemical garments and our bodies are the instruments through which our souls play their music.

—ATTRIBUTED TO ALBERT EINSTEIN

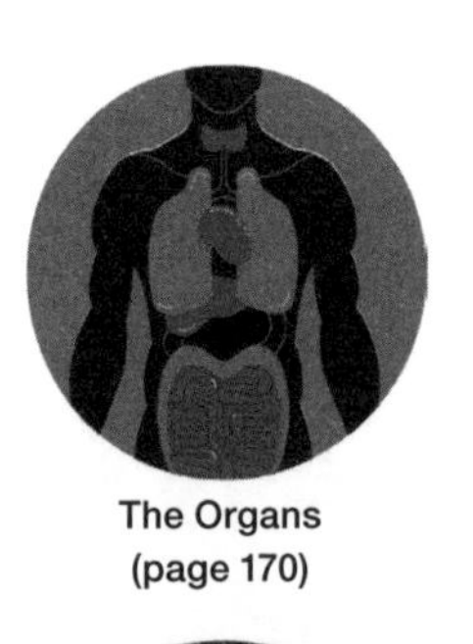

The Organs
(page 170)

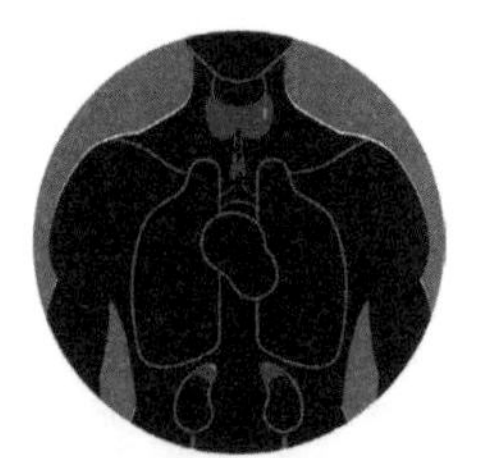

The Glands
(page 189)

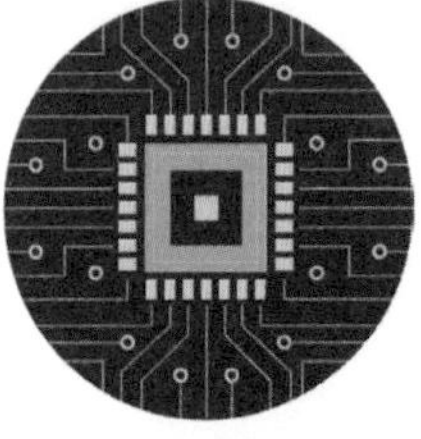

Systems
(page 205)

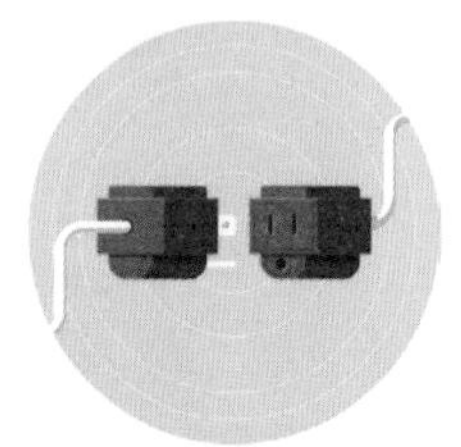

Disconnections
(page 223)

This category of imbalances pertains to the organs and glands as well as to their related systems. In addition, this category includes the various energetic connections between the organs, glands, and muscles.

11

CIRCUITS

We store our issues in our tissues.

—ANONYMOUS

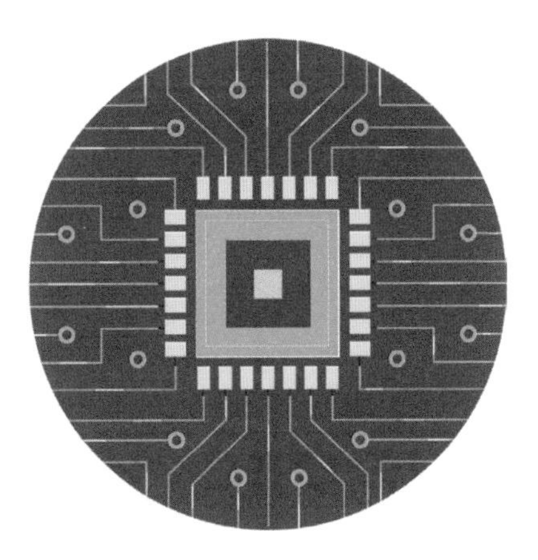

ORGANS, GLANDS, AND MUSCLE CONNECTIONS

There is a unique and largely unknown energetic connection between various organs and glands and specific muscles. Put simply, if an organ is imbalanced, a certain muscle or muscles will also be imbalanced.

For example, when I was in the student clinic, I had a particular patient who came to see me every week. He was a middle-aged man who suffered from chronic pain between his shoulder blades, which was being caused by misaligned vertebrae in his spine. I would realign this area of his spine once a week, to his great relief. However, after a few days the pain would reappear, and the next week I would realign his spine again, and this cycle repeated for months.

I was left to wonder, "What is going on here? Is there something wrong with me, as his doctor? Is there something wrong with him? Why won't these bones stay aligned?"

Many years passed before I realized that this man probably had an imbalance in his liver, since the liver is energetically connected to the rhomboid muscle, which connects the inside of the right shoulder blade to the spine.

Every organ and many glands have connections to muscles like this. I'd like to share a couple of other stories with you to help you understand how important these connections are.

JAZZERCISE

One day, a new patient named Joan came to me complaining, "My knees are killing me. I've been to the doctor; he tells me I have an overuse injury. As you can see, I'm overweight. I've been going to Jazzercise classes to lose weight. The doctor told me that I have to stop Jazzercising because of my knees, but I'm afraid that if I don't keep at it, I'm not going to be able to lose the weight, and if I can't lose the weight, I'm afraid my husband is going to leave me."

I knew that left knee pain is very often associated with an imbalance of the left adrenal gland, because it has energetic connections to muscles that cross the left knee joint. And I knew that right knee pain is often associated with an imbalance of the gallbladder, because of its muscle connections that cross the right knee joint. So I had somewhere to begin.

I had her hold out one arm parallel to the floor and I began testing the organs and glands in her body to see how balanced they were. When I said, "gallbladder," her arm suddenly went weak. Something was not right with her gallbladder. When I asked her if she had any trouble with her gallbladder, she replied, "No, not that I'm aware of."

I asked, "Do you have a trapped emotion imbalancing your gallbladder? When I pressed down on her arm now, her arm was strong, indicating a yes answer. I was able to find a couple of trapped emotions that were affecting her gallbladder and released them. When I was done, her gallbladder was strong on muscle testing, indicating that it was balanced again.

I said, "Why don't you walk around for a moment, and let's see how your right knee is doing now."

She took a few steps, looked at me, and said, "I don't feel any pain in my right knee at all. Wow!"

So far so good. I continued checking her organs and glands and testing her muscle strength for each one. When I got to her left adrenal gland, her arm went weak again. Having learned in my work with patients that most imbalances of organs and glands are caused by trapped emotions, I asked, "Is there a trapped emotion that we can release that is imbalancing this gland?" Her arm tested strong, and again I found a few trapped emotions at the root of this imbalance and released them. Again, I asked her to walk around my office a bit and test out her left knee.

After a few steps she turned to me and exclaimed, "How is this possible? I don't feel any pain in either knee now!"

CIRCUITS

To understand the phenomenon of how circuits work, let's compare your body to your home. Have you ever blown a fuse in your home? If you plug too many appliances into a single electrical outlet, you will draw too much power, which will blow a circuit. Suddenly the lights and all the electrical appliances in that room will turn off, or the power may go out in that entire section of the house. If the lights go out in the room you are in at the time, is it possible that in the next room the television may suddenly shut off as well? How could that happen? It can only happen if the television is on the same circuit as the electrical outlet you just overloaded.

In the body, if you overload any organ or gland, you overload its circuit and blow a "fuse," in a sense. Here's how this can happen in our bodies. Let's use the liver for this example. The liver's job is to detoxify the body. One of the ways that you might overload the liver is by taking things into your body that are toxic. If you have trapped emotional energies that lodge in the liver, or if you are exposed to pesticides or herbicides, or if you drink too much alcohol or consume toxic food additives, you can overload the liver, which may blow its "fuse." The liver will no longer be able to function at its full capability until its imbalances are corrected.

Although our organs and glands don't have a literal "fuse," it's the easiest way to explain and understand how the organs and glands and muscles are connected energetically. Besides reducing an organ's function, overloading an organ will imbalance certain muscles that are connected, because they are on the same circuit. Every organ and most of the glands have this connection with a muscle or muscles in the body.

Imbalance in an organ or gland will usually cause pain in the joints or the areas served by its muscle connections. It can also cause muscle weakness, making that particular part of the body vulnerable and prone to injury. For example, right knee injuries are common in people who have imbalanced gallbladders, because the gallbladder is on the same circuit as a particular muscle in the back of the right knee, as Tracey found in the following story.

Ghost of Her Gallbladder

I've been watching every webinar I can about the Emotion Code and the Body Code. You were discussing how having a gallbladder imbalance can cause right knee pain. I don't have *The Body Code* yet, but I decided just to ask my body if I had an imbalance in my gallbladder. The answer was yes, and I released two emotions. My knee feels great now! (My doctor said it was arthritis.) Why this is so amazing is that my daughter was born in 1990 and I had my gallbladder removed two weeks later. The physical organ has been gone for twenty-two years, but the energy (spirit) organ is still there!

—Tracey B., Wisconsin, United States

If your left knee hurts, it's probably because you have an imbalance in your adrenal gland.

If your right knee hurts, it's probably because of an imbalance in your gallbladder.

If you have a nagging pain between your shoulder blades, it's probably because of an imbalance in your liver.

If your lower back hurts, it's probably because your kidneys are imbalanced, and so on.

When you understand that every organ and most of the glands are connected energetically to muscles that are connected to joints, you realize that the first place to look when there is joint pain is to the organs or glands that are associated.

Of course, the organs and glands are not physically touching the muscles they are energetically connected to. Instead, they are simply on the same "electrical circuit." Think of the analogy of the electrical wiring in your home and blowing a fuse.

THE "USUAL SUSPECTS"	
Low Back Pain	Kidney—Ileocecal Valve—Uterus—Adrenal Glands
Knee Pain	Adrenal Glands (Left Knee) Gallbladder (Right Knee)
Upper Back Pain	Liver—Spleen—Gallbladder
Mid-Back pain	Kidney—Gallbladder
Wrist/Elbow	Gallbladder—Stomach—Spleen—Pancreas
Shoulder	Thyroid—Gallbladder (right shoulder)—Heart (left shoulder)
Temporomandibular Joint (TMJ)	Kidney

Over the years I have learned that the most common organ and gland imbalances that create discomfort can be arranged into a table like that shown here. This can be useful in knowing which organs or glands to check if you are attempting to address a specific problem. For example, let's say your friend is suffering from low back pain. You might begin by checking the balance of the kidneys, both left and right. If they are testing okay, you might check the ileocecal valve, then the uterus and the adrenals. You can test these organs and glands in any order you want, but the organs and glands are arranged here by frequency or likelihood of your finding them to be part of the problem. In other words, kidney imbalance is the most common cause of low back trouble, followed by the ileocecal valve, followed by the uterus, followed by adrenals. Remember that this is not cast in stone, this order simply reflects my own experience, and I share it here to save you time. This list is not all-inclusive, but it gives you a great place to start.

TESTING FOR CONTENTEDNESS

A wonderful way to determine imbalance in organs and glands is what I like to call testing for contentedness. If you simply ask an organ or gland or any part of the body if it is "happy" or "balanced," the body will tell you through muscle testing. This can reveal imbalances that otherwise may not show up for a long time, because an organ may be imbalanced for years before it begins to manifest serious problems.

To understand how this works, you need to understand the nature of things, at least as I see it. I think this may make sense to you too. I believe that all things were created spiritually before they were created physically. I believe that all things are designed for joy, and I believe that joy is the ultimate purpose of our existence, to learn to live joyfully.

HAPPY ORGANS

The ancient physicians looked upon the organs and glands as separate "officials" in the "kingdom" of the body. Some organs and glands were subservient to others and some were dominant over others, and there were intricate relationships between them all, and each organ and gland was viewed as a separate *intelligence*. If you simply ask an organ or gland or any part of the body if it is "contented" or "happy," the body will tell you. This can reveal imbalances that otherwise may not show up for a long, long time, because an organ may be "unhappy" or "discontent" for years before it finally manifests disease.

If an organ or gland shows up as being "unhappy," you might turn to the Body Code Map in part III (page 101) and ask, "Is this because of an imbalance on the right side of the chart?" If it's not, then you know it's an imbalance on the left side of the chart. Asking questions in this way will lead you to the reason for the imbalance. Whenever you find an organ that's imbalanced, there is always a reason for it, and all of the categories of imbalances are listed on the chart.

It may be a pathogen. It could be some kind of a nutritional deficiency. It could be a structural imbalance. It could be a trapped emotion. It could be a trauma. It could be some kind of toxicity. If an organ is unhappy, I guarantee you that you will be able to find the reason why in short order if you use the Body Code Map. In this way, you may be able to find and correct imbalances that otherwise might not show up for many, many years.

PAIRED ORGANS AND GLANDS

The paired organs and glands are those that have the same organ on each side of the body, such as the kidneys, lungs, adrenals, ovaries, breasts, and testicles. The organ or gland on the left side is usually the main or primary organ of the two, with the right side as the backup or reserve organ or gland. As a result, the left-side organ or gland will usually become imbalanced first, because it is bearing a heavier load than its right-sided sibling. The left-side organ or gland is directly connected with the associated muscle or muscles on the left side of the body. Therefore, when the left organ or gland becomes overloaded and blows its "fuse," the related muscles on that same side of the body will immediately become imbalanced.

Accordingly, when the right organ or gland becomes overloaded, the related right muscle or muscles on that same side of the body will become imbalanced.

For example, let's take a look at the adrenal glands. When a person is under too much stress for too long, it will overload the adrenal glands, which are the "stress glands" of the body. The left adrenal gland will tend to become imbalanced first, since the left-sided organs and glands are primary.

As a result, the muscles that cross the left knee joint, which are energetically connected to the left adrenal gland, will become imbalanced the moment the left adrenal gland becomes imbalanced. The result will eventually be discomfort or pain in the left knee because of the muscular imbalance that now exists. This imbalance increases the probability of injury and may ultimately lead to osteoarthritis of the knee joint. If the stress continues, the right adrenal gland may also become imbalanced as well, resulting in right knee pain. In this case, we can see the inner workings of the body and now understand a little better why one of the very first signs of too much stress is left knee pain.

CARPAL TUNNEL SYNDROME

I remember seeing a particular patient who was referred to me by another doctor's office. She had been suffering from carpal tunnel syndrome for an entire year, with absolutely no relief for her painful condition, even though she was being regularly treated by the doctors in this chiropractic office, since she was their office manager.

The first thing that I found when I examined her was that her gallbladder was imbalanced. Not only does the gallbladder connect energetically to a muscle behind the right knee, it also connects with the deltoid muscle in the right shoulder. This muscle imbalance in her shoulder proved to be the whole cause of her persisting carpal tunnel syndrome. The muscle imbalance was secondary to her gallbladder having become imbalanced due to the emotional energies that were trapped there. After releasing these trapped emotions, her gallbladder returned to a state of energetic balance, the associated muscle became balanced as well, and the carpal tunnel syndrome disappeared in short order and never returned. One session at my office was all it took to resolve her chronic problem.

In the next two chapters I will explain how to find and correct imbalances in organs and glands that may need help.

12

THE ORGANS

The human heart was such a complex organ, fragile and sturdy all at once.

—SUSAN WIGGS

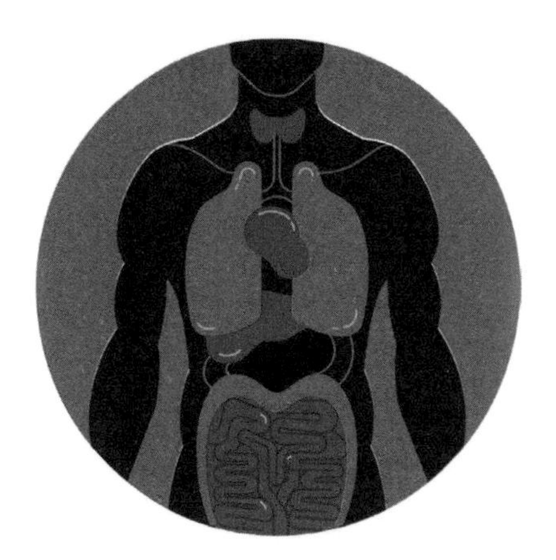

In this chapter I outline each organ, including its functions, its connection with various muscles, and the most common symptoms of imbalance. If you discover an imbalanced organ through testing, you can look up the organ in this chapter to read more about it and follow these instructions to correct the imbalance.

There are two ways to find an organ that is imbalanced or unhappy. If you suspect that an organ may need some help, you can simply ask, "Is the [organ name] balanced?" For example, "Is my heart happy?" or, "Is my liver balanced?"

When you ask, "Is my ____ happy (or balanced)?" and perform a muscle test, you'll get a yes or a no answer. If the muscle response is strong, this indicates a congruent or a yes answer, which means

ORGAN CHART

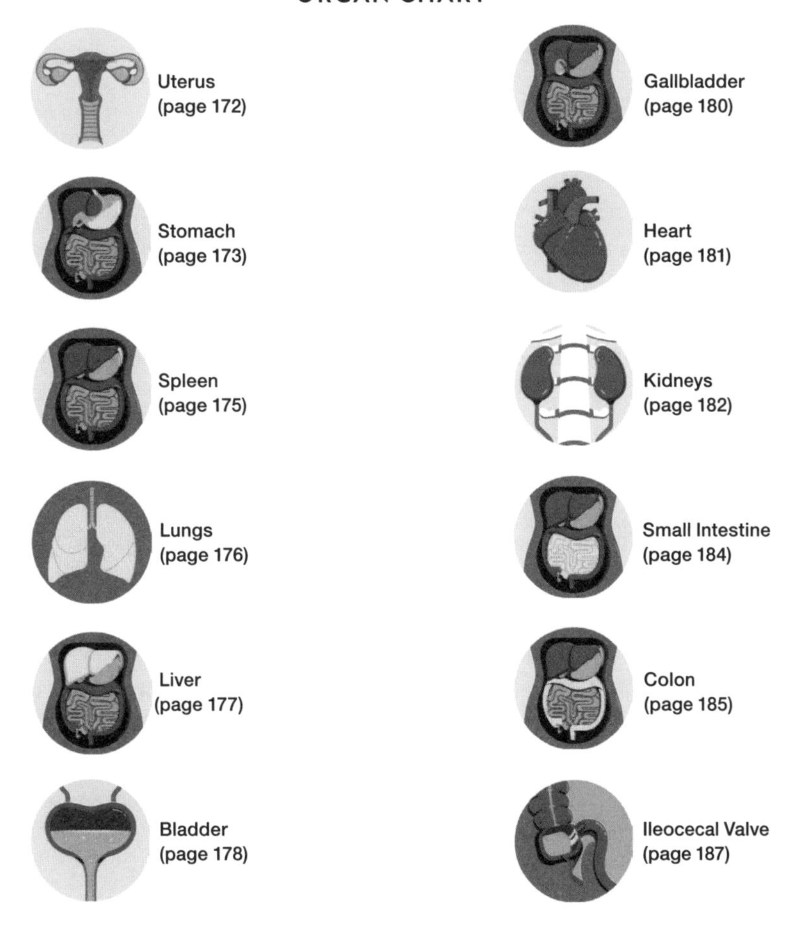

that the organ is likely doing fine. If the muscle response is weak, indicating no, this indicates that the organ is asking for help. If you have arrived at this point in your testing and have identified an organ that is imbalanced, proceed to Step 3 in the following process.

Another way to find an imbalanced organ is to use the organ chart by following these steps.*

*Note that this chart has been modified for this book, and does not include the brain or interstitium. These are found in detail in the app. In addition, the ileocecal valve is not typically classified as an organ, but its importance earns it a place in this list for our purposes.

STEP 1.

Ask: "Do I [or you] have an imbalanced [or unhappy] organ?"

- If yes, ask, "Is the organ on the right side of the organ chart?"
  - If yes, move to Step 2.
  - If no, it is on the left side. Move to Step 2.

STEP 2.

Start at the top of the side identified and ask, "Is the ____ imbalanced?" For example, let's say you received a yes answer in Step 1, so you know the organ is on the right side of the chart. Since the bladder is at the top of the chart on the right side, you would then ask, "Is the bladder imbalanced?" If you receive a no answer, you would continue down that column to the next organ and ask, "Is a gallbladder imbalanced?" and so on until you receive a yes answer.

STEP 3.

Once you've identified an imbalanced organ, follow these instructions to find and correct any imbalances affecting that organ.

STEP 4.

(Association) Ask: "Is there an associated imbalance that needs to be decoded?"

- If no, simply swipe three times with a magnet or your hand on any length of the governing meridian, while holding the intention to reset the organ.
- If yes, return to the Body Code Map, then decode and address any associated imbalances, then return here and repeat the above question. (Note that most of the time, organs are imbalanced by trapped emotions or other energies.)

STEP 5.

Ask: "Is the organ balanced [or happy] now?" When the answer to this question is yes, you have successfully rebalanced that organ.

UTERUS

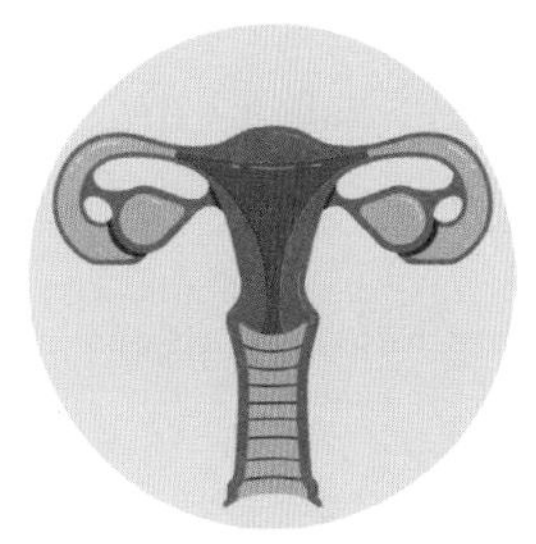

EXPLANATION

The uterus is a muscular organ located in the lower abdomen and the center of the pelvic cavity. The uterus is part of the female reproductive system.

PURPOSES OF THE UTERUS

- To provide a growth environment for the fetus
- To provide the muscular force needed for labor and delivery
- To produce sexual response by directing blood flow to the other parts of the female system

COMMON SYMPTOMS OF UTERUS IMBALANCE

- Discomfort in the lower back, lower abdomen, or left hip
- Discomfort during or after intercourse
- Infertility

UTERUS EMOTIONS

The uterus emotions are listed in row 6 on the Emotion Code Chart.

UTERUS-MUSCLE CONNECTIONS

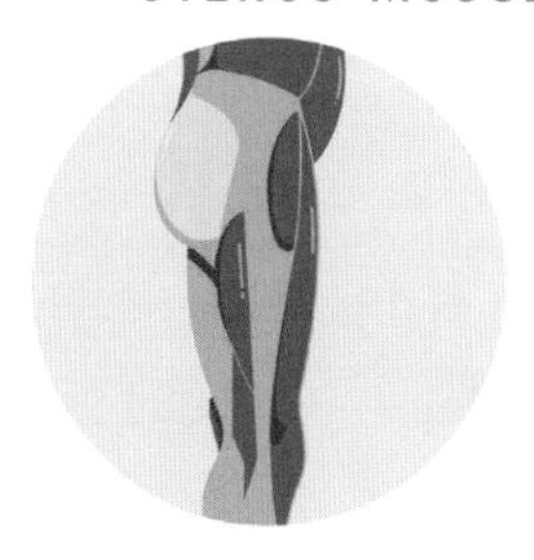

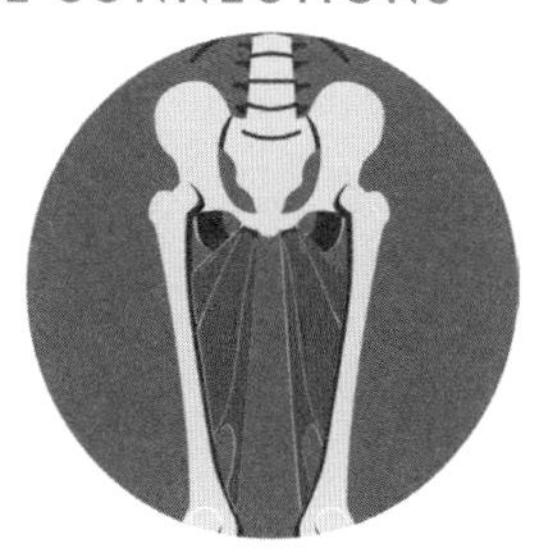

- Gluteal or buttock muscles
- Adductor muscles of the inner thighs

STOMACH

EXPLANATION

The stomach is a hollow muscular organ located in the abdominal cavity. It is part of the digestive system.

PURPOSE OF THE STOMACH

- To secrete protein-digesting enzymes, hydrochloric acid, and mucus
- To churn up swallowed food and begin the digestive process

COMMON SYMPTOMS OF STOMACH IMBALANCE

- Discomfort in the neck, shoulders, elbows, and wrists
- Hiatal hernia

- Acid reflux
- Stomach pain
- Ulcers
- Gas
- Bloating
- Diarrhea
- Constipation

Hiatal hernia is a condition in which part of the stomach protrudes upward through an opening in the diaphragm. This can cause stomach pain, acid reflux, belching, and other unpleasant symptoms. Contrary to popular belief, surgery is rarely needed to correct a hiatal hernia. It is very common for stomach imbalance to create a hiatal hernia, so often, correcting the stomach imbalance will also correct a hiatal hernia.

To find a hiatal hernia, simply ask, "Do I [or you] have a hiatal hernia?" If the answer is yes, find and correct any associated imbalances, then correct the hiatal hernia energetically by swiping a few times on the governing meridian with intention.

STOMACH EMOTIONS

The stomach emotions are listed in row 2 on the Emotion Code Chart.

STOMACH-MUSCLE CONNECTIONS

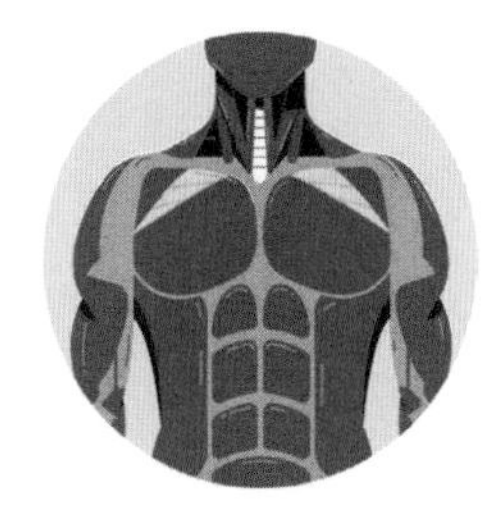
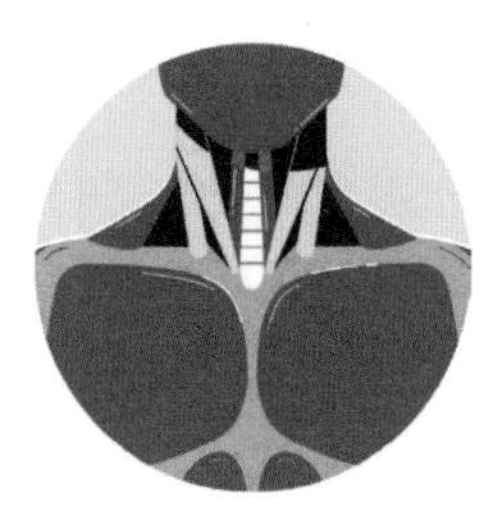
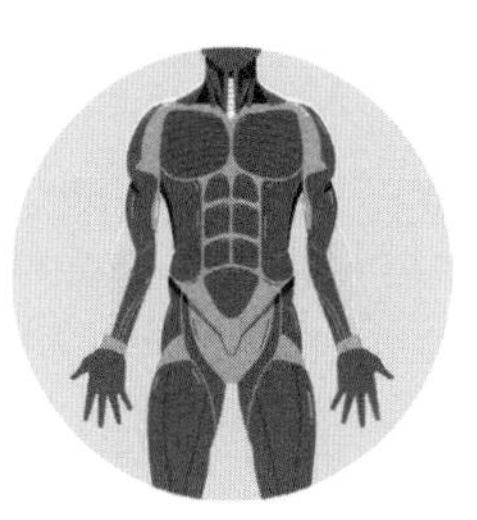
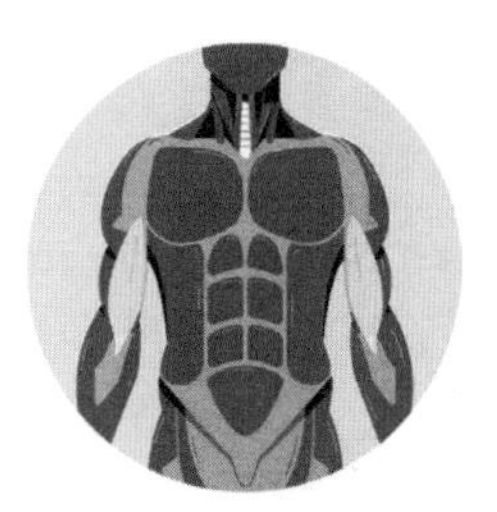

- Pectoralis major clavicular muscles are the uppermost section of the pectoralis muscles that attach to the clavicle, or the collarbone.
- Neck flexor muscles are located deep within the neck. Collectively they are made of two groups of several little muscles called the longus capitis muscles and the longus colli muscles.

- Brachioradialis muscles are located in the forearms and elbows. Imbalance in these muscles will tend to affect the elbow and/or the wrist on either or both sides. The brachioradialis muscles, when imbalanced, will tend to cause painful and persistent problems such as carpal tunnel syndrome.
- The biceps muscles are located at the front of the upper arms.

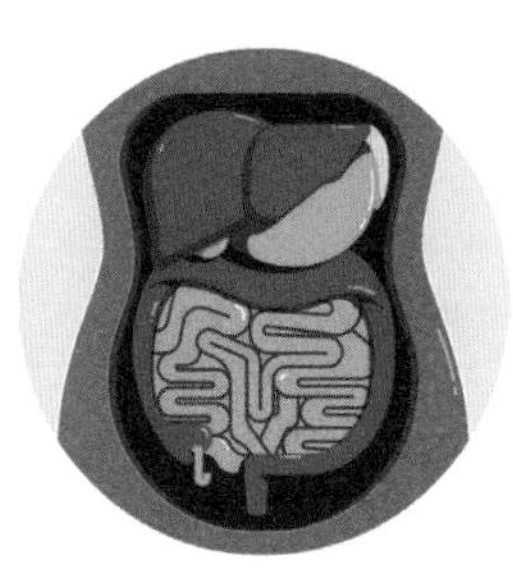

SPLEEN

EXPLANATION

The spleen is located in the upper abdominal cavity, at the left side of the stomach. It is part of the immune system as well as the lymphatic system. When the spleen is imbalanced or has been removed, it tends to create increased susceptibility to infection and anemia.

PURPOSE OF THE SPLEEN

- To dispose of old red blood cells
- To perform important immune functions such as removing pathogens from the blood
- To hold a reserve of blood
- To recycle iron

COMMON SYMPTOMS OF SPLEEN IMBALANCE

- Discomfort in the mid back or left shoulder
- Lowered immunity
- Pain in the upper left abdomen
- Repeated bouts of infection
- Excessive bleeding
- Anemia
- Dizziness
- Fatigue
- Headaches

SPLEEN EMOTIONS

Emotions produced by the spleen are in row 2 on the Emotion Code Chart.

SPLEEN-MUSCLE CONNECTIONS

- Trapezius muscle, specifically the mid and the lower parts of the trapezius

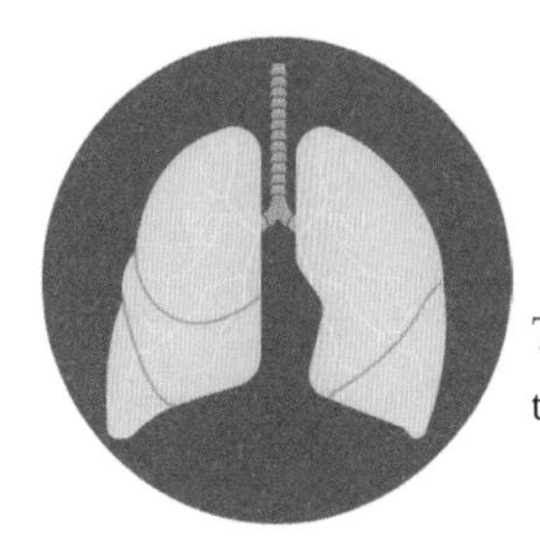

LUNGS

EXPLANATION

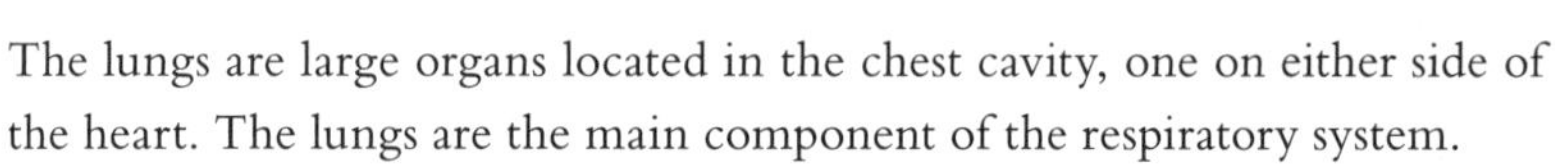

The lungs are large organs located in the chest cavity, one on either side of the heart. The lungs are the main component of the respiratory system.

PURPOSE OF THE LUNGS

- To bring oxygen into the body to oxygenate the blood
- To eliminate carbon dioxide

SYMPTOMS OF LUNG IMBALANCE

- Discomfort between the shoulders, in the ribs, or upper back
- Asthma
- Shortness of breath
- Decreased ability to exercise
- A persistent cough
- Pain or discomfort when breathing

LUNG EMOTIONS

The lung emotions are listed in row 3 on the Emotion Code Chart.

LUNG-MUSCLE CONNECTIONS

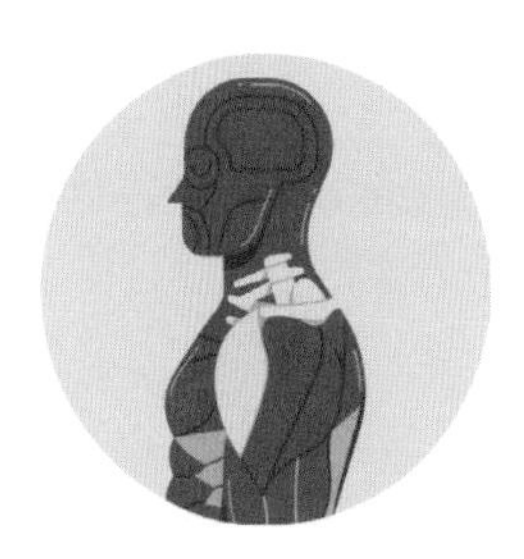
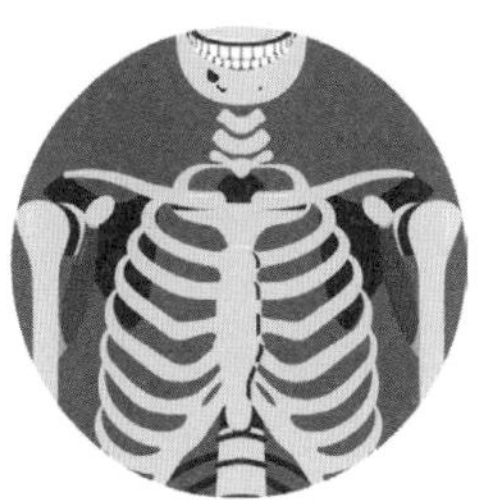
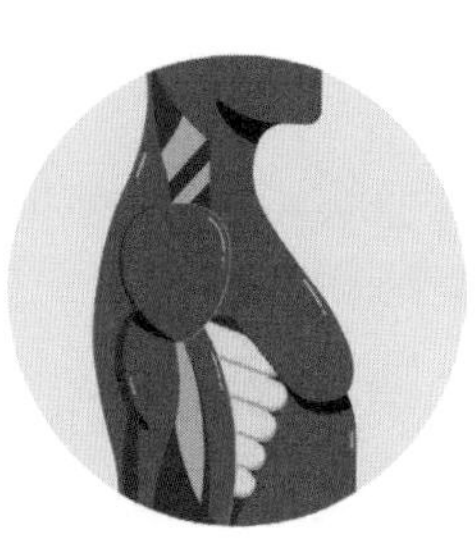
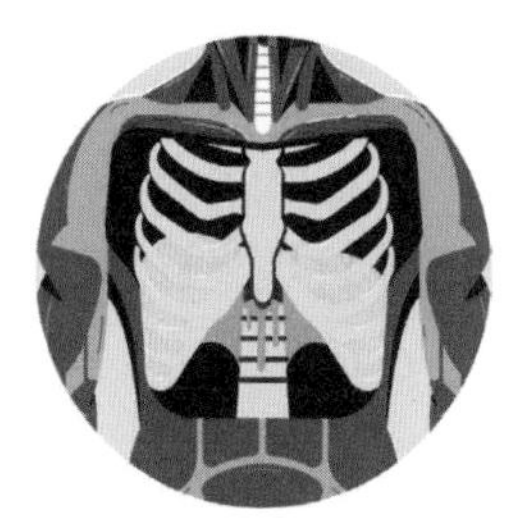

- Deltoid muscles of the outer shoulders
- Coracobrachialis muscles under the arms, which draw the humerus forward toward the torso
- Serratus anterior muscles, which are in the sides of the chest and ribs
- The diaphragm, a dome-shaped muscle that is located below the lungs and is the major muscle of respiration

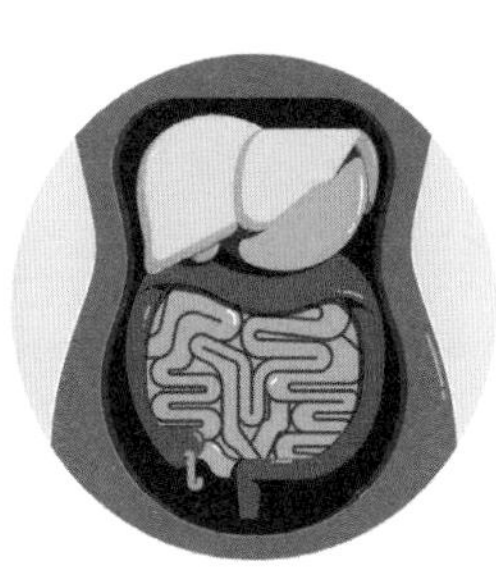

LIVER

EXPLANATION

The liver is a very large organ located under the rib cage on the right side, just above the gallbladder. It is part of both the digestive and immune systems.

PURPOSE OF THE LIVER

- To support the immune system
- To cleanse and detoxify the blood from foreign substances
- To break down chemicals and toxins

COMMON SYMPTOMS OF LIVER IMBALANCE

- Discomfort between the shoulder blades or in the right shoulder
- Headaches

In severe cases, you may also see:

- Jaundice (a yellowish tint to the skin and eyes)
- Loss of appetite leading to weight loss
- Swelling under the right lower ribs

The last three items are a sign of serious liver malfunction. If you notice any of these symptoms, it's time to see a medical doctor.

LIVER EMOTIONS

The liver produces the emotions listed in row 4 on the Emotion Code Chart.

LIVER–MUSCLE CONNECTIONS

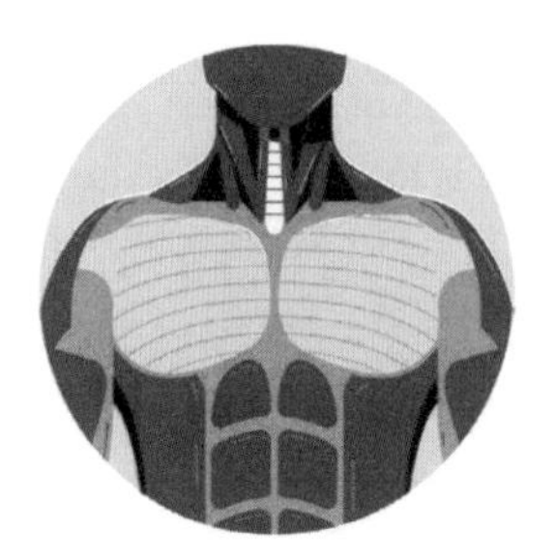

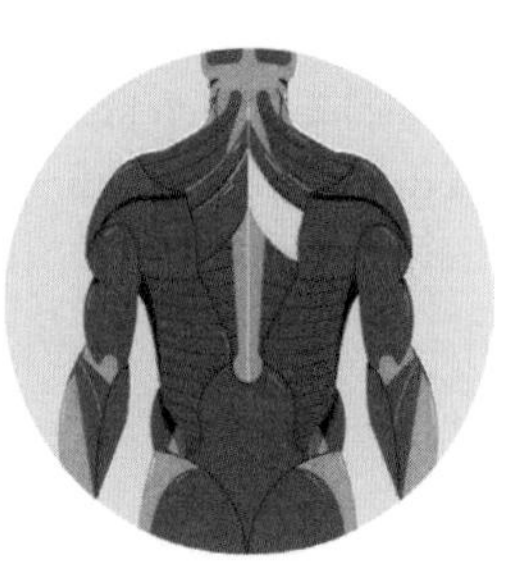

- Pectoralis major muscles in the middle of the chest
- Rhomboideus major or the rhomboid muscle on the right side. The rhomboid muscle goes from the thoracic vertebrae in the center of the spine (the second, third, and fourth thoracic vertebrae) and travels right at an oblique angle and connects to the inside edge of the shoulder blade.

BLADDER

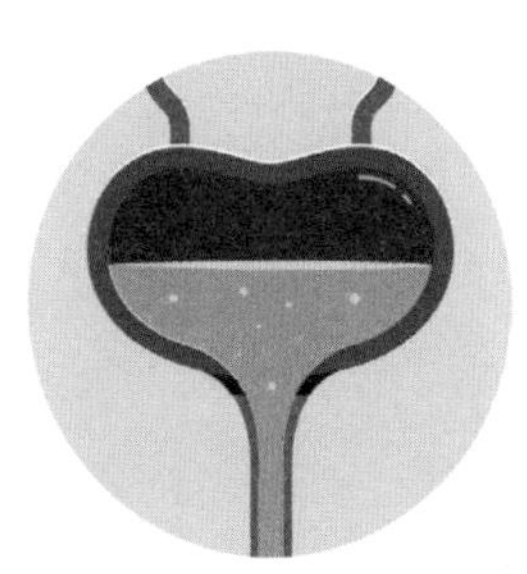

EXPLANATION

The bladder is a very muscular and elastic hollow organ, located in the lower abdomen. It is part of the urinary system.

PURPOSE OF THE BLADDER

- To store urine that is produced by the kidneys
- To eliminate urine through urination

COMMON SYMPTOMS OF BLADDER IMBALANCE

- Discomfort in the low back, knee, ankle, or foot
- Nocturia, or interrupted sleep, due to frequent urination
- Urgency, frequent urination
- Bed-wetting
- Incontinence
- Urinary tract infection
- Bleeding with urination (blood in urine is the number-one sign of bladder cancer)

BLADDER EMOTIONS

Emotions produced by the bladder are in row 5 on the Emotion Code Chart.

BLADDER-MUSCLE CONNECTIONS

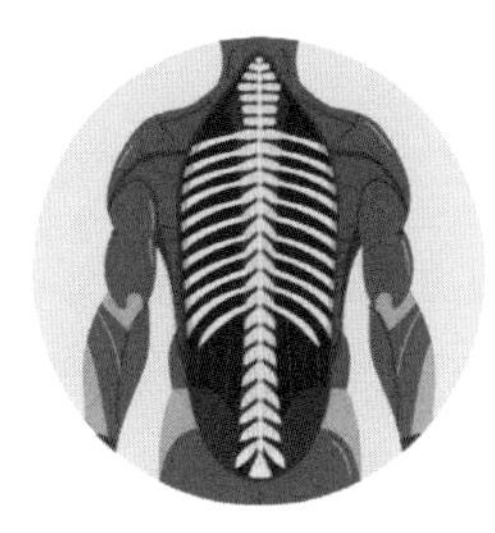
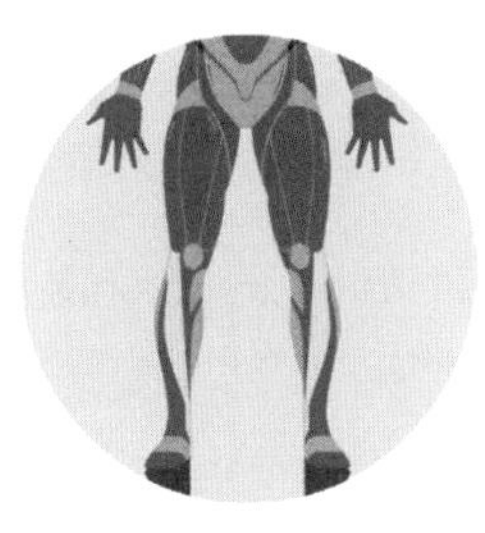
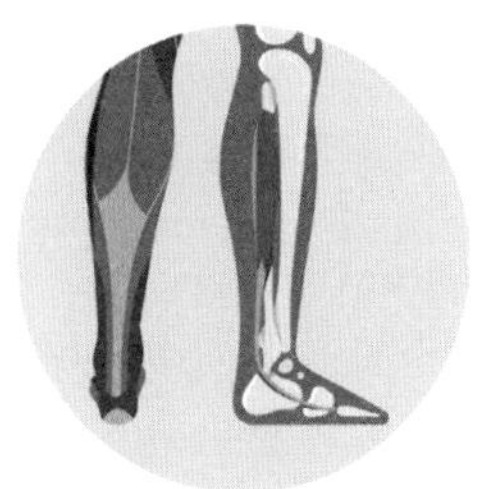
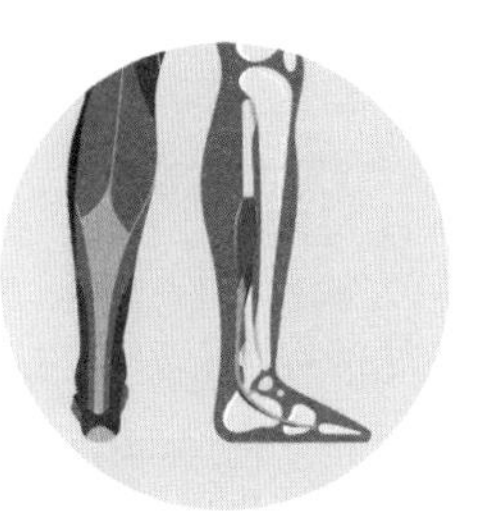

- Paraspinal muscles are several muscles that lie along the entire length of the spine on both sides, from the base of the skull all the way down to the very bottom of the lumbar spine.
- Tibialis anterior muscles are the muscles that become painful with shin splints.
- Peroneus longus and peroneus brevis muscles are also in this same area in the lower legs, controlling balance in the ankles.

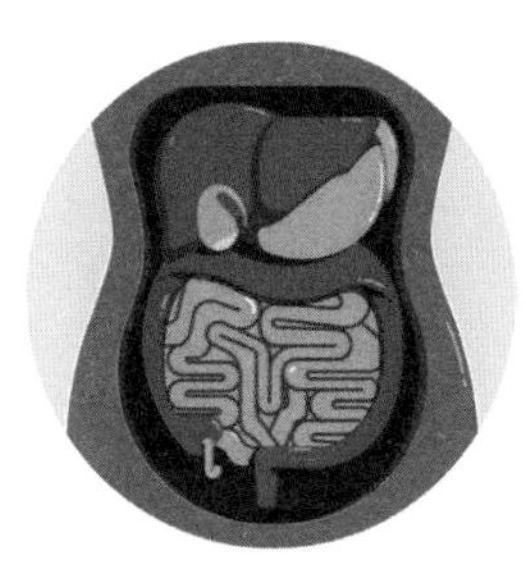

GALLBLADDER

EXPLANATION

The gallbladder is located in the right side of the abdomen under the rib cage, nestled into the underside of the liver. It is part of the digestive system.

PURPOSE OF THE GALLBLADDER

- To secrete bile, which helps to absorb and digest fat

Bile could be considered the body's detergent. If you've ever put a drop of detergent into a sink full of greasy or oily water and noticed how it breaks up the grease or oil immediately, you will understand this. When we take fat into our body, the gallbladder injects bile into the intestine. There the bile breaks down the fat so it can be absorbed into the bloodstream.

COMMON SYMPTOMS OF GALLBLADDER IMBALANCE

- Discomfort in the right knee, right shoulder, or under the right rib cage
- Pain in the right side of the chest
- Nausea
- Vomiting
- Gas
- Bloating

Typically, these symptoms will become worse after eating foods that are high in fat. Discomfort under the right rib cage, nausea, and vomiting are more rare than the other symptoms and usually result from stones, inflammation, or congestion in the gallbladder, indicating a more severe or long-term imbalance.

GALLBLADDER EMOTIONS

The gallbladder produces the emotions listed in row 4 on the Emotion Code Chart.

GALLBLADDER-MUSCLE CONNECTIONS

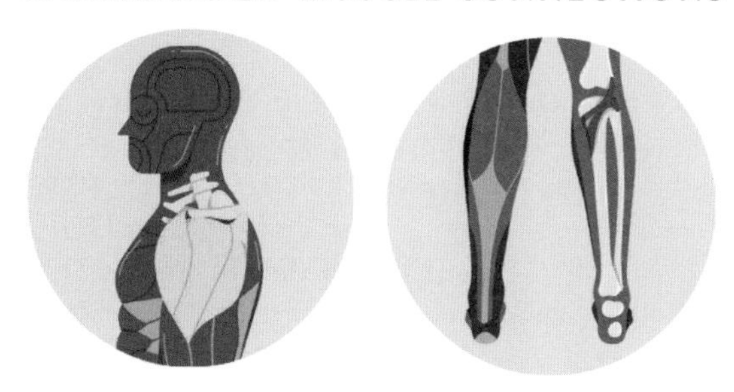

- Anterior deltoid muscle in the right shoulder
- Popliteus muscle located on the back of the right knee

When the gallbladder becomes imbalanced, these muscles also become imbalanced, destabilizing the right knee and the right shoulder. Right knee trouble is the most common symptom of gallbladder imbalance, followed by discomfort in the right shoulder.

HEART

EXPLANATION

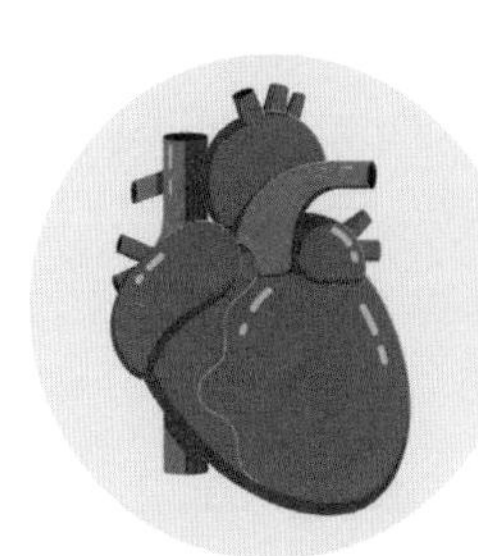

The heart is a muscular pump located in the chest, about the size of a clenched fist. It is the powerhouse behind the circulatory system, keeping the body tissues well supplied with blood and vital nutrients. The heart not only pumps blood but many consider it to be a second brain. Ancient societies believed the heart was the seat of the soul, the source of romance and creativity, and the core of our being. For more information see *The Emotion Code* chapter titled "The Walls Around Our Hearts."

PURPOSE OF THE HEART

- To pump blood throughout the body
- To be the center of your being, the core of who you really are!

COMMON SYMPTOMS OF HEART IMBALANCE

- Low energy or exhaustion
- Skipped beats, racing or pounding heart (palpitations)
- Discomfort in the chest and shoulders
- Trouble giving and receiving love (usually indicates a Heart-Wall)

People who have a very difficult time just walking up a flight of stairs often have an imbalance in the heart.

HEART EMOTIONS

The heart emotions are listed in row 1 on the Emotion Code Chart.

HEART-MUSCLE CONNECTIONS

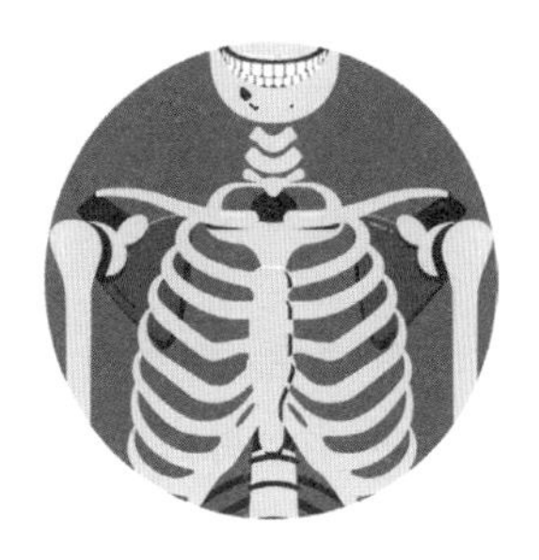

- Subscapularis muscles, which lie on the underside of the shoulder blades

KIDNEYS

EXPLANATION

There are two kidneys, left and right. The kidneys are retroperitoneal, meaning they are located behind the peritoneum and the rest of the abdominal organs and are closer to the back of the body than the front. They are part of both the urinary and endocrine systems.

PURPOSE OF THE KIDNEYS

- To cleanse and filter the blood (Most toxins end up in the kidneys as they are filtered out of the blood.)
- To create urine
- To regulate blood pressure
- To store energy (In Chinese medicine, the kidneys are known as energy reservoirs.)

COMMON SYMPTOMS OF KIDNEY IMBALANCE

- One of the most common reasons why people have back pain is because of kidney imbalance.
- Discomfort in the low back (most common), mid back, lower rib area, lower neck, or hip (usually associated with kidney imbalance on that side)
- TMJ (temporomandibular joint) pain
- Fatigue

MORE SERIOUS SYMPTOMS OF KIDNEY MALFUNCTION

- Leg pain
- Swelling in the ankles or face
- A foul or metallic taste
- Lack of urine production (Seek medical care in this case.)

Kidney imbalance can also cause discomfort in the lower neck because of the connection with the upper trapezius muscles. In addition, I have found that the TMJ can be imbalanced and aggravated by a kidney imbalance, apparently due to the connection of the trapezius muscles and the function of the cervical spine and the TMJ.

KIDNEY EMOTIONS

Emotions produced by the kidneys are in row 5 on the Emotion Code Chart.

KIDNEY–MUSCLE CONNECTIONS

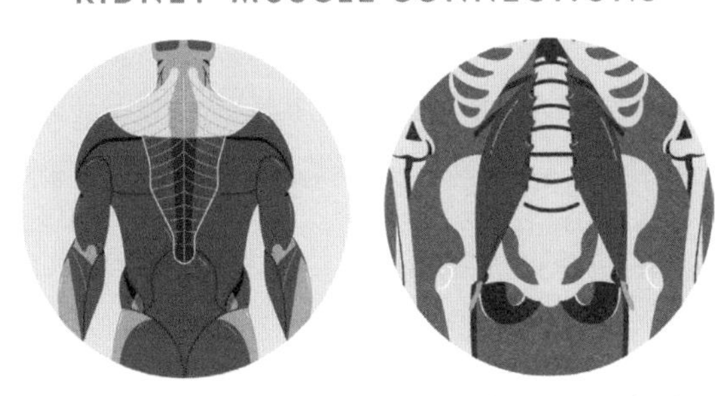

- Upper trapezius muscles (on both the right and left) are attached to the base of the skull and then come down and are attached to the shoulder blades on both sides. Imbalance in either of these muscles will tend to create trouble in the shoulders or in the neck.
- Psoas muscles are located deep in the lower back and the pelvis. They originate near the lumbar vertebrae and then connect with the pelvis, attaching to the upper femur below the hip joint.

When either of the psoas muscles becomes imbalanced, it can have a severe effect on the stability of the lower body. Disc injuries and disc problems are much more likely to occur with kidney–psoas imbalance. In all the years that I practiced in my brick-and-mortar chiropractic business, I saw hundreds of patients with low-back and disc pain. Every single disc patient that I ever saw had a kidney imbalance. When we corrected the kidney imbalances, we were able to help every patient get well, except for two cases that were too far gone, who we had to send out for surgical intervention.

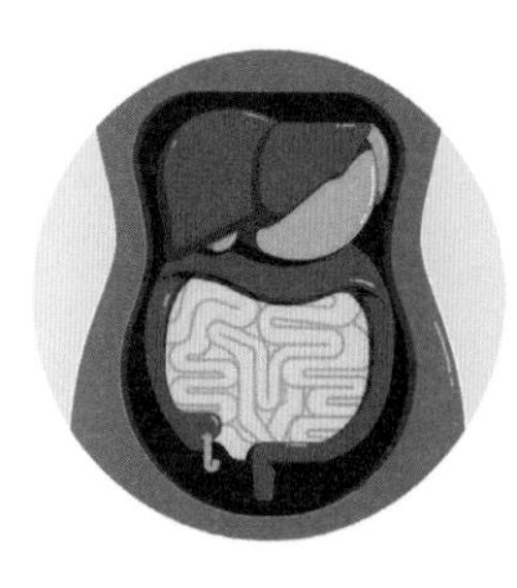

SMALL INTESTINE

EXPLANATION

The small intestine is a very long, skinny organ located in the abdomen. Due to the special nature of its lining, the small intestine has a surface area about the size of a tennis court. It is part of the digestive system.

PURPOSE OF THE SMALL INTESTINE

- To absorb nutrients from food. The food that you eat travels from the stomach into the small intestine, where it is further digested and the nutrients absorbed into the bloodstream.

COMMON SYMPTOMS OF SMALL-INTESTINE IMBALANCE

- Pain in the low back or knees
- Bloating
- Gas
- Diarrhea
- Nausea
- Skin problems due to lack of nutrients. When the small intestine is imbalanced, it is often less able to absorb nutrients that the rest of the body tissues need in order to function optimally. The skin is one of the last organs to receive the nutrients absorbed by the small intestine, and because of this, the skin may show symptoms of nutrient deficiency in the form of a rash, dryness, flaking, and/or cracking.

SMALL-INTESTINE EMOTIONS

The small-intestine emotions are listed in row 1 on the Emotion Code Chart.

SMALL INTESTINE–MUSCLE CONNECTIONS

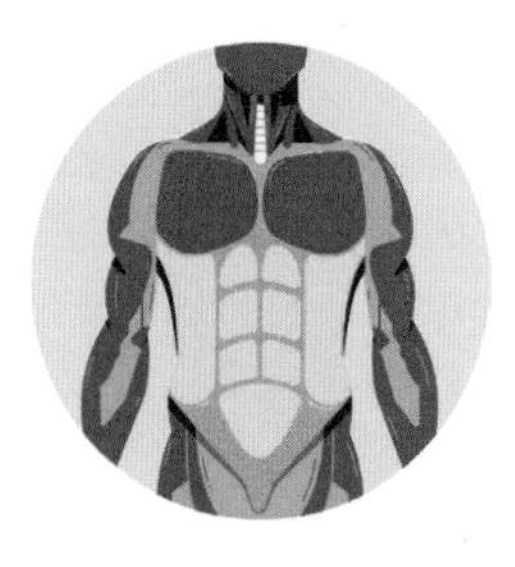
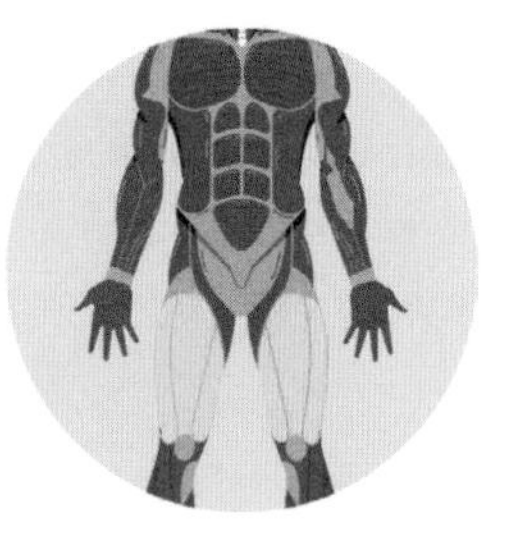

- Abdominal muscles
- Quadriceps femoris muscles, the large muscles in the front of the thighs. Both of these muscles can lead to trouble in the knees and the low back if they are imbalanced.

When the small intestine becomes imbalanced, all of the abdominal muscles also become imbalanced because they are on the same circuit. Any personal trainer will tell you that you need to have strong abdominal muscles in order to have a stable core. Having a small-intestine imbalance will automatically create weakness in the abdominal muscles, destabilizing the core, which can lead to lower-back pain.

COLON

EXPLANATION

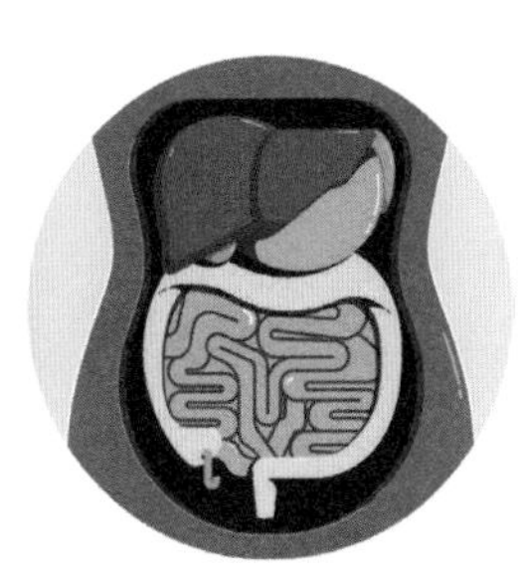

The colon is also known as the large intestine, and is a large organ located in the abdomen. It is part of the digestive system. There are different sections of the colon: The ascending colon begins on the right side of the body in the lower abdomen, just above the appendix, and then travels up to just below the liver. The transverse colon swoops across from the right to the left side of the body. Then the descending colon travels down the left side of the body and becomes the sigmoid colon. The last section of the colon or large intestine is known as the rectum, which terminates in the anus, where fecal matter is eliminated from the body.

PURPOSE OF THE COLON

- To absorb water and electrolytes from fecal matter, dehydrating fecal matter, and forming stool
- To eliminate fecal matter

I read a story once about some people who were stranded in a desert. The only water they could find was very brackish water that they could not drink. They were able to survive by introducing the undrinkable water into their colon through an enema device, because their colons could absorb it. A good thing to remember, perhaps.

COMMON SYMPTOMS OF COLON IMBALANCE

- Discomfort in the low back or hips
- Diarrhea
- Constipation
- Change in bowel habits or stool quality or consistency
- Stools with mucus
- A feeling of incomplete defecation or a reduction in the caliber of feces
- Bloody stools, black stools, or rectal bleeding

Bloody stools, black stools, or rectal bleeding are definitely indications that it's time to see a doctor!

Colon imbalance that is prolonged or severe also tends to cause common conditions such as colitis, irritable bowel syndrome (IBS), diverticulosis (small bulging pouches that develop), and diverticulitis (inflammation and/or infection of these pouches).

COLON EMOTIONS

The emotions produced by the colon are in row 3 on the Emotion Code Chart.

COLON–MUSCLE CONNECTIONS

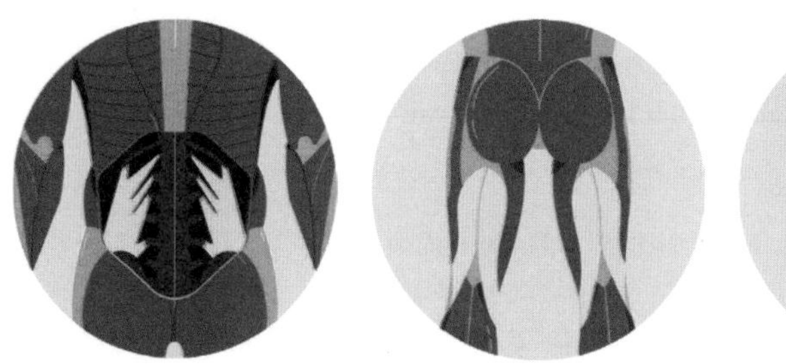

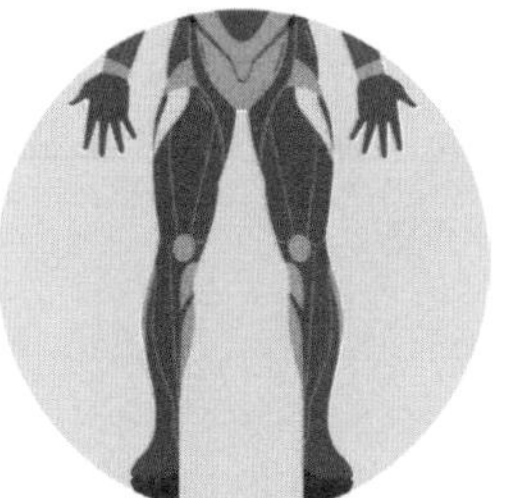

- The quadratus lumborum muscle, the deepest abdominal muscle, is located in your lower back on either side of the lumbar spine.
- The hamstring muscles are the large muscles at the backs of the thighs.
- The tensor fasciae latae muscle runs along the outside of each of the legs, starting at the hip area and then traveling down to the outside of the knee.

ILEOCECAL VALVE

EXPLANATION

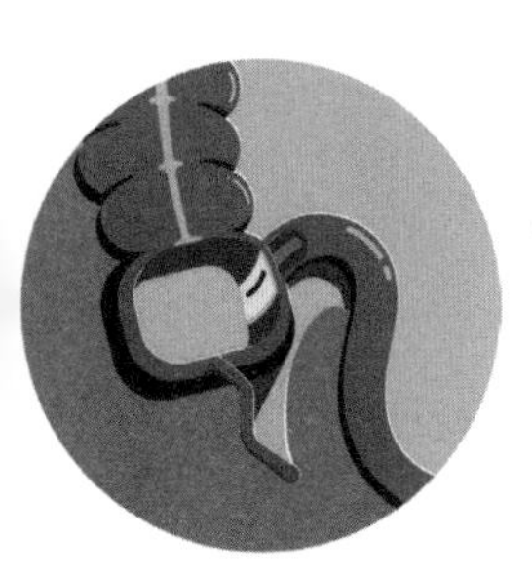

The ileocecal valve is a sphincter muscle at the connection of the small intestine and the colon. The reason it's called the ileocecal valve is because it joins the cecum, or beginning part of the colon, to the ileum, the last part of the small intestine. The ileocecal valve is perhaps the most easily imbalanced "organ" in the body and is often a location where trapped emotions lodge. The ileocecal valve is not generally considered to be a separate organ, but I include it here because of its importance, and because it is often problematic.

PURPOSE OF THE ILEOCECAL VALVE

- To control and regulate the flow of fecal matter from the small intestine into the colon

COMMON SYMPTOMS OF ILEOCECAL-VALVE IMBALANCE

- Discomfort in the appendix area, low back, or right hip
- Sinus problems and drainage
- Irritable bowel syndrome (IBS)
- Diarrhea
- Constipation
- Bloating and gas

Discomfort in the appendix area is very often caused by ileocecal-valve imbalance, but it's hard to spot unless you know what you are looking for. In fact, a lot of people end up having the appendix taken out because of an ileocecal-valve irritation. These are the occasions of appendicitis you hear about where the doctor comes back and says, "We didn't find anything. Your appendix looked okay. We took it out anyway, but it didn't seem to be infected." I believe that the culprit here is often an irritated ileocecal valve.

When the ileocecal valve becomes imbalanced, poor elimination of toxins (metabolic waste) is the result. Toxins from fecal matter will start to be reabsorbed into the bloodstream, so the body will try to get rid of them by shedding them through the nasal sinuses. The result is postnasal drip or sinus problems (including recurring sinus infections). Sinus drainage due to ileocecal valve imbalance is what I call "false allergies." Typically, when people have sinus problems like this, they'll go to their doctor, who will diagnose them with allergies and prescribe allergy medication. But if you correct the imbalance in the ileocecal valve, these sinus drainage problems will go away, often immediately or within hours. I've seen cases where people's sinuses simply dried up and the problems were gone within thirty seconds! It is very likely that about 20 percent of people who take allergy medication actually don't have allergies at all, just an ileocecal-valve imbalance.

ILEOCECAL VALVE–MUSCLE CONNECTIONS

- Right iliacus muscle

The ileocecal valve is on the same circuit as the iliacus muscle on the right side. Keep in mind, however, that the colon and/or the small-intestine circuits can also become imbalanced when the ileocecal valve is imbalanced. This means that imbalance in the ileocecal valve could potentially lead to several different muscles becoming imbalanced.

ILEOCECAL-VALVE EMOTIONS

The emotions produced by the ileocecal valve are listed with the small intestine in row 1 on the Emotion Code Chart.

This concludes the organs section. Next, we will discuss the glands.

13

THE GLANDS

All thinking is done with the glands. Logic is added later to tidy things up.

—JOHN MACDONALD

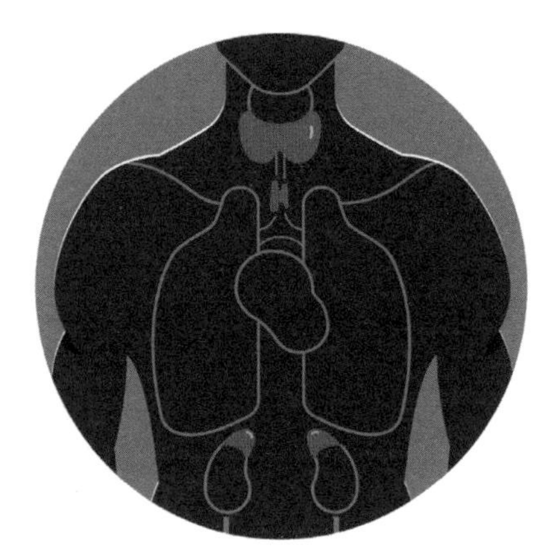

In this chapter I outline each gland, including its functions, its connection with various muscles, and the most common symptoms of imbalance. If you discover an imbalanced gland through testing, you can look up the gland in this chapter to read more about it and follow the instructions to correct the imbalance.

There are two ways to find a gland that is imbalanced or unhappy. If you suspect that a gland may need some help, you can simply ask, "Is the [gland name] balanced?" For example, "Is my pancreas balanced?" or, "Is my thyroid balanced?"

When you ask, "Is my ____ balanced?" and perform a muscle test, you'll get a yes or a no answer. If the muscle response is strong, this indicates a congruent or a yes answer, which means that the gland is likely doing fine. If the muscle response is weak, indicating no, this indicates that

GLAND CHART

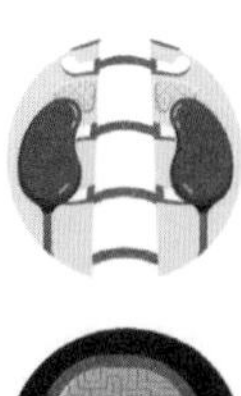
Adrenal Glands (page 191)

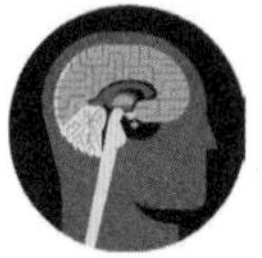
Hypothalamus (page 193)

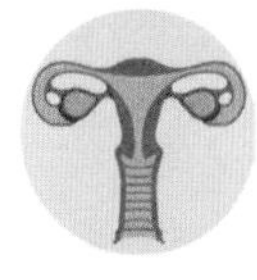
Ovaries (page 194)

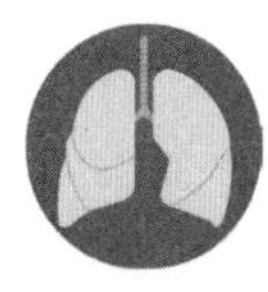
Pancreas (page 195)

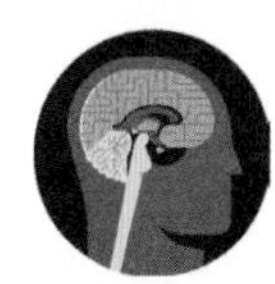
Pineal Gland (page 196)

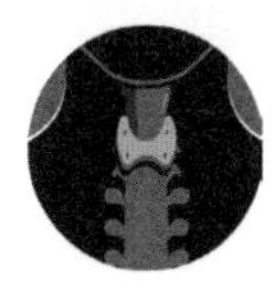
Parathyroid Glands (page 197)

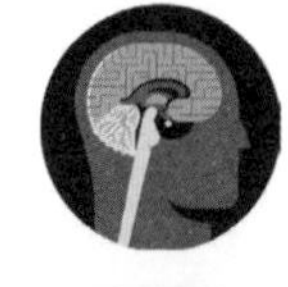
Pituitary Gland (page 198)

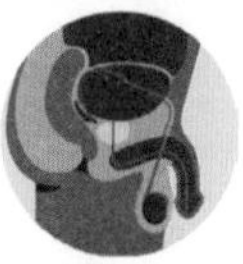
Prostate Gland (page 199)

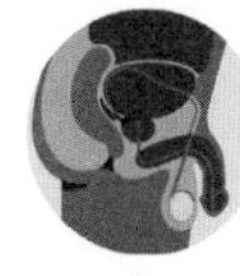
Testicles (page 200)

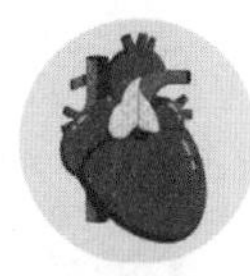
Thymus Gland (page 201)

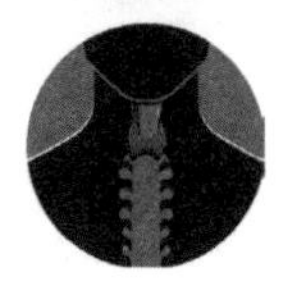
Thyroid Gland (page 202)

the gland is asking for help. If you have arrived at this point in your testing and have identified a gland that is imbalanced, proceed to Step 3 in the following process.

Another way to find an imbalanced gland is to use the Gland Chart by following these steps.

STEP 1.

Ask: "Do I [or you] have an imbalanced [or unhappy] gland?"

- **If yes, ask, "Is the gland on the right side of the gland chart?"**
  - **If yes, move to Step 2.**
  - **If no, it is on the left side. Move to Step 2.**

STEP 2.

Start at the top of the side identified and ask, "Is the ____ imbalanced?" For example, let's say you received a yes answer in Step 1, so you know the gland is on the right side of the chart. Since the pituitary gland is at the top of the chart on the right side, you would then ask, "Is the pituitary gland imbalanced?" If you receive a no answer, you would continue down that column to the next gland and ask, "Is the prostate gland imbalanced?" and so on, until you receive a yes answer.

STEP 3.

Once you've identified an imbalanced gland, follow these instructions to find and correct any imbalances affecting that gland.

STEP 4.

(Association) Ask: "Is there an associated imbalance that needs to be decoded?"

- If no, simply swipe three times with a magnet or your hand on any length of the governing meridian, while holding the intention to reset the gland.
- If yes, return to the Body Code Map, then decode and address any associated imbalances, then return here and repeat the above question. (Note that most of the time, glands are imbalanced by trapped emotions or other energies.)

STEP 5.

Ask: "Is the gland balanced [or happy] now?" When the answer to this question is yes, you have successfully rebalanced that gland.

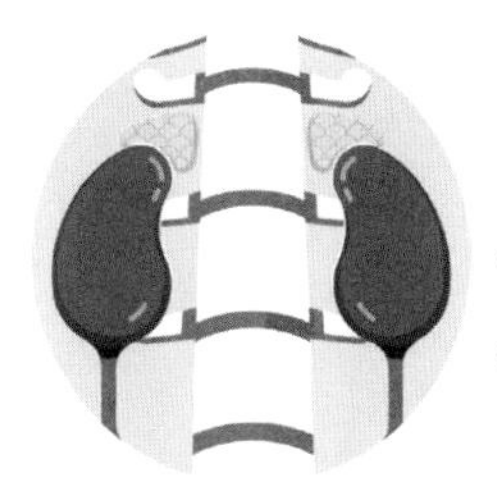

ADRENAL GLANDS

EXPLANATION

The adrenal glands are the "stress glands" of the body. There are two, each situated atop one of the kidneys. They form part of the endocrine system.

PURPOSE OF THE ADRENAL GLANDS

- To produce the stress hormones adrenaline and cortisol

When you're under stress, the body responds through its "fight or flight" reaction and the adrenal glands kick into gear, producing these hormones. This reaction is very appropriate in the short term, especially if you need to fight or run away. Most of the time we experience a reaction to everyday stresses that don't require such a drastic response. If the body is under too much stress for too long, the adrenals can become overloaded.

COMMON SYMPTOMS OF ADRENAL-GLAND IMBALANCE

- Pain in the left knee
- Pain in the low back
- Low immune function
- Fatigue
- Sensitivity to light
- "Joint noise"
- Inability to cope with stress
- Brain fog

ADRENAL EMOTIONS

The adrenals emotions are listed in row 6 on the Emotion Code Chart.

ADRENAL GLAND–MUSCLE CONNECTIONS

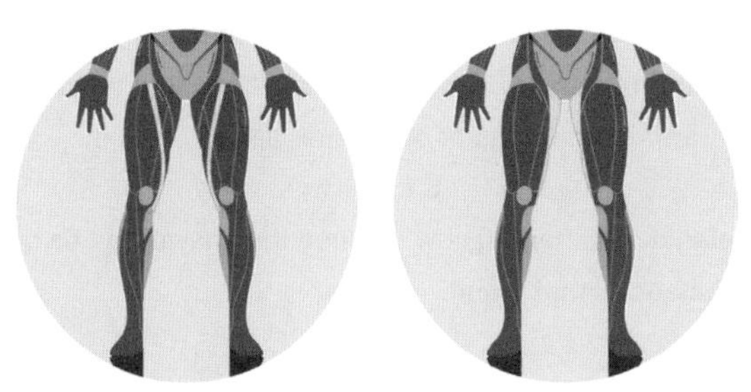

- Sartorius muscles, left and right
- Gracilis muscles, left and right
- Posterior tibial muscles located deep in the posterior compartment of the lower leg and situated between the flexor digitorum longus and the flexor hallucis longus. It is a key stabilizing muscle supporting the medial arch of the foot.
- The soleus is a powerful muscle in the back part of the lower leg (the calf). It runs from just below the knee to the heel and is involved in standing and walking.

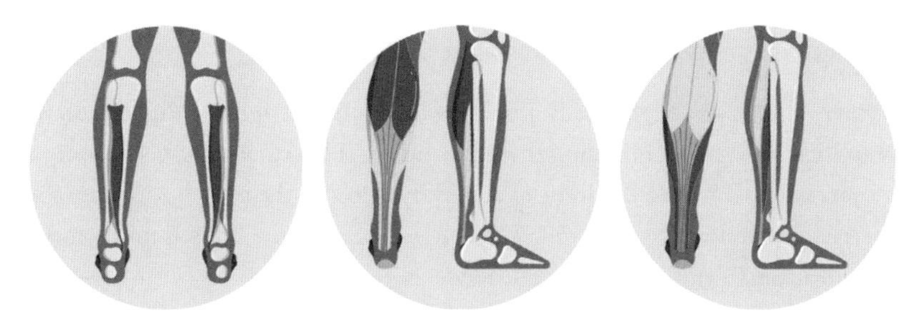

- The gastrocnemius, also called the leg triceps, is the large posterior muscle of the calf of the leg. It originates at the back of the femur (thighbone) and patella (kneecap) and, joining the soleus (another muscle of the calf), is attached to the Achilles tendon at the heel.

All these muscles keep the legs stable. The sartorius and gracilis muscles cross the knee joint; when imbalanced they create instability in the knee. The pelvis can also be affected by imbalance in these muscles.

The left adrenal is likely to become imbalanced before the right side is affected. Therefore, the left side muscles will typically become imbalanced more often, resulting in left knee pain and sometimes lower-back pain stemming from pelvic imbalance on the left side. Of course, if the stress continues, eventually the right adrenal may become imbalanced as well, most often resulting in pain in both knees. It is also possible for the right adrenal to become imbalanced before the left one does, especially if a trapped emotion or other energy lodges in the area. So you may need to ask which side is imbalanced, the left side or the right side.

HYPOTHALAMUS

EXPLANATION

The hypothalamus is a gland located in the brain between the left and right thalamus. It is part of the endocrine system as well as the central nervous system.

PURPOSE OF THE HYPOTHALAMUS

To secrete hormones that:

- Regulate body temperature
- Regulate hunger mechanism
- Regulate thirst mechanism
- Regulate circadian rhythm (the sleeping and waking rhythms of the body)

COMMON SYMPTOMS OF HYPOTHALAMUS IMBALANCE

- Insomnia
- Chilling, or inability to stay cool or warm
- Disruption of the thirst mechanism (never feeling thirsty)

HYPOTHALAMUS EMOTIONS

There are no known emotions that are produced by the hypothalamus.

HYPOTHALAMUS-MUSCLE CONNECTIONS

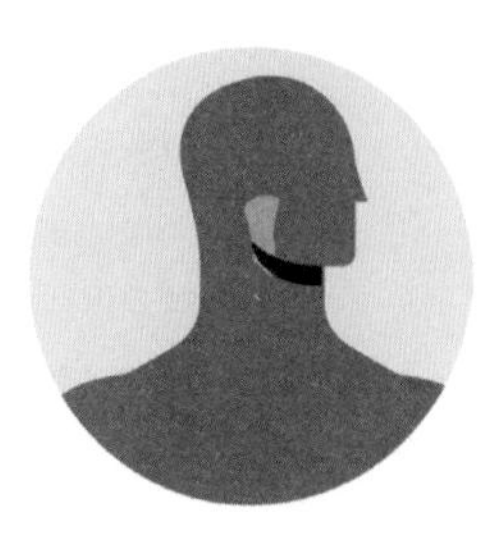

The hypothalamus is connected energetically with the muscles of the pharynx. These are the muscles that control swallowing, and also have an effect on breathing and vocalization.

OVARIES

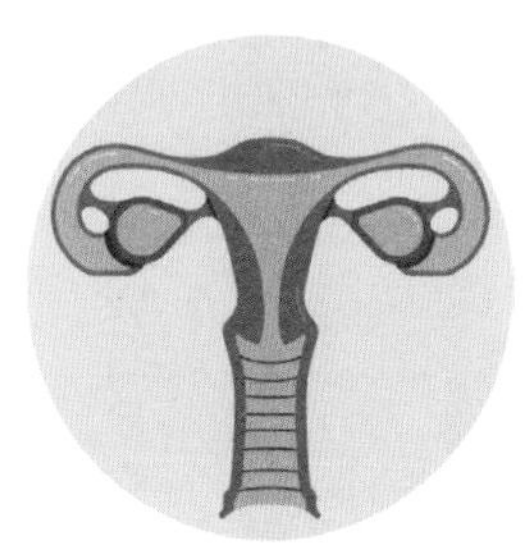

EXPLANATION

There are two ovaries, left and right, located in the lower abdomen on either side of the uterus, at the upper ends of the fallopian tubes. They are part of the female reproductive system as well as the endocrine system.

PURPOSE OF THE OVARIES

- To produce ova, or eggs (which can then be fertilized by a male's sperm and grow into a fetus)
- To secrete estrogen and progesterone (which are the primary female hormones)

COMMON SYMPTOMS OF OVARY IMBALANCE

- Difficult or irregular menstruation (due to hormonal fluctuations)
- Pain in the lower abdomen (between navel and hip on either side)
- Ovarian cysts
- Infertility
- Ectopic pregnancy (a medical emergency)
- Lowered sex drive
- Lowered initiative

OVARY-MUSCLE CONNECTIONS

There are no known muscle connections between the ovaries and the muscles.

OVARY EMOTIONS

Emotions produced by the ovaries are in row 6 on the Emotion Code Chart.

You can work on one ovary at a time or both if the body allows. Keep in mind that imbalances such as trapped emotions can certainly imbalance a large enough area as to affect both ovaries, and the same is true for other problems, like pathogens or nutritional deficiencies.

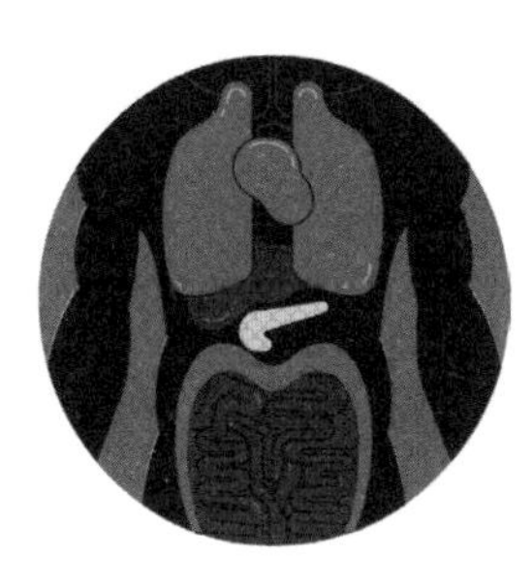

PANCREAS

EXPLANATION

The pancreas is located beneath the liver and sits between the liver and the stomach. It is a part of the endocrine system as well as the digestive system.

PURPOSE OF THE PANCREAS

- To secrete insulin, which regulates blood sugar
- To secrete digestive enzymes

Insulin is a necessary hormone for our bodies because it allows sugar to absorb into our cells. If the pancreas malfunctions, we may end up with diabetes (type 1), caused by the pancreas not producing enough insulin to help us digest and metabolize sugar. The pancreas also secretes enzymes that help us digest our food.

COMMON SYMPTOMS OF PANCREAS IMBALANCE

- Discomfort in the mid back, left shoulder, low back, neck, wrist, or thumb
- Indigestion
- Bloating and gas
- Peptic ulcers
- Diabetes (major malfunction)

PANCREAS EMOTIONS

Emotions produced by the pancreas are in row 2 on the Emotion Code Chart.

PANCREAS-MUSCLE CONNECTIONS

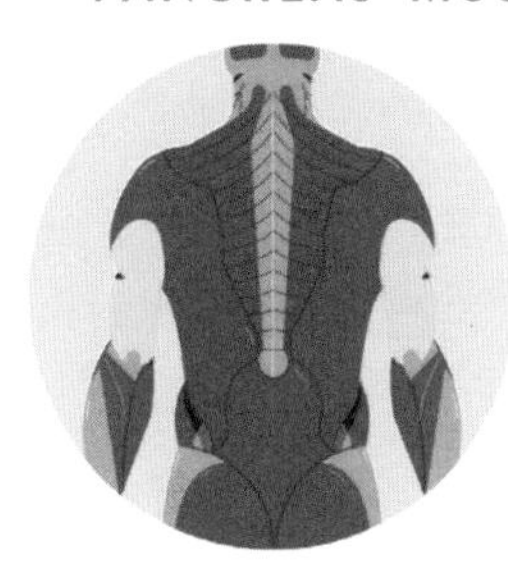

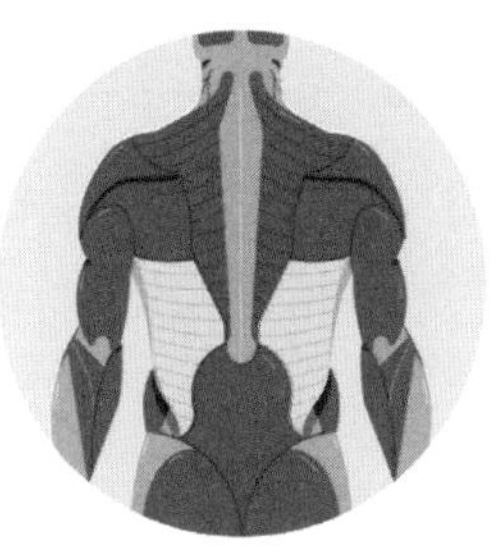

- Triceps muscles are located in the back of the upper arms.
- Latissimus dorsi muscles are located in the lower and mid-back area.

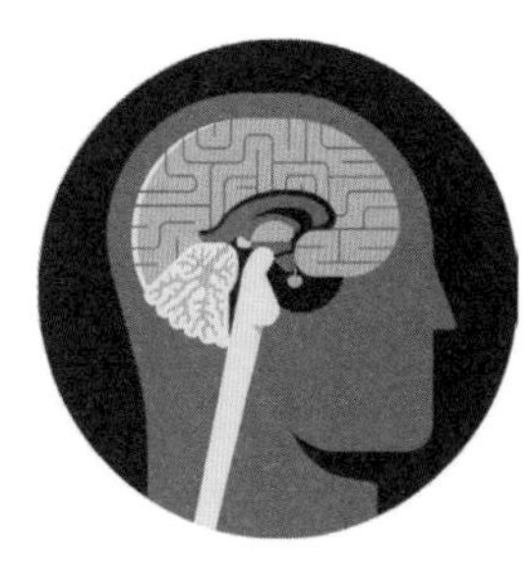

PINEAL GLAND

EXPLANATION

The pineal is a very small gland located near the center of the brain. It is part of the endocrine system as well as the central nervous system.

PURPOSE OF THE PINEAL GLAND

- To produce melatonin (a hormone that helps stabilize the circadian rhythm and facilitates proper sleep)
- To connect to the brow chakra and function as the "third eye"

COMMON SYMPTOMS OF PINEAL-GLAND IMBALANCE

- Insomnia
- Difficulty planning ahead
- Eye pain
- Vision problems

The pineal gland is very much affected by the amount of sunlight we receive. People who live in the far northern or southern latitudes sometimes suffer from SAD, or seasonal affective disorder, which is caused by long dark winters and not enough sunlight. This can be helped by getting more sunlight, of course, but you can also achieve the same balancing effect by using light therapy, directed at the center of the forehead.

Fluoride and other metals can cause the pineal gland to become calcified, reducing its functionality and increasing the symptoms listed previously.

PINEAL-GLAND EMOTIONS

There are no known emotions that are produced by the pineal gland.

PINEAL GLAND–MUSCLE CONNECTIONS

The small muscles that control eye movement are connected on the same circuit with the pineal gland. An imbalance in the pineal gland will tend to imbalance these muscles.

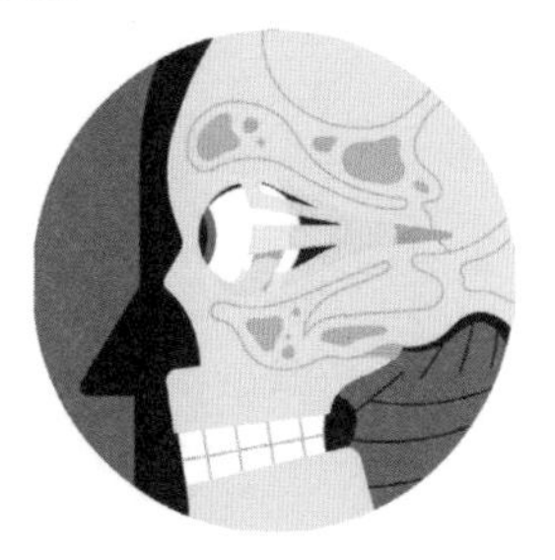

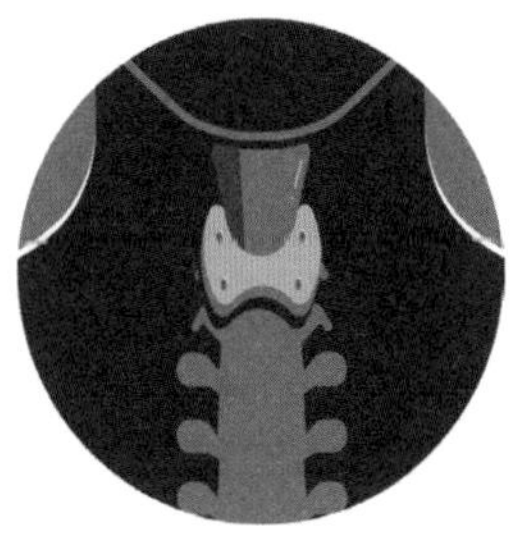

PARATHYROID GLANDS

EXPLANATION

The parathyroid glands consist of four small glands situated on the back side of the thyroid gland.

PURPOSE OF THE PARATHYROID GLANDS

- To produce parathyroid hormone (a hormone that controls the amount of calcium in the blood and bones)

COMMON SYMPTOMS OF PARATHYROID-GLAND IMBALANCE

The symptoms of parathyroid gland imbalance vary, depending on whether the parathyroid is overproducing parathyroid hormone or underproducing it.

COMMON SYMPTOMS OF HYPOPARATHYROIDISM (UNDERPRODUCTION)

- Low blood calcium levels
- Muscle spasms, especially in hands and feet
- Tetany
- Fatigue
- Headaches
- Insomnia
- Tingling around mouth or extremities

COMMON SYMPTOMS OF HYPERPARATHYROIDISM (OVERPRODUCTION)

- Kidney stones
- Excessive urination
- Gallstones
- Fatigue
- Nausea
- Bone pain
- Abdominal pain
- Low energy or weakness
- Depression
- Heart issues
- Short-term memory loss

- Vomiting
- Osteoporosis
- Elevated blood calcium levels

In addition, because the parathyroid gland connects to the levator scapulae muscle, any imbalance in the parathyroid will tend to result in neck or shoulder discomfort.

PARATHYROID-GLAND EMOTIONS

The parathyroid produces the emotions listed in row 6 on the Emotion Code Chart.

PARATHYROID GLAND–MUSCLE CONNECTIONS

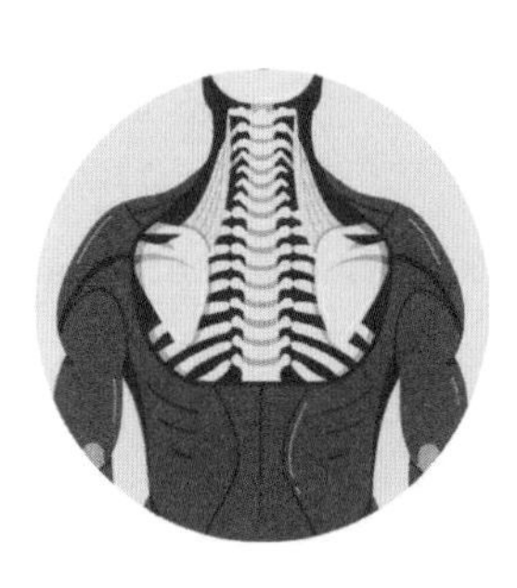

The parathyroid gland is energetically connected to the levator scapulae muscle.

This muscle is activated when a person shrugs the shoulders.

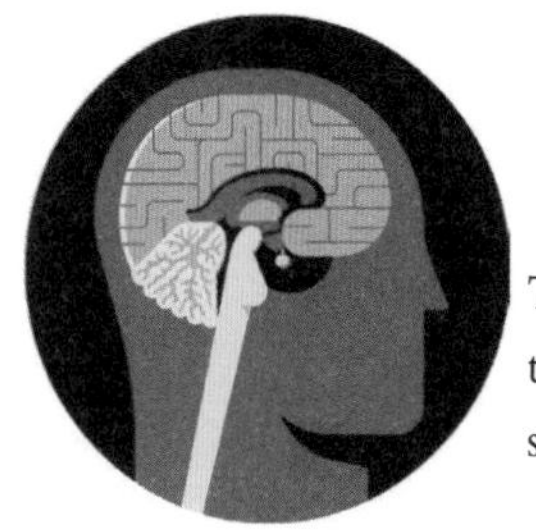

PITUITARY GLAND

EXPLANATION

The pituitary is a brain gland located in the lower part of the front half of the brain. It is part of the endocrine system as well as the central nervous system.

PURPOSE OF THE PITUITARY GLAND

- To secrete hormones that regulate overall body balance, or homeostasis
- To secrete hormones that influence other glands, to control:
  - Growth
  - Blood pressure
  - Thyroid-gland function
  - Metabolism
  - Water and hydration regulation
  - Water absorption by the kidneys
  - Temperature regulation
  - Sex-gland function in both sexes

- Aspects of childbirth and pregnancy
- The production of breast milk

As you can see, the pituitary gland is very important and has a large influence over the body.

COMMON SYMPTOMS OF PITUITARY-GLAND IMBALANCE

- Hormonal imbalances
- Thyroid problems (see "Thyroid Gland" section)
- Dehydration
- Fatigue
- High blood pressure
- Weight gain (usually due to thyroid-gland imbalance)

PITUITARY-GLAND EMOTIONS

There are no known emotions that are produced by the pituitary gland.

PITUITARY GLAND–MUSCLE CONNECTIONS

There are no known muscle connections.

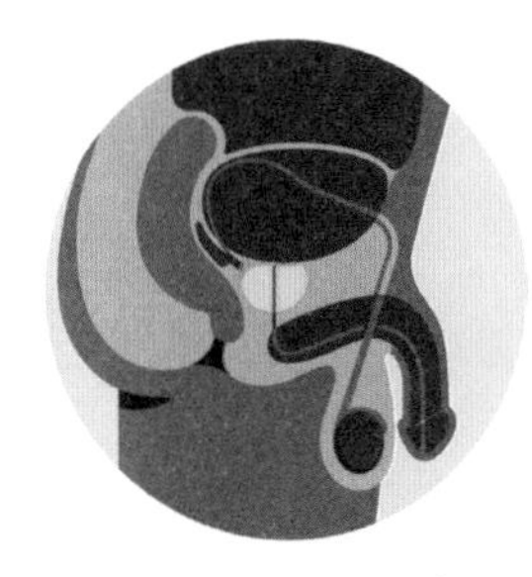

PROSTATE GLAND

EXPLANATION

The prostate gland is a small muscular gland about the size of a chestnut located just below the bladder. It is part of the male reproductive system.

PURPOSE OF THE PROSTATE GLAND

- To produce prostatic fluid (a thin zinc-containing opaque secretion that helps to nourish the sperm cells)
- To propel ejaculate fluid via muscular contractions

COMMON SYMPTOMS OF PROSTATE-GLAND IMBALANCE

- Sterility
- Pain in the low back
- Pain in the left hip
- Decreased urine flow

As men age past fifty they often begin to suffer from benign prostatic hypertrophy, or BPH, which tends to reduce the flow of urine. It's one of the reasons why, when men get older, they will often report that they have to get up a number of times every night to urinate and that their urine flow is also reduced. One of the reasons for this is zinc deficiency, because every time a man ejaculates, he loses a good deal of zinc contained in the prostatic fluid.

PROSTATE EMOTIONS

The prostate produces the emotions listed in row 6 on the Emotion Code Chart.

PROSTATE GLAND–MUSCLE CONNECTIONS

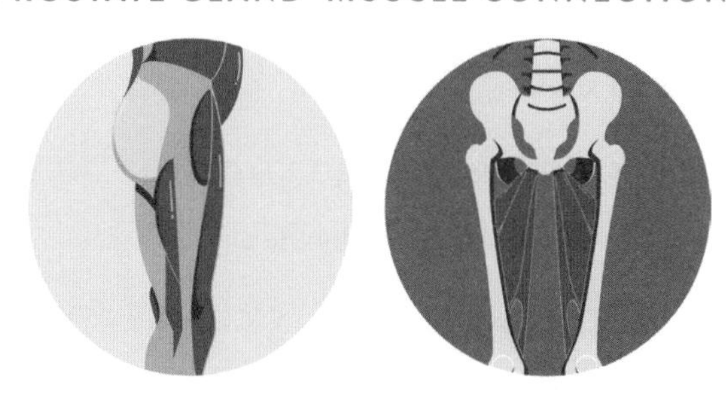

- Gluteal or buttock muscles
- Adductor muscles of the inner thighs

TESTICLES

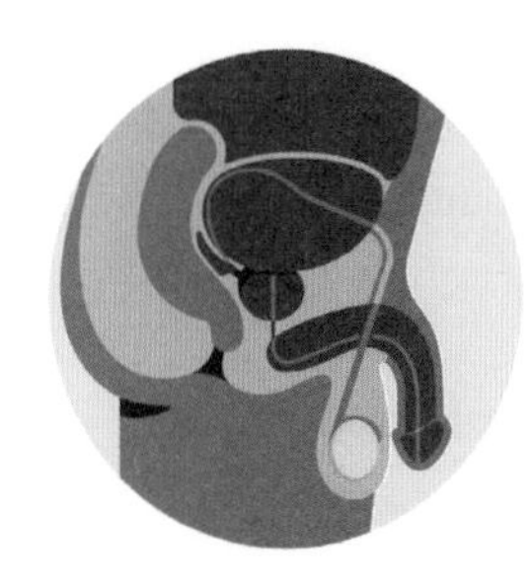

EXPLANATION

The testicles (aka testes) are two glands (right and left) located in the scrotal sac between the legs, where it's a little bit cooler, as sperm function better in cooler temperatures. The testicles are part of the male reproductive system and the endocrine system.

PURPOSE OF THE TESTICLES

- To produce sperm
- To produce male hormones (especially testosterone, the most significant of the male hormones)

COMMON SYMPTOMS OF TESTICLE IMBALANCE

- Sterility
- Lowered sex drive
- Lowered initiative (due to reduction in testosterone)

TESTICLE EMOTIONS

The testicles produce the emotions in row 6 on the Emotion Code Chart.

TESTICLE-MUSCLE CONNECTIONS

There are no known muscle connections between the testicles and the muscles.

You can work on one testicle at a time or both if the body allows. Keep in mind that imbalances such as trapped emotions can certainly affect a large enough area to include both testicles.

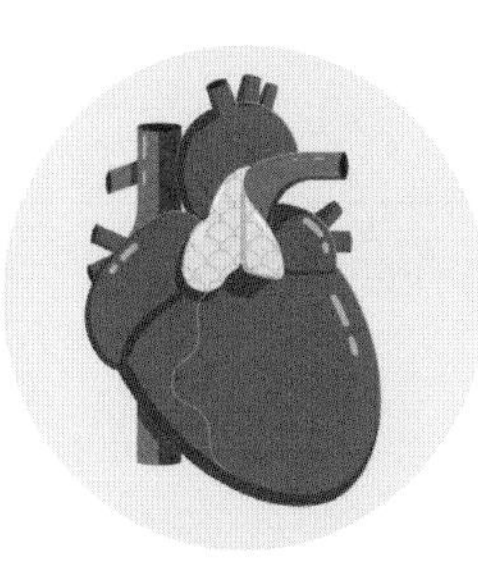

THYMUS GLAND

EXPLANATION

The thymus gland is located in the chest and sits right on top of the heart. In a newborn baby, the thymus is quite large in relation to the heart. As the heart grows, the thymus stays the same size. It is an important part of the immune system.

Note that the thymus gland will suffer energetically when a Heart-Wall is present, and this is another reason for lowered immune function in Heart-Wall cases.

PURPOSE OF THE THYMUS GLAND

- To help T-cells to mature. (The T in T-cell actually stands for thymus.) T-cells protect the body from infection. These cells help to protect against autoimmune disease as well.

COMMON SYMPTOMS OF THYMUS IMBALANCE

- Discomfort in the shoulder
- Lowered immunity
- Autoimmune problems

THYMUS-GLAND EMOTIONS

The thymus produces the emotions in row 6 on the Emotion Code Chart.

THYMUS GLAND–MUSCLE CONNECTION

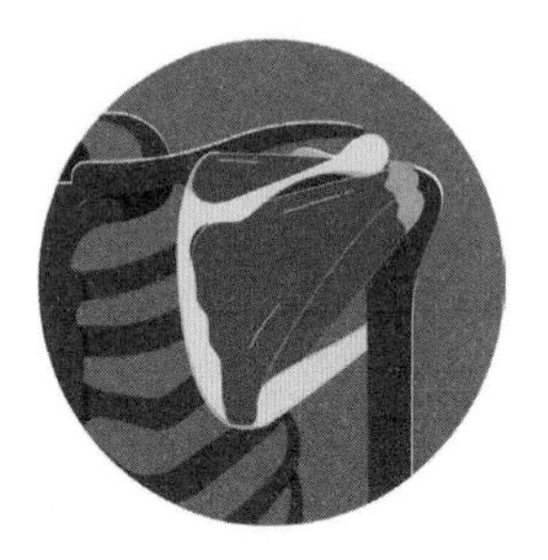
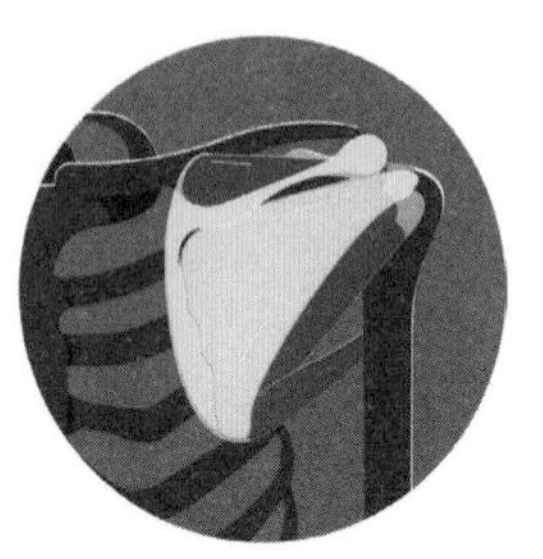

- The teres major muscles, which lie on the bottom half of the shoulder blades and connect the shoulder blades to the shoulder, help to rotate the shoulder externally and also bring the shoulder and the arm backward.
- The infraspinatus muscle, a thick triangular muscle, occupies the chief part of the infraspinatous fossa. As one of the four muscles of the rotator cuff, the main function of the infraspinatus is to externally rotate the humerus and stabilize the shoulder joint.

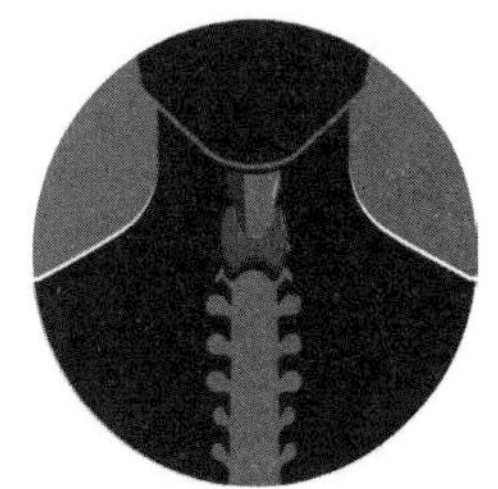

THYROID GLAND

EXPLANATION

The thyroid gland is situated in the lower part of the front of the throat. It is part of the endocrine system.

PURPOSE OF THE THYROID GLAND

- To control metabolism, growth, and development
- To control blood calcium
- To stimulate digestion
- To maintain cardiovascular health
- To regulate many other body functions

The thyroid produces a hormone called thyroxine. When the thyroid is imbalanced and is not producing enough thyroxine, it creates symptoms that are grouped together as a condition known as hypothyroidism. Overproduction of thyroxine is known as hyperthyroidism, the most common cause being Grave's disease, an autoimmune condition.

COMMON SYMPTOMS OF THYROID-GLAND IMBALANCE

HYPOTHYROIDISM (LOW THYROID FUNCTION)

- Weight gain
- Fatigue
- Thin, brittle nails
- Cold intolerance

HYPERTHYROIDISM (HIGH THYROID FUNCTION)

- Fatigue
- Frequent bowel movements or diarrhea
- Goiter, an enlarged thyroid that may cause your neck to look swollen, which may cause trouble with breathing or swallowing.
- Mood swings
- Muscle weakness
- Nervousness or irritability
- Rapid and irregular heartbeat
- Tremor, usually in your hands
- Trouble sleeping
- Trouble tolerating heat
- Weight loss

OTHER MINOR SYMPTOMS OF THYROID IMBALANCE

Other signs of general thyroid imbalance (either high or low function) may be the following:

- Discomfort or weakness in the shoulder
- Discomfort or weakness in the wrist
- Discomfort or weakness in the elbow
- More easily dislocated shoulders

Many people have thyroid imbalances that are not so extreme as to show major symptoms; more often, the symptoms will be on a more minor scale.

THYROID-GLAND EMOTIONS

The thyroid produces the emotions listed in row 6 on the Emotion Code Chart.

THYROID GLAND–MUSCLE CONNECTION

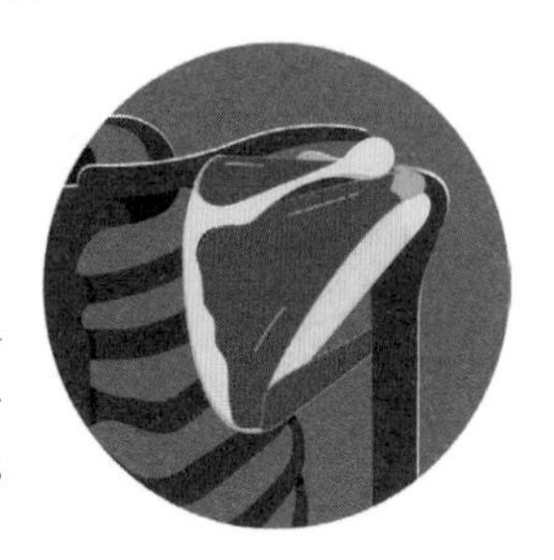

- Teres minor muscles (in both the right and left shoulders) cross from the bottom side of the shoulder blade over to the shoulder joint itself, to the head of the humerus bone.

When the thyroid becomes imbalanced, the teres minor muscle on either or both sides may also become imbalanced. This can create weakness, tension, and/or pain in either or both shoulders. Shoulder injury is also common because the stability of the joint has been compromised.

This concludes the glands section. Next, we will cover the systems.

14

SYSTEMS

The body maintains balance in only a handful of ways. At the end of the day, disease occurs when these basic systems are out of whack.

—MARK HYMAN

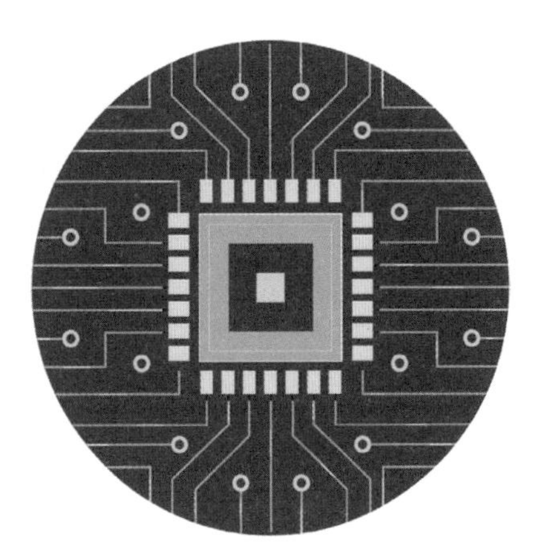

In this area of the Body Code you will find the various systems of the body that most people are familiar with, at least to some degree. For example, most of us have heard of the circulatory system and the digestive system. Perhaps a little less well known are the integumentary system, urinary system, and endocrine system. All of the muscles of the body form the muscular system. The brain and nerves comprise the nervous system. The lungs and their associated components make up the respiratory system. The reproductive organs form the reproductive system, and so on.

The body is made up of multiple different systems, with some parts playing roles in more than one system. For example, if a person has a problem with the skin, he or she might be guided by the subconscious mind to the immune system, and then to the liver, since the skin is an organ of detoxification that may manifest symptoms such as acne if the liver is overwhelmed.

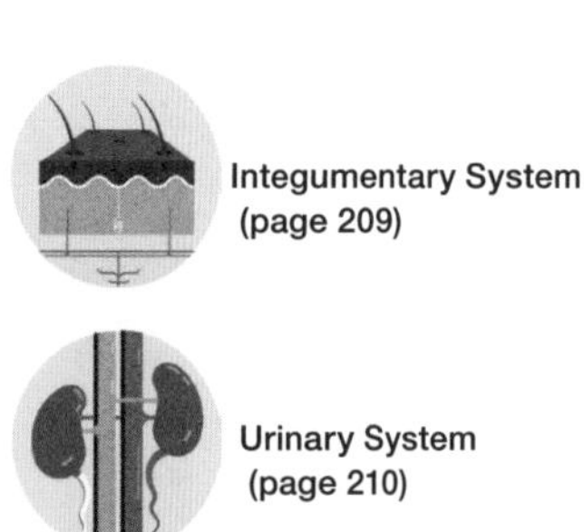

Integumentary System
(page 209)

Urinary System
(page 210)

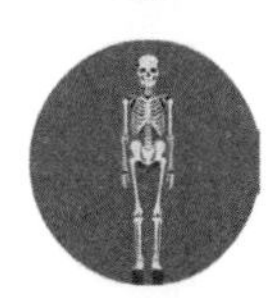

Skeletal System
(page 211)

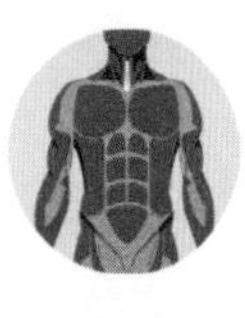

Muscular System
(page 214)

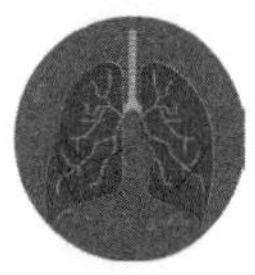

Respiratory System
(page 215)

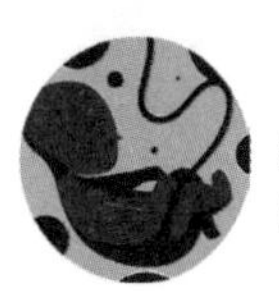

Reproductive System
(page 215)

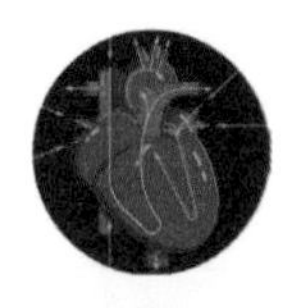

Circulatory System
(page 217)

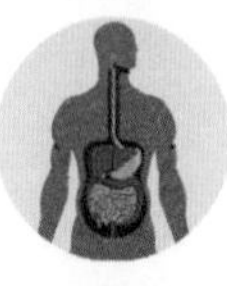

Digestive System
(page 217)

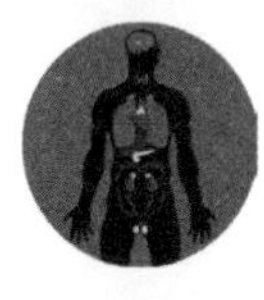

Endocrine System
(page 218)

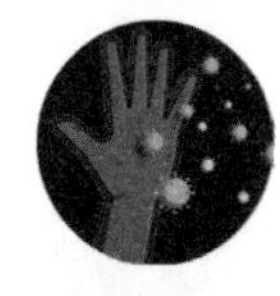

Immune/Lymphatic System
(page 219)

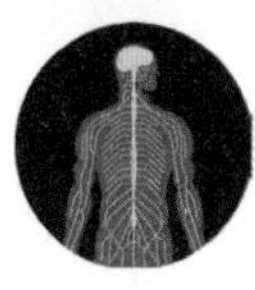

Nervous System
(page 220)

When you're using the Body Code, it's important to realize that there is more than one way to arrive at a particular imbalance.

For example, let's say that you are working on your mother, who is not feeling well. Let's assume for the sake of this example that your mother's problem is actually an imbalance in her liver, which is, in turn, being caused by toxicity and a trapped emotion.

There are several ways you might arrive at the solution to your mother's problem. Her subconscious mind might take you to the toxicity area of the Body Code, or it might take you to the trapped emotions area of the Body Code, or it might take you straight to the liver. It doesn't really matter how the subconscious mind takes you where you need to go. However, it's important to realize that the subconscious mind is always trying to communicate when it is giving answers to questions.

For example, at some point you might be taken to a place in the Body Code that may cause you to scratch your head and wonder what the subconscious mind is trying to tell you. Open your heart and mind to the possibilities without making any assumptions.

Let's say that you are trying to help a friend who seems to be suffering from allergies. Your first question to your friend's subconscious mind might be, "Is there an underlying reason for your allergies?"

After obtaining a yes answer using muscle testing to this first question, and looking at the Body Code Map in part III (page 101), you might ask, "Is this imbalance on the right side of the chart?" Let's say the answer is no. That means the underlying imbalance you're looking for must be on the left side of the chart. So, starting at the top you ask, "Is this imbalance in energies?" No. "Is this imbalance in circuits and systems?" Yes.

You turn to the "Circuits and Systems" section (page 161) and use the chart found there to ask, "Is this imbalance on the right side of this chart?" No. "Is it in a system?" Yes.

You turn to the system chart at the beginning of this chapter and continue testing in this way, and ultimately land on "digestive system." You may be thinking, "But, wait a second. . . . Shouldn't I be taken to the allergies area of the Body Code? Why am I being taken to the digestive system?"

You decide to go wherever the subconscious mind wants to take you, and continuing to muscle test, you are taken to the ileocecal valve chart icon.

You turn to the ileocecal valve information, again, wondering what in the world the subconscious mind is doing.

You begin reading the explanation, when suddenly your mouth drops open as you read that an imbalance in this valve will cause sinus problems!

The ileocecal valve is a valve at the very end of the small intestine; it controls the flow of fecal matter from the small intestine into the large intestine. When the valve becomes imbalanced, toxic fecal matter is not eliminated efficiently from the body. Toxins begin to back up and are reabsorbed into the bloodstream. A side effect of this increased blood toxicity is sinus drainage, as these toxins begin to overflow and shed through the nasal mucosa.

As you continue with the exercise instructions, you are directed to ask your friend's subconscious mind, "Is there an associated imbalance that needs to be decoded?"

Let's say the answer is yes, and that you are directed to release a few trapped emotions that are imbalancing your friend's ileocecal valve. After releasing the trapped emotions you recheck her ileocecal valve and ask, "Is your ileocecal valve balanced now?" Let's say the answer is yes. At this point you might ask your friend to take a deep breath in through her nose and see if her sinus drainage is as bad as it was before. Don't be surprised if your friend's sinuses have become much more open. It may be that your friend's symptoms were not allergies at all, but instead were the effort of her body doing its best to eliminate toxins any way it could.

If you're looking for the solution to a particular problem, you must have an open mind that the solution might be anywhere within the Body Code. Anything can cause anything.

Don't make the mistake of thinking a certain complaint is caused by a certain imbalance. Just because the migraine headaches that your father was suffering from were being caused by a kidney imbalance doesn't mean that the next person with migraine headaches will have the same underlying cause or causes. Be open to any possibility.

For this next exercise, you will use the systems chart at the beginning of this chapter to identify the system and component that is imbalanced.

EXERCISE: FIND AND CORRECT AN IMBALANCE IN A SYSTEM

STEP 1.

Ask: "Do I [or you] have an imbalanced [or unhappy] system?"

- If yes, ask, "Is the system on the right side of the systems chart?"
  - If yes, move to Step 2.
  - If no, it is on the left side. Move to Step 2.

STEP 2.

(Decoding) Start at the top of the side identified and ask, "Is the ____ system imbalanced?" For example, let's say you received a yes answer to Step 1, so you know the system in question is on the right side of the chart. Since the circulatory system is at the top of the list on the right side, you would then ask, "Is the circulatory system imbalanced?" If you receive a no answer, you would continue down that column to the next system and ask, "Is the digestive system imbalanced?" and so on until you receive a yes answer.

- Turn to the page indicated in the chart to view the system components.
- Identify the system component (if needed).
  - Ask: "Do I need to identify which component of this system is imbalanced?"

If no, continue to Step 3 (Association).

- If yes, find the system in the following pages and test the components in that system until you find the one that is imbalanced by using the chart of components that belongs to that system, asking, "Is the imbalanced component on the left side of this chart?" and narrowing down the possibilities.

Once you've identified the component, continue to Step 3 (Association).

STEP 3.

(Association) Ask: "Is there an associated imbalance that needs to be decoded?"

- If no, move to Step 4 (Intention).
- If yes, return to the Body Code Map and decode and address any associated imbalances, then return here and repeat the Step 3 (Association) question.

STEP 4.

(Intention) Swipe three times with a magnet or your hand on any length of the governing meridian, while holding the Intention to reset and balance the system or the system component you have identified.

STEP 5.

Ask: "Is the [system or component] balanced?"

- If yes, you can start at the beginning on Step 1 and repeat the process to find another imbalanced system, if one exists.
- If no, refocus, say a prayer for help, allow your heart to feel love and gratitude that this is going to help, and swipe three times once again with intention.

HELPFUL TIPS FOR CORRECTING A SYSTEM IMBALANCE

Another way to do this is if you know something is not quite right within a certain system, you can simply ask, "Is the ____ system balanced?" For example, let's say you have eczema and you want to find the underlying causes for it. You might ask directly, "Is my integumentary system balanced?" or, "Is my skin balanced (or happy)?"

By asking directly about the system you know is having issues, you can skip the identifying steps.

In the following pages I have listed the systems of the body along with graphic charts of their various components.

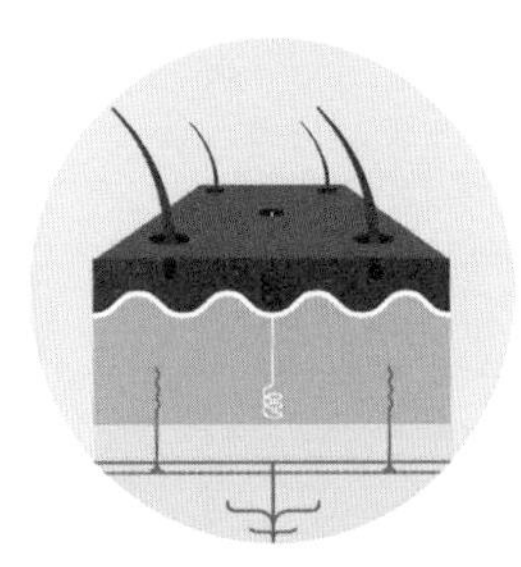

INTEGUMENTARY SYSTEM

EXPLANATION

The integumentary system serves as a protective barrier between the external environment and the remainder of the body. It includes the skin, nails, and hair.

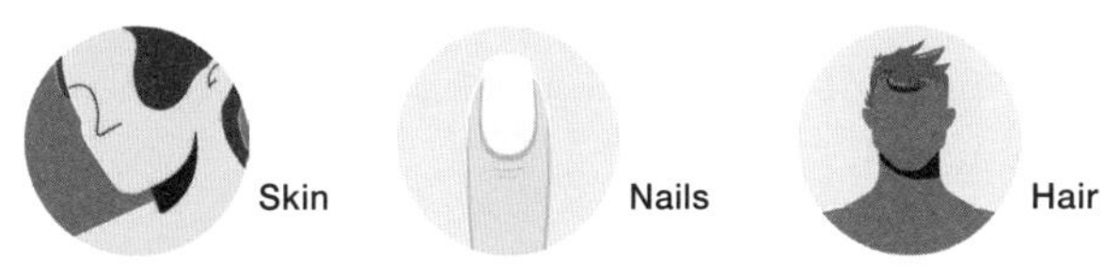

SKIN

The skin is comprised of three different layers, the hypodermis, dermis, and epidermis. The hypodermis is the deepest layer of skin, which connects the skin to the underlying fascial tissue surrounding the muscles and bones, as well as housing most of the adipose tissue or fat in the body.

The dermis, the middle layer of the skin, contains connective tissue and blood vessels that nourish the skin and carry away waste products. The glands and hair follicles originate in the dermis.

The epidermis is the outermost layer of skin, the layer that forms the protective barrier between us and the harsh world around us. It consists of many layers of epithelial cells that replace themselves every two to two and a half months.

NAILS

Fingernails and toenails are made of keratin, the same material that horns are made of. A nail has three main parts: the root, plate, and free margin. Other structures around or under the nail include the nail bed, cuticle, and nail fold.

HAIR

Hair is made of a tough protein called keratin. A hair follicle anchors each hair into the skin. The hair bulb forms the base of the hair follicle. In the hair bulb, living cells divide and grow to build the hair shaft.

Once you've identified the system component, you can return to the exercise at the beginning of this chapter and continue to Step 3 (Association).

URINARY SYSTEM

EXPLANATION

The urinary system is responsible for eliminating waste products from the body in the form of urine. All the blood in the body passes through the kidneys every few minutes. The kidneys filter the blood and form urine, which is then passed down the ureters into the urinary bladder. When the bladder becomes full, urine is then passed through the urethra and is eliminated.

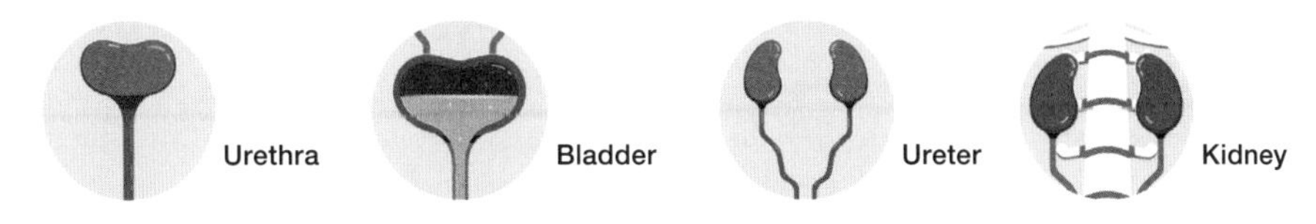

Once you've identified the component part, you can return to the exercise at the beginning of this chapter and continue to Step 3 (Association).

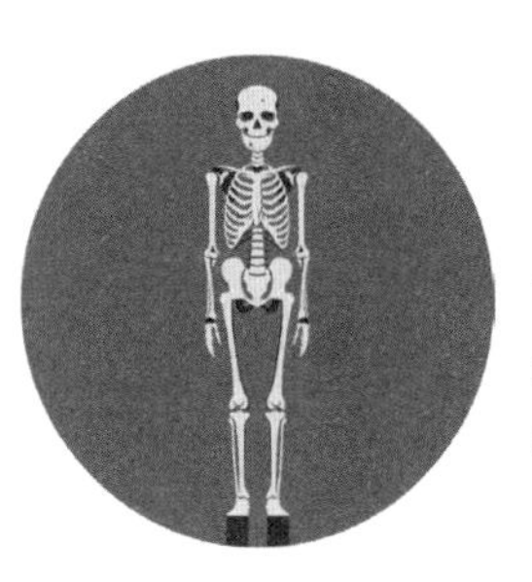

SKELETAL SYSTEM

EXPLANATION

The skeletal system is made up of bones and connective tissue, such as ligaments and tendons, which shape the body and protect the organs. The skeletal system works with the muscular system to help the body move.

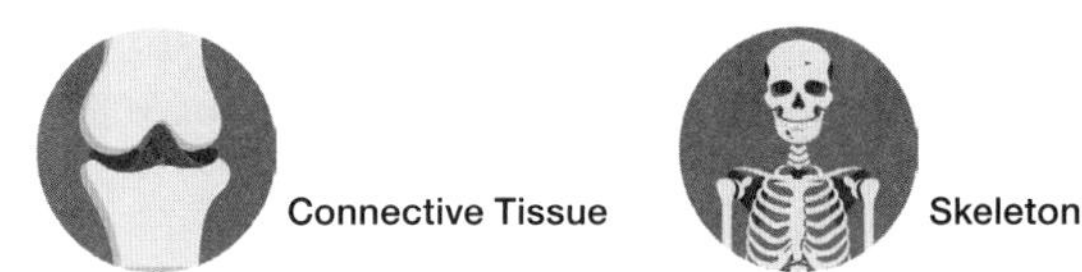

You can test even further if you want to by reading about each of these component parts below and testing the categories within each part. If you do not wish to identify the specific part, you can return to the exercise at the beginning of this chapter and continue to Step 3 (Association).

CONNECTIVE TISSUE

If you find that the connective tissue is imbalanced, ask if you need to know which component part is imbalanced. If yes, test the following one by one until you get a yes answer.

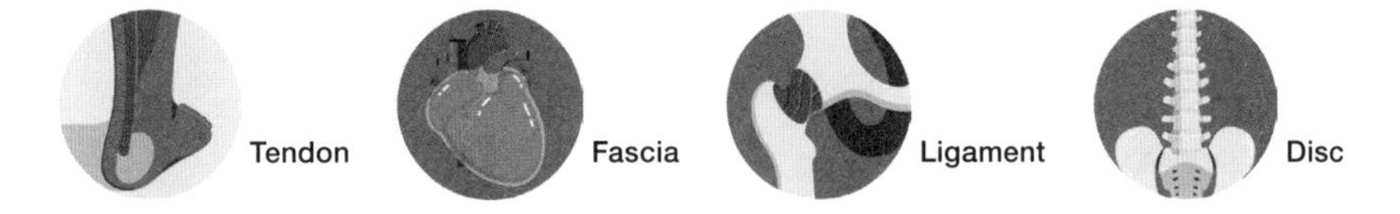

Tendons connect muscle to bone and are found on both ends of every muscle in the body. The fascia covers and separates all the muscles in the body, one from another. In addition, the fascia provides a protective coating for every bone, organ, artery, vein, and tissue of the body. Ligaments connect bone to bone and are found throughout the body, wherever two bones adjoin.

Discs are the shock absorbers of the body. You can think of each disc as being like a "jelly doughnut" made of concentric layers of cartilage, surrounding a gelatinous center called the nucleus pulposus. It's a brilliant design, because the gelatinous center acts like a ball bearing between each vertebra, transferring weight down the spine in a very efficient way.

Sometimes discs bulge. When they do so, they invariably put pressure on the spinal nerve nearby. When the nerve is compressed, the result is usually either pain or some sort of numbness or tingling, usually in the arm or leg. The general rule of thumb is that the more pressure there is on a nerve, the worse the numbness or tingling will be. If the pressure gets bad enough, there will be total anesthesia, or complete lack of feeling. This is never something to play around with, of course. If you or someone you are working on is dealing with this problem or having these symptoms, if they don't improve right away from what you do, you should refer them to a chiropractor or other health provider.

There are all kinds of things that can make a disc bulge. In my experience, the most common thing is actually some sort of organ imbalance. The reason for this is that the organ imbalance will always cause muscle imbalance. The biggest culprits here are the kidneys because of their connection with the psoas muscles, which support the lumbar spine. Just remember that anything can cause anything. I have seen infections and trauma energies in discs before, as well as trapped emotions and other energies that can imbalance the spine, causing the spinal discs to bulge and cause pain, tingling, and numbness.

SKELETON

If you are guided to the skeleton, ask if you need to know which part is imbalanced. If yes, the skeleton can be broken down into two main divisions, referred to as the appendicular skeleton and the axial skeleton. Ask in which of these two the imbalance can be found.

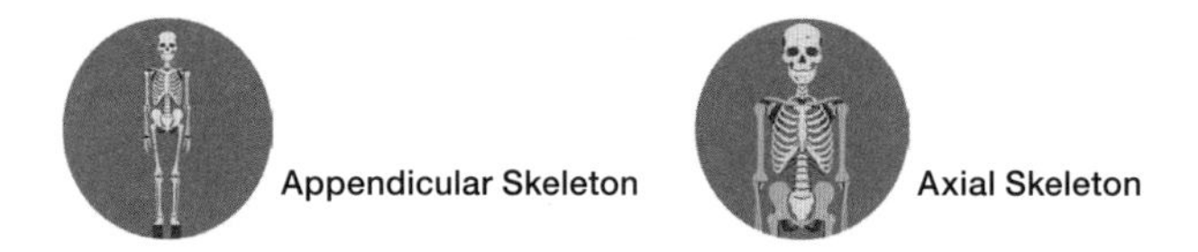

APPENDICULAR SKELETON

Because there are so many bones in the body, some areas are referred to simply by region.

If you find that the appendicular skeleton is imbalanced, ask if you need to know which region is imbalanced. If yes, test the following regions one by one until you get a yes answer.

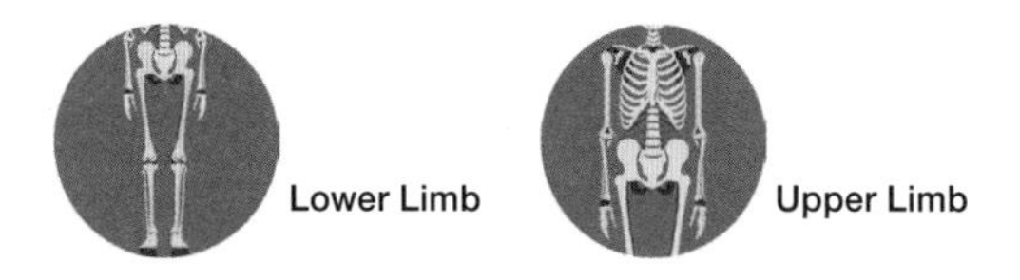

The appendicular skeleton includes the bones of the upper limbs, including the shoulder blades, or scapulae, and the collarbones, or clavicles, as well as the bones of the upper and lower arms, wrists, and hands. In addition, it includes the bones of the pelvis and the bones of the lower limbs, including the femur bones, tibia, fibula, and the bones of the ankle and foot. You can test each of these bones or areas if you would like to identify the exact bone that is imbalanced.

AXIAL SKELETON

If you find that the connective tissue is imbalanced, ask if you need to know which component part is imbalanced. If yes, test these one by one until you get a yes answer.

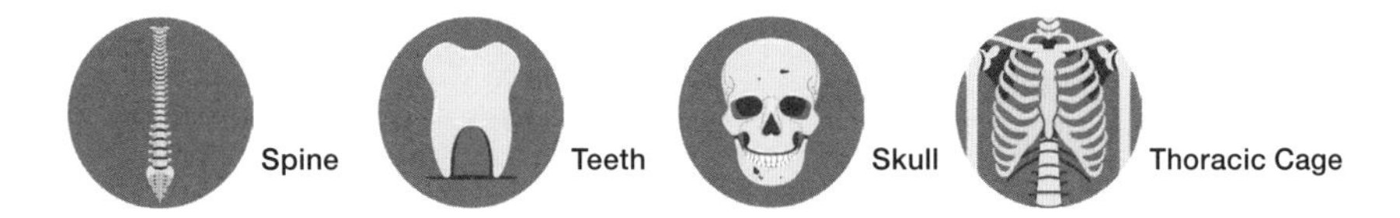

In the axial skeleton, the skull is a dynamic, amazing structure that is capable of far more movement than the medical or dental profession believes. As the skull expands and contracts between six and fourteen times per minute, each cranial bone moves very slightly. Sometimes cranial bones become misaligned very slightly. Sometimes the movement between one cranial bone and another becomes impinged. The biggest underlying cause of this sort of problem is trapped emotions. As a lifelong student of craniopathy, the branch of healing that addresses the craniosacral respiratory mechanism and its importance in controlling the central nervous system, I understand the dramatic difference that it can make to have all of the bones of the skull functioning normally.

Alignment of the spinal vertebrae is especially important because the spinal column houses the spinal cord, which is like the freeway connecting the brain to the rest of the body. If a vertebra is out of alignment, it can impede the communication between the brain and the body.

MUSCULAR SYSTEM

EXPLANATION

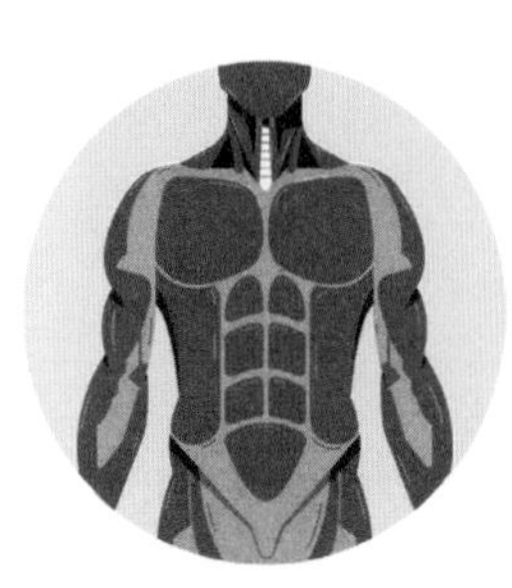

The muscular system includes smooth muscle, cardiac muscle tissue, and skeletal muscle. Smooth muscle is considered to be an involuntary type of muscle, since you can't consciously make it contract like you can a skeletal muscle. It's found in the walls of blood vessels, lymphatic vessels, the bladder, uterus, male and female reproductive tracts, the digestive system, the respiratory system, the skin (tiny muscles in the skin make your hair stand on end when you get gooseflesh), and the iris of the eye.

Cardiac muscle tissue is a highly specialized type of muscle that only exists in the heart. It's designed to contract automatically and relax in a continuous cycle that lasts your whole life.

Skeletal muscle, unlike the first two types, is under conscious control and is what moves the skeleton, enabling us to run and jump and walk, comb our hair, and do everything else we do.

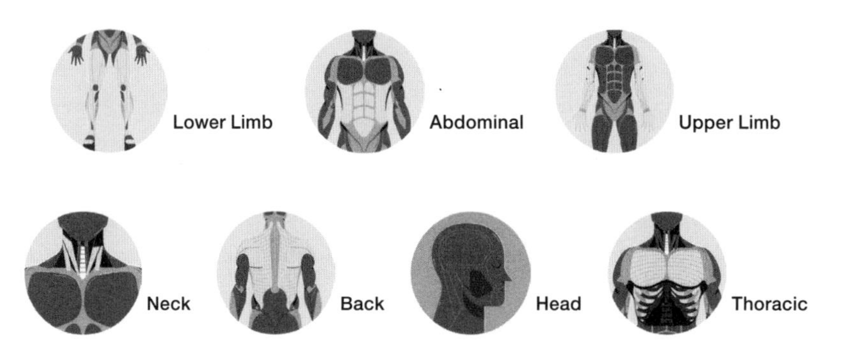

You can return to the exercise at the beginning of this chapter and continue to Step 3 (Association).

Note that most muscle imbalances are actually the result of an imbalance in an organ or gland. In other words, an organ or gland becomes overloaded and imbalanced, and the muscle that is energetically connected to that organ or gland also becomes imbalanced.

RESPIRATORY SYSTEM

EXPLANATION

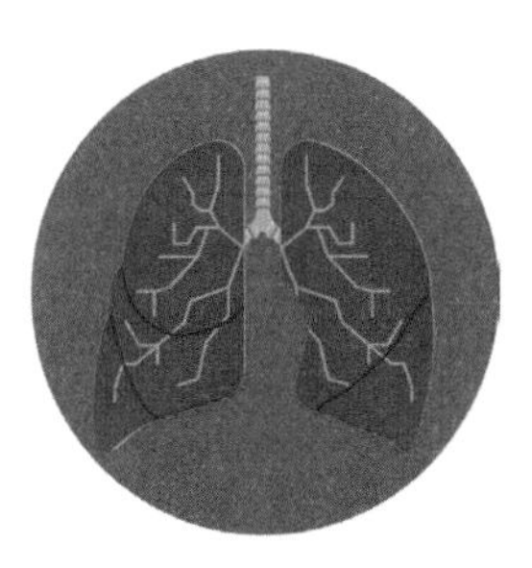

The respiratory system brings oxygen into the body and removes carbon dioxide through the act of breathing. Air enters the body through the nose and mouth, passes down the trachea, or windpipe, is diverted into either the left or right bronchial tube, and passes into progressively smaller tubules, referred to as bronchioles. Eventually it ends up in the alveoli, where oxygen is actively absorbed across the alveolar membrane into the blood, and carbon dioxide passes from the blood and is exhaled.

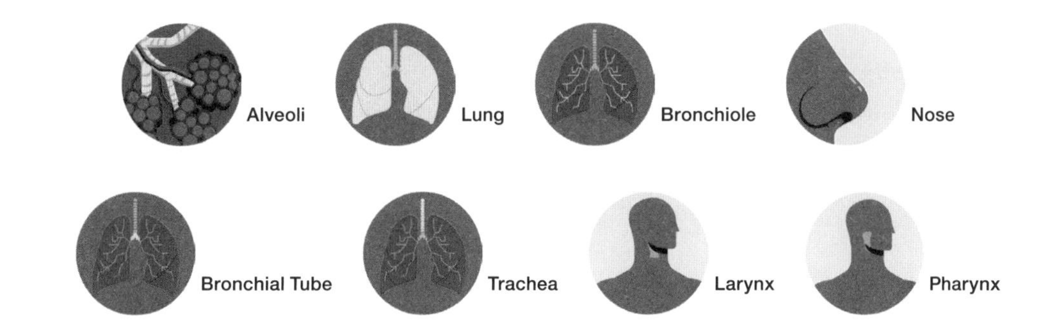

REPRODUCTIVE SYSTEM

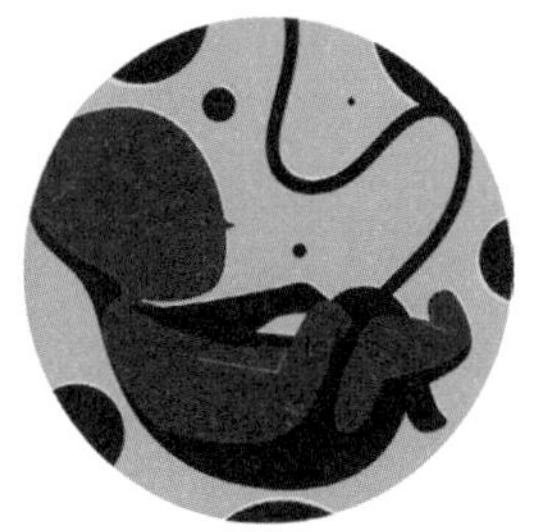

EXPLANATION

The reproductive system is what ensures our survival as a species. Sperm from the male may fertilize the female's egg, or ovum, in the fallopian tube. The fertilized egg then travels from the fallopian tube to the uterus, where it may implant itself in the uterine wall. The fetus would then develop over a period of nine months.

The reproductive system also works closely with other organs and organ systems. For example, the hypothalamus and pituitary gland help regulate the production and release of hormones such as estrogen and testosterone.

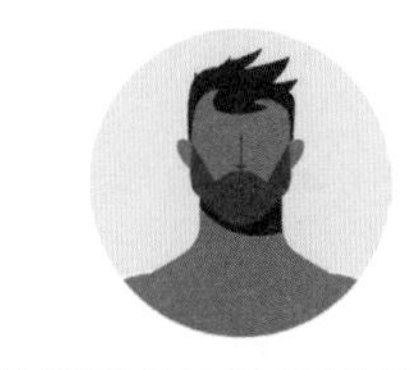

MALE REPRODUCTIVE SYSTEM

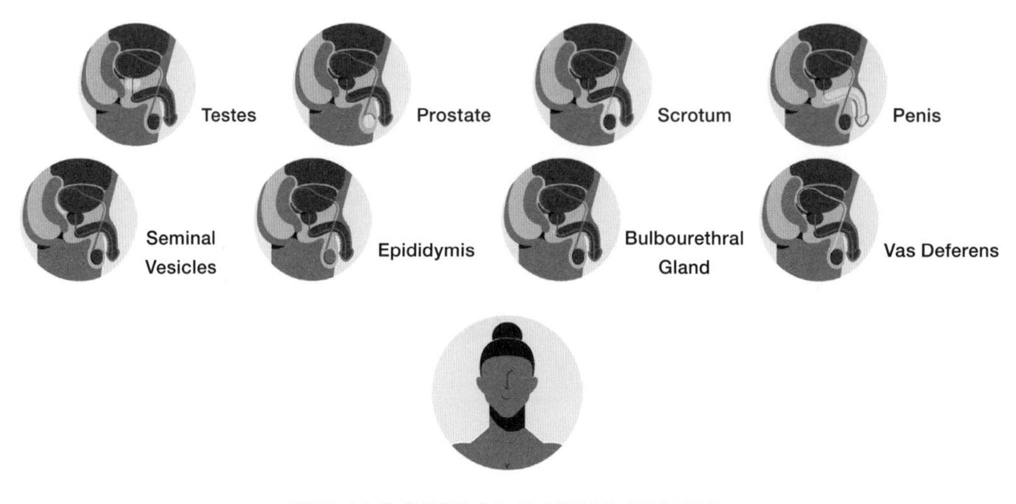

FEMALE REPRODUCTIVE SYSTEM

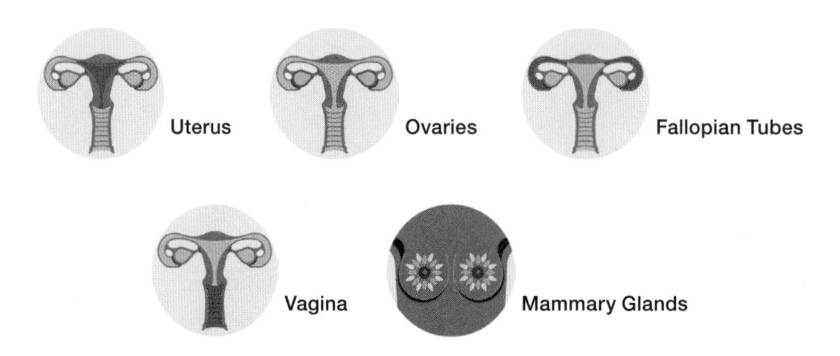

Once you've identified the component part, you can return to the exercise at the beginning of this chapter and continue to Step 3 (Association).

CIRCULATORY SYSTEM

EXPLANATION

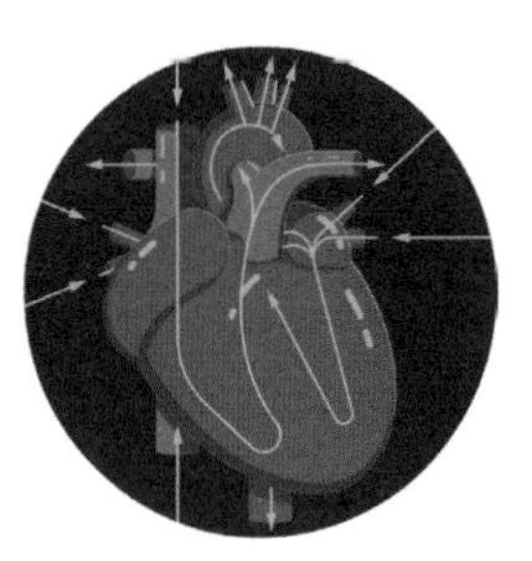

The circulatory system facilitates the movement of blood, lymph, and nutrients throughout the body. This helps to provide nourishment to the body tissues, fight infection, regulate body temperature, and maintain homeostasis. The circulatory system includes not only the heart, but also all of the miles of vessels, including arteries, veins, and capillaries that carry blood to and from all parts of the body.

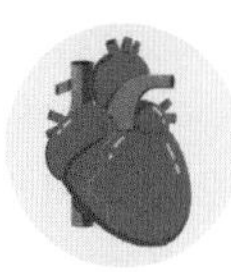

Heart

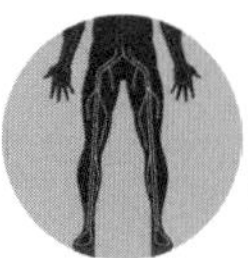

Lower Limb Vessel

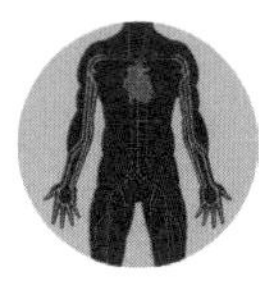

Upper Limb Vessel

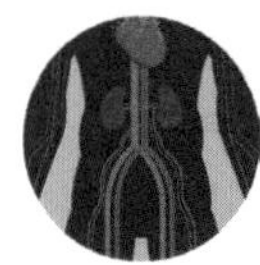

Abdominal Vessel

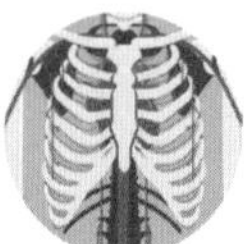

Thoracic Vessel

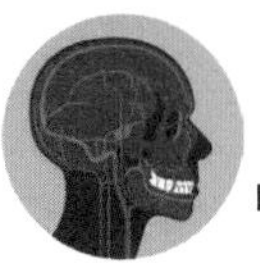

Head or Neck Vessel

Once you've identified the component part, you can return to the exercise at the beginning of this chapter and continue to Step 3 (Association).

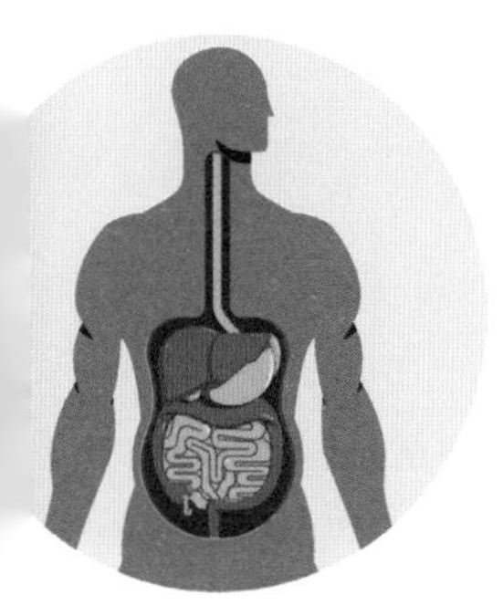

DIGESTIVE SYSTEM

EXPLANATION

The digestive system is responsible for the breakdown and extraction of nutrients from the food and drink that we consume. Digestion begins in the mouth, where the teeth grind up the food and mix it with saliva, which contains salivary amylase, an enzyme that begins to break down and digest starch that we've eaten.

The muscular action induced by swallowing propels the food down the esophagus, through the cardiac sphincter, which relaxes to allow the food to pass, and into the stomach. Churning of the stomach and secretion of hydrochloric acid and pepsin, an enzyme that digests protein, continues the digestive process.

Hydrochloric acid in particular can be very damaging to the walls of the stomach, so the stomach secretes a layer of mucus to act as a barrier to its contents. After an hour or two, the stomach contents (now referred to as chyme) pass through the pyloric sphincter and enter the small intestine, where digestive enzymes from the pancreas are secreted into the mix. About 95 percent of nutrient absorption occurs in the small intestine, while water and minerals are reabsorbed back into the blood from the colon. The next step is for the fecal matter to be eliminated from the colon through the rectum and the anus.

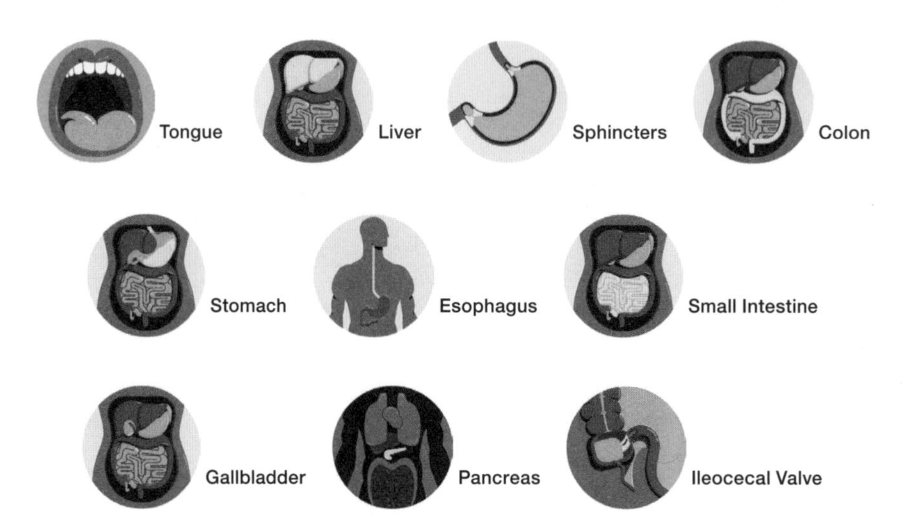

You can read more about most of these in chapter 12, "The Organs." Once you've identified the component part, you can return to the exercise at the beginning of this chapter and continue to Step 3 (Association).

ENDOCRINE SYSTEM

EXPLANATION

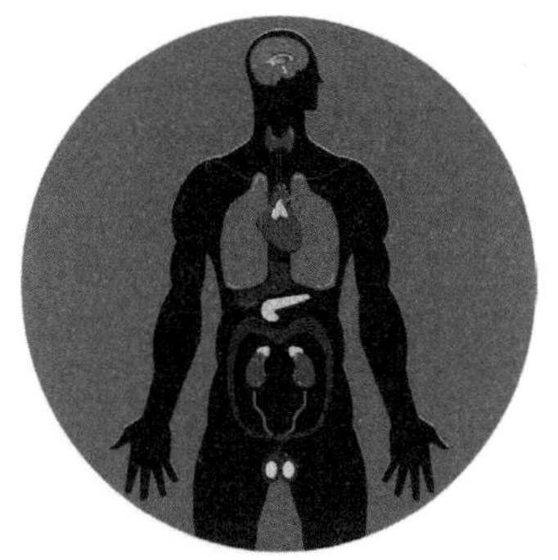

The endocrine system is a series of glands that secrete hormones directly into the bloodstream. Hormones are responsible for regulating all sorts of functions in the body, including metabolism, growth and development, tissue function, sleep, and mood.

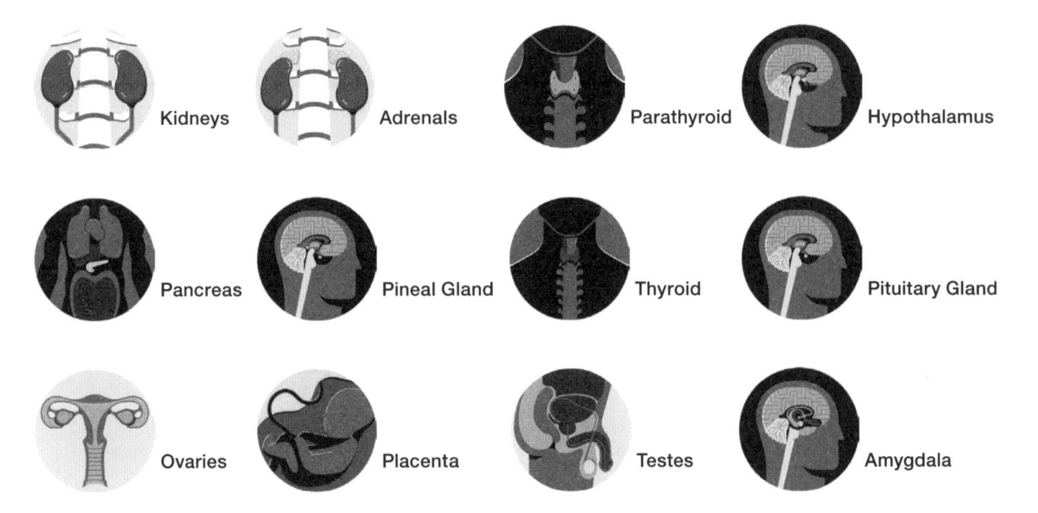

You can read more about all of these glands individually in chapter 13, "The Glands." Once you've identified the component part, you can return to the exercise at the beginning of this chapter and continue to Step 3 (Association).

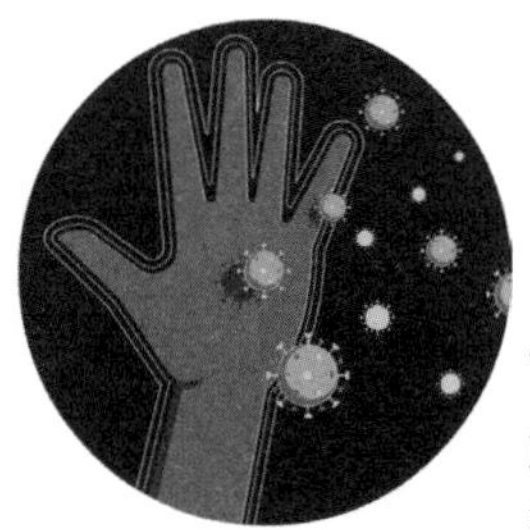

IMMUNE/LYMPHATIC SYSTEM

EXPLANATION

The function of the immune system is to protect the body against disease, particularly against disease caused by outside invaders, such as bacteria, viruses, molds, fungi, and parasites.

I've always believed that determining how well the immune system is actually functioning is a wonderful indicator of how healthy a person really is. During the years that I was in practice, I found that people who had been diagnosed with some sort of major problem, such as fibromyalgia, chronic fatigue, lupus, cancer, etc., would typically have an immune system that was functioning below 10 percent.

This is easy to determine through muscle testing, and it's also fascinating to watch the immune system improve as you make corrections using the Body Code. I have seen the release of a single trapped emotion improve a person's immune function by as much as 20 percent. It's important to note that any imbalance that is listed in the Body Code will have the effect of lowering immune function, and conversely, the correction of any imbalance will serve to improve immune function.

The lymphatic system filters out disease-causing organisms, produces white blood cells, and generates disease-fighting antibodies. It consists of a network of ducts and glands that carry a clear fluid known as lymph. Lymph fluid is actually formed from blood plasma, which filters into the lymph system from the circulatory system. The lymphatic system plays an important role in immune function, as it produces different types of white blood cells, or lymphocytes, and is important for the removal of toxic waste products from cells.

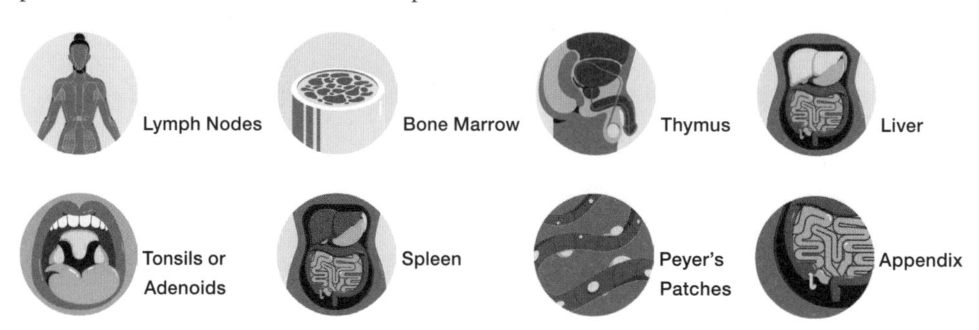

Once you've identified the component part, you can return to the exercise at the beginning of this chapter and continue to Step 3 (Association). If you are unfamiliar with Peyer's Patches, they are small egg-shaped lymph nodes that line the outside of the small intestine, helping the immune system to respond to pathogenic organisms in the gut.

NERVOUS SYSTEM

EXPLANATION

The nervous system is the body's communication system. It coordinates all of the activities of the body, whether voluntary or involuntary, and enables communication and the relay of information between different parts of the body. It consists of the central nervous system (the brain and spinal cord) and the peripheral nervous system (the nerves that connect the central nervous system to the rest of the body).

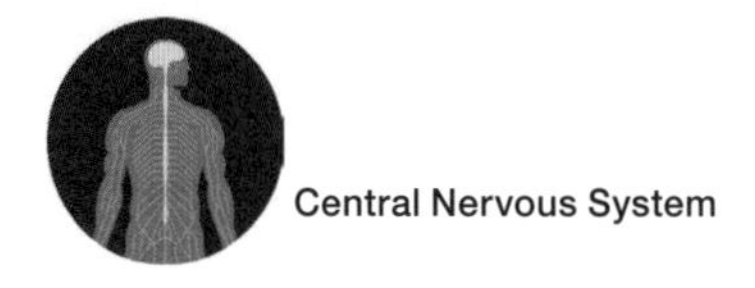

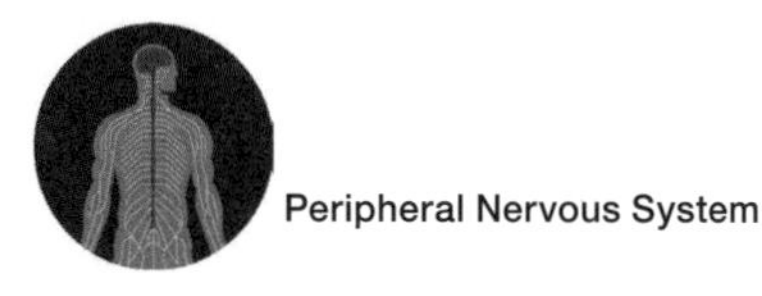

THE CENTRAL NERVOUS SYSTEM

The central nervous system is divided into the brain and the spinal cord.

THE BRAIN

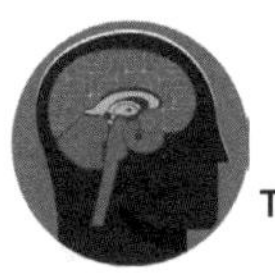
The Brain

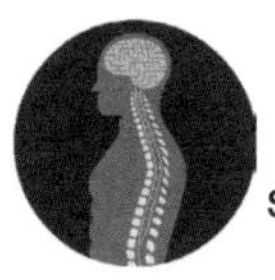
Spinal Cord

If the body can be compared to a machine, the brain is the computer within that machine. An adult brain weighs around three pounds and consists of more than 100 billion nerves that communicate with each other over trillions of junctions called synapses. The brain is the hardware interface for the physical body and the spirit. Through the brain you are able to live and move. It regulates all the functions of your physical body including hunger, temperature control, heartbeat, digestion, breathing, vision, motor skills, and more, and controls memory, thought, touch sensation, and all the other processes that are needed to keep your body alive and functioning.

THE SPINAL CORD

The spinal cord is the brain's information superhighway that enables it to communicate with all the organs, glands, muscles, and tissues of the body. Communications are constantly traveling to and from the brain and all parts of the body by way of the spinal cord. Extending from the base of the skull to the lower back, the spinal cord is protected by the spinal vertebra. Thirty-one pairs of spinal nerves branch out from the spinal cord, connecting the brain with all the tissues of the body.

THE PERIPHERAL NERVOUS SYSTEM

The peripheral nervous system is divided into the somatic nervous system and the autonomic nervous system.

SOMATIC NERVOUS SYSTEM

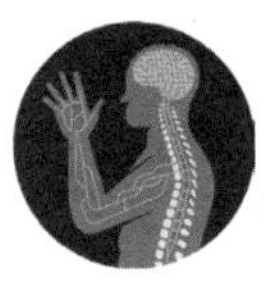
Somatic Nervous System

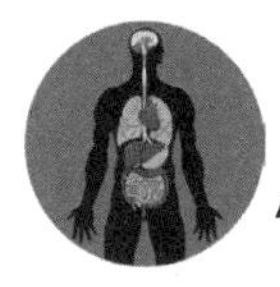
Autonomic Nervous System

The somatic nervous system is responsible for carrying impulses and information to and from the central nervous system to all the muscles and other tissues of the body.

AUTONOMIC NERVOUS SYSTEM

The autonomic nervous system is divided into three parts, the sympathetic, enteric, and parasympathetic nervous systems.

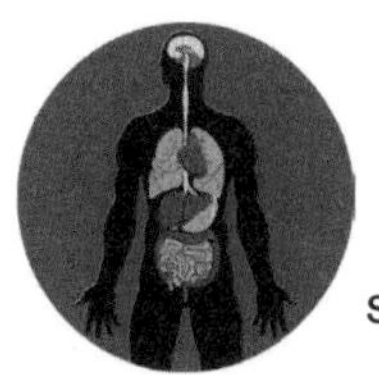

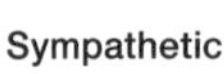

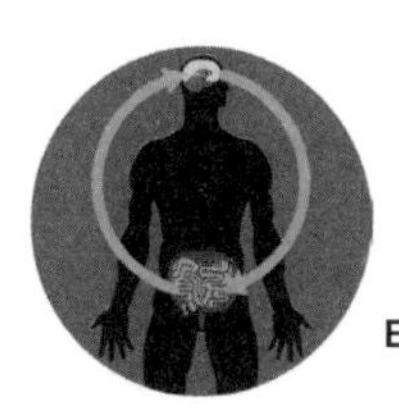

Enteric

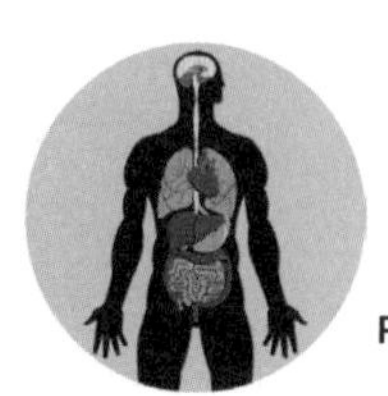

Parasympathetic

Sympathetic Nervous System

The sympathetic nervous system is most responsible for the "fight or flight" response, but it's also responsible for helping us to maintain homeostasis, and thus it is always active to some degree.

Enteric Nervous System

The enteric nervous system is responsible for both secretion and motility and is basically considered a separate, stand-alone nervous system that belongs solely to the digestive system. Although it functions on its own, it may be modified by the sympathetic or parasympathetic nervous systems.

Parasympathetic Nervous System

The parasympathetic nervous system is the division of the autonomic nervous system that is responsible for the activities that occur in the body when we are relaxed, resting, or eating, including digestion, sexual activities, urination, salivation, defecation, lacrimation (crying), and so on.

You can return to the exercise at the beginning of this chapter and continue to Step 3 (Association).

This concludes the systems section. Next, we will discuss disconnections between the physical and energy body, or spirit.

15

DISCONNECTIONS

Nature is the source of all true knowledge. She has her own logic, her own laws; she has no effect without cause nor invention without necessity.

—LEONARDO DA VINCI

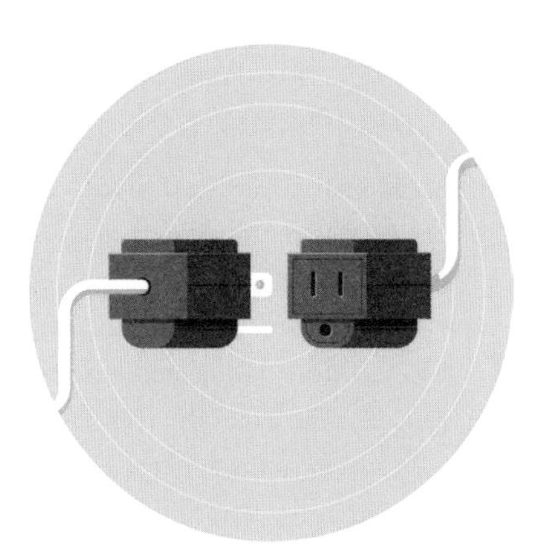

Disconnections refer to interruptions in energetic communication that occur between the spirt and body, as well as between various components of the body.

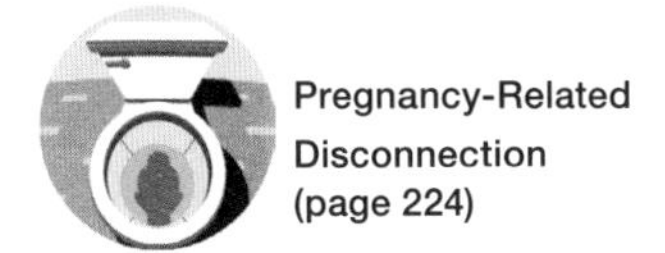

Pregnancy-Related Disconnection (page 224)

Spiritual/Physical Disconnection (page 225)

Spirit Out of Body (page 229)

PREGNANCY-RELATED DISCONNECTION

EXPLANATION

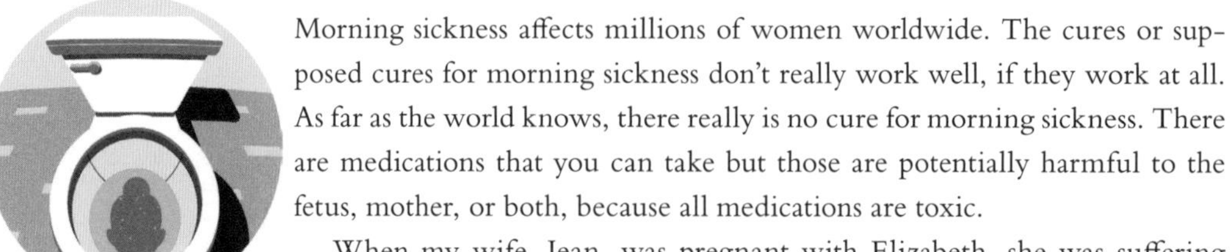

Morning sickness affects millions of women worldwide. The cures or supposed cures for morning sickness don't really work well, if they work at all. As far as the world knows, there really is no cure for morning sickness. There are medications that you can take but those are potentially harmful to the fetus, mother, or both, because all medications are toxic.

When my wife, Jean, was pregnant with Elizabeth, she was suffering with morning sickness. She asked me to help her, and I immediately started thinking of all the things that I knew that were supposed remedies; things that I had tried before with her or with other patients that had never really worked, but that might take the edge off the morning sickness, like ginger, wristbands, etc.

DISCONNECTION

Without any real viable options that I knew of, I decided to turn to the Higher Power and ask for some help. The answer that came to me was that morning sickness is caused by a disconnection between the brain of the mother and her growing fetus.

What I found was the brain is sometimes not initially connected with this new life that is growing within. Essentially, the brain has to be connected energetically with the fetus, with the umbilical cord, with the amniotic fluid (the fluid that the baby floats in), and the placenta (the lining of the uterus that connects the baby to the mother). Until the brain is connected with these four different parts, there will be morning sickness. The moment that the connection is made between these parts and the brain, the morning sickness disappears, usually instantly.

TESTING FOR DISCONNECTION

Here's the process. Simply ask the following questions: "Is your brain connected to the fetus?" If the answer is yes, then you go to the next question. "Is your brain connected to the umbilical cord?" If that's a yes, go to the next question. "Is your brain connected to the amniotic fluid?" And if that's a yes, you'd ask, "Is your brain connected to the placenta?" If any of these questions test weak, you reconnect the brain to that particular component by swiping a magnet or your hand over any length of the governing meridian three times.

Then you would retest by asking these same questions again, correcting any imbalances until they all test strong. If you have trouble correcting any particular connection, the reason will most often be a trapped emotion that can easily be found and released.

I found that this communication is a two-way process. In other words, the communication flows from the brain down to these parts, and from these parts up to the brain. So once you have corrected any imbalances from the brain down to these parts, then you need to reverse the process and ask the following, starting with: "Is the fetus connected to your brain?" If that tests strong, go to the next one. "Is the umbilical cord connected to your brain? Is the amniotic fluid connected to your brain? Is the placenta connected to your brain?" If any of these questions test weak, reconnect by swiping *up* the governing meridian three times and then retest. In other words, if you ask, "Is the fetus connected to your brain?" and you get a weak muscle test or you sway backward, then that answer is no and you'd swipe up the governing meridian.

Let me clarify here. When you swipe up the governing meridian, you might start on the low back and swipe a magnet or your hand up from the low back area toward the head three times. If you were doing this on yourself, to swipe up the governing meridian you would start at the back of the neck and go over the top of the head to the forehead three times.

I've seen a good number of morning-sick women over the years since I was led to this knowledge, and I haven't had anyone yet that this has not helped. Often the effect is immediate and quite dramatic.

As soon as you make those connections, typically the morning sickness will be gone instantly. What women most often say is, "I feel better, I'm going to go eat something." I think that you'll enjoy this one, it's something that you won't find anywhere else but the Body Code.

SPIRITUAL/PHYSICAL DISCONNECTION

EXPLANATION

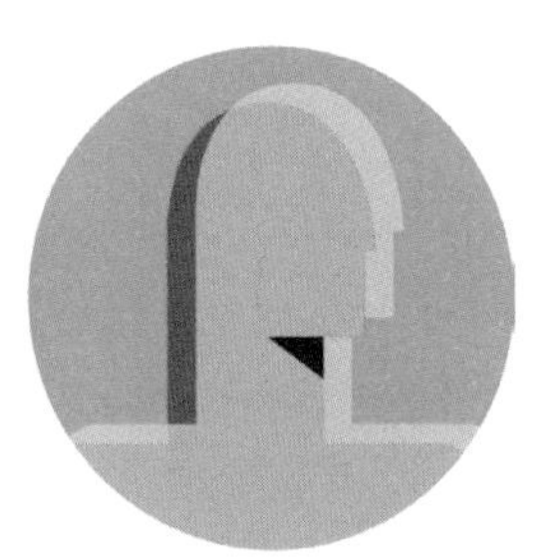

To understand spirit/physical disconnection, you have to understand a little bit about our dual nature. I personally believe that each of us have always existed as separate and distinct intelligences, without beginning. I believe that we have always existed and that we will always exist. I also believe that ages ago, God, our Heavenly Father, organized our intelligences into spirit bodies for us and he gave us our agency, or our freedom to choose. This earth was created to provide a place for us to be able to progress, and our physical bodies are in the express perfect image of our spirit bodies. In other words, if you could take the spirit out of your body right now and put it right next to you, I believe that it would look exactly like you, in the most minute detail.

THE SPIRIT-BODY TEMPLATE

This is the template that our physical body grows into, I believe. I also believe that having a physical body is a critical part of our progression in this world and in the worlds to come.

The questions that I had for many years were "How does it work? What is the connection? How does the physical body connect with the spirit body and vice versa, and is it possible that this interface itself is susceptible to imbalance?" Although we still do not understand the interface, it can indeed break down.

Any part of the physical body can become disconnected from the spirit body. Now, of course if your spirit disconnects from your physical body completely, we call that death, and they're going to be planning your funeral. But it is possible for the spirit and the physical body to be disconnected to quite a large degree sometimes, and you will still be alive. However, you may not be feeling very well if this happens, as the physical body definitely needs the intelligence of the spirit to operate efficiently.

Shortly after I discovered a way to correct disconnections of this type, a woman came into my office who had pain from the base of her skull all the way down to her low back, which she described as 9.5 on a 0 to 10 scale. When I checked her, her entire physical body, her head and her neck, her chest, and her abdomen were all completely disconnected from the spirit within her.

By simply reconnecting the spirit to the physical body, her pain level went from a 9.5 to about a 2 immediately.

The result of disconnection between the spirit body and the physical body is misalignment of bones, lowered immunity, organ and gland malfunction, and I believe it can be a contributing factor in cancer as well. I believe one of the reasons why we get cancer is because of disconnection between the spirit and the physical body. Think about it this way: the spirit is the intelligence within you, the physical body is really just the hardware; it's the walking, talking computer system, if you will, and if there is a disconnection that occurs so that the physical body and the spirit are no longer communicating, then it can create a situation where cancer may arise.

TESTING FOR DISCONNECTION

So, to check for this problem you might ask something like this:

"Is your spirit fully communicating with your body?" If the answer is no, to dig deeper you might ask, "Is your spirit fully communicating with your head or your neck? Is your spirit fully communicating with your thorax? Is your spirit fully communicating with your abdomen? Or the right arm? The left arm? The left leg? The right leg?"

These seem to be the regions that the spirit and body use as far as communication. It's broken down into these areas. Head, neck, thorax, abdomen, right arm, left arm, left leg, and right leg.

RECONNECTING THE SPIRIT/PHYSICAL BODY

I remember when I had a patient once who came to see me who had pain in her right foot. I tested to see what was wrong and found a misaligned bone in her foot. But she also had a disconnection between the spirit and the body, and it just so happened that it was that entire leg that was disconnected. I reconnected it by simply swiping down the back, down the governing meridian three times, and immediately she was able to walk with no limp. When she'd walked in, she had a pronounced limp and it just took a matter of seconds to make this reconnection. Suddenly she was able to get up and walk without any limp at all. After taking a few steps she whirled around and exclaimed, "How did you do that? What did you do?" All I had done was pass a magnet down her back three times with an intention to fix this disconnection, but the result was an instant reconnection of her spirit with her physical leg, resulting in immediate self-correction of the misalignment in her foot!

You see, when the spirit and the physical body become disconnected, it allows misalignments to continue and to remain uncorrected. If the brain really wanted to, couldn't it reconnect or realign bones that are out of alignment? Why doesn't it do it? I believe that one of the big reasons why it doesn't do it is because of this phenomenon of disconnection.

TESTING FOR COMMUNICATION

To check for communication problems in the other direction, you might simply ask these questions in reverse. Is your body fully communicating with your spirit? In other words, this is a two-way communication. Your spirit has to communicate to your physical body and your physical body has to communicate to your spirit.

RECONNECTING THE SPIRIT/PHYSICAL BODY

As we saw with morning sickness, you may need to correct this sort of communication breakdown in two directions. In other words, If you find imbalances between the spirit and the physical body, if it's the spirit that is disconnected from the physical, then you'll correct by swiping a magnet or your hand down the governing meridian three times. If it's the physical that is disconnected from the spirit, it's corrected by swiping up the governing meridian.

Just think of the spirit as being a higher vibration. So to connect spirit to body you are going from a higher vibration (spirit) to a lower vibration (physical body) and so you roll down the governing meridian. And by the same token, if some part of the body is not communicating with the spirit then you'd roll up from the physical body to the spirit.

So if you ask the question, "Is your body fully communicating with your spirit?" and if the answer is no, you might ask, "Is your head fully communicating with your spirit? Is your spirit fully communicating with your head? Is your thorax fully communicating with your spirit?" and so on. You could also ask, of course, about the left and right arm and the left and right leg.

FINDING SPECIFIC DISCONNECTIONS

Sometimes a region of the body will contain a smaller area of tissue that is disconnected. For example, a specific muscle, organ, gland, bone, or other tissue may be disconnected. If disconnection shows up while scanning the body but no specific region seems to be the problem, you might ask, "Is this a disconnection of something within the head (or within the neck or within the abdomen or the chest)?" and so on. This will lead to this specific tissue that is disconnected.

For example, if you're working with someone who has a low back problem you might ask, "Is there a disconnection between spirit and abdomen or between the spirit and your low back?" Or, "Is there a disconnection between this region of the body and the spirit?" And if you get an answer that is affirmative to that question, then you'd simply either roll up or roll down depending on if you're trying to reconnect that part of the body to the spirit or the spirit to that part of the body.

FULL-DUPLEX COMMUNICATION

Most often, you will find disconnections like this when you are using the Body Code Mind Map.

Remember that this is a full-duplex communication. What does that mean? A walkie-talkie, for example, is not a full-duplex communication device because only one person can talk at a time. A telephone, on the other hand, is a full-duplex communication device, meaning two people can talk at the same time. This needs to be checked both ways. You need to check for spirit communication to the physical and then if that one is blown or imbalanced, you would roll down the governing meridian three times to correct it. You also need to check for physical connection to spirit. You roll up the governing meridian three times, and again, if you're doing this on yourself and you need to roll down the governing meridian, you'd simply go from the forehead in that direction. Go from the forehead toward the back of the neck, just like releasing a trapped emotion three times, and if you're going the opposite direction, you just start at the back of the neck and go over the head to the forehead.

SPIRIT OUT OF BODY

EXPLANATION

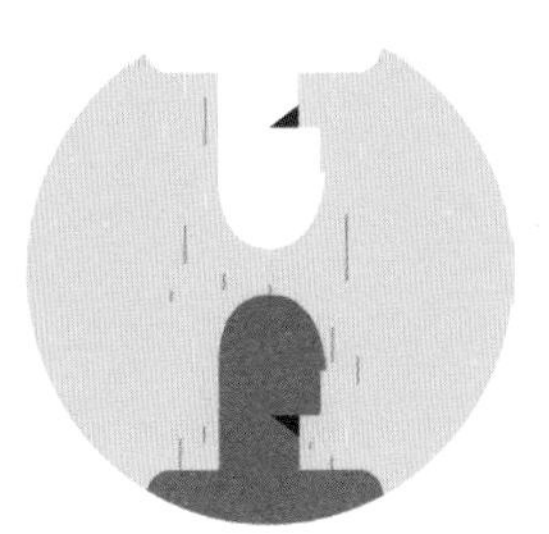

The next thing we're going to talk about is how the spirit can sometimes actually leave the body to some degree. Of course, death is the complete separation of the spirit and the body, but what about partial separation of spirit and body? This is different from a disconnection in that in this case, the spirit actually comes out of the body or is displaced out of the body to some degree.

The spirit may actually become dislodged from the physical body due to some kind of a physical trauma such as a fall, a car accident or some other kind of injury, or from some intense emotional stress, such as combat or torture and extremes of that sort.

SPIRIT/BODY SEPARATION

If a portion of the spirit is outside of the physical body, the result will be similar to a disconnection of spirit and body. The distinction involves the location of the spirit. In simple disconnection, the spirit body is where it should be, but it's not communicating to the physical body for some reason. But if the spirit is actually displaced out of the physical body to some degree, communication difficulties will be apparent in that case as well.

TESTING FOR SPIRIT/BODY SEPARATION

You can simply ask, "Is 100 percent of your spirit within your physical body?" If not, ask how much of the spirit is within the physical body, and determine a percentage. To correct it, simply roll down the governing meridian while you say, "I now bring your spirit back 100 percent into your physical body where it belongs." Then retest.

SECTION 4

MISALIGNMENTS

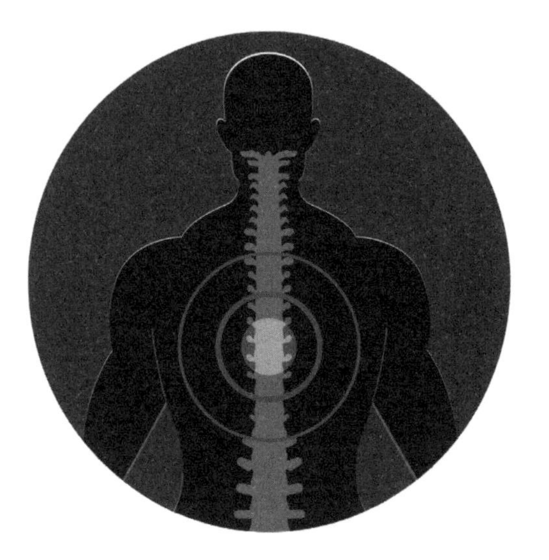

The physical concerns and misalignment we experience in the spinal vertebrae of our body are often directly correlated with the spiritual energetic ability to flow freely.

—DASHAMA KONAH GORDON

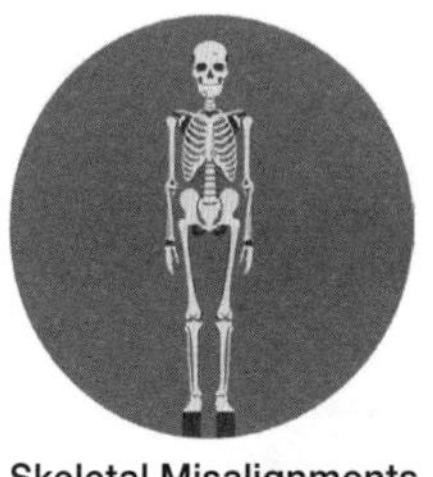

Skeletal Misalignments
(page 233)

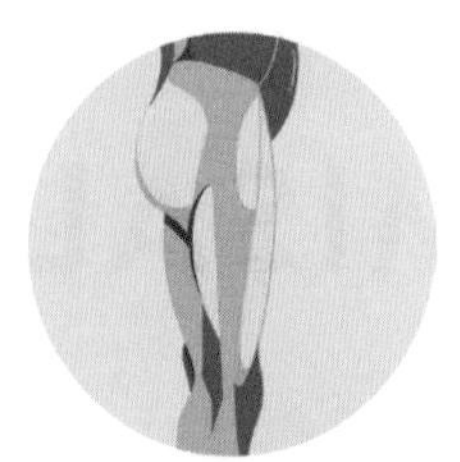

Soft Tissue Misalignments
(page 241)

The purpose of this next chapter is to help you to understand misalignments of bones and other tissues, how to identify them, and what to do to correct them.

16

SKELETAL MISALIGNMENTS

I feel it my bounden duty to not only replace displaced bones, but also teach others, so that the physical and spiritual may enjoy health, happiness, and the full fruition of our earthly lives.

—DANIEL DAVID PALMER

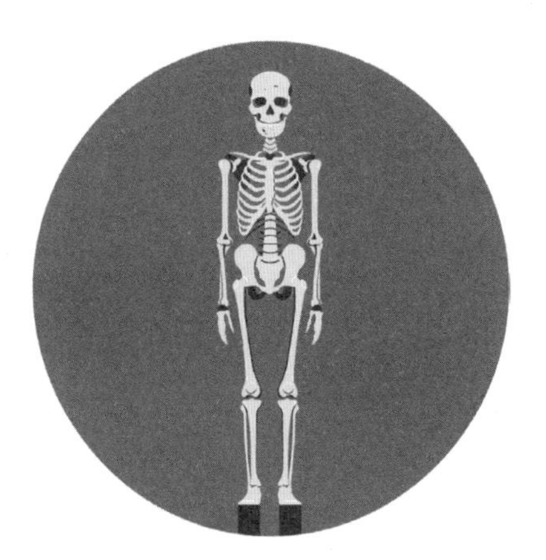

Structural misalignments are a major source of imbalance in the body because structure affects function. You probably know that doctors of chiropractic specialize in aligning bones, but did you know that any part of the physical and energetic body can become misaligned? I've found misalignments in bones, muscles, tendons, ligaments, nerves, organs, teeth, and even the eyeballs, chakras, and meridians, just to name a few.

To include all the tissues that can become misaligned is beyond the scope of this book, but they're included in the Body Code System app. Visit discoverhealing.com/app for more information.

The purpose of this chapter is not to teach you how to be a chiropractor or how to replace proper chiropractic care, but instead to teach you how to help your body attain and retain proper alignment and balance. I practiced for many years as a doctor of chiropractic starting in 1988, and

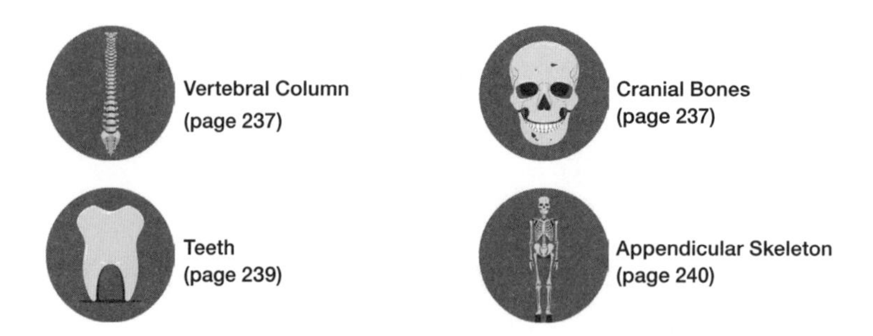

I have seen how profoundly important and life changing chiropractic care can be. When you use the Body Code you will find that your chiropractic adjustments last much longer by helping you to find and eliminate the underlying causes of misalignments.

STRUCTURE AFFECTS FUNCTION

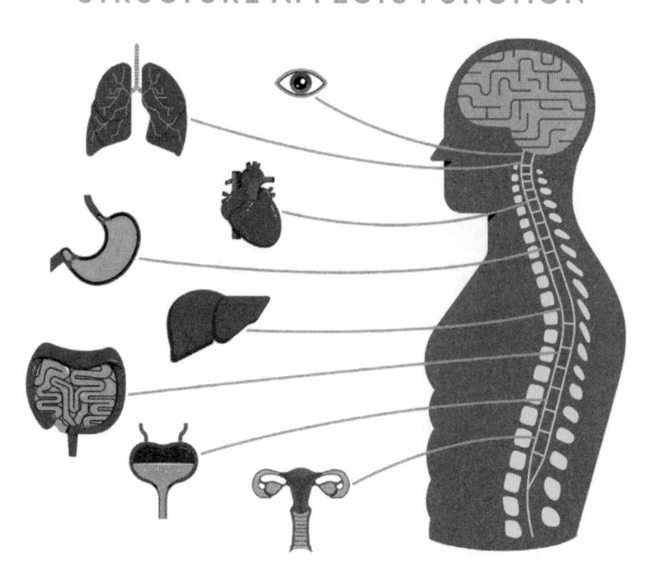

Take a look at this image of the spine, brain, and organs.

The lines represent the nerves that are carrying communications between the brain and the organs shown in the image. Messages originating in the brain travel down the spinal cord and ultimately along the nerves to their destination. The spinal cord is housed and protected by the vertebrae in the spinal column.

SPINAL MISALIGNMENT

Proper alignment of the spinal vertebrae allows nerve impulses to flow freely, but misalignment of these bones, known as subluxation, can result in reduced nerve transmission. This results in reduced communication between the brain and the organs and tissues of the body. When organs and tissues do not have good communication with the brain, the result may include reduced function, pain, and eventual disease.

It's important to realize how essential it is to have good communication between the brain and all of the parts of the body. For example, if you develop a misalignment in the upper back, it may create interference in the nerves that are traveling from the brain to the lungs. What symptoms might you eventually notice from nerve interference like this? If your lungs begin to malfunction, you may be more prone to respiratory infections and other lung problems. The following story shows how important it is to have good communication between the brain and the lungs.

ASTHMA AT THREE YEARS OLD

A woman brought her three-year-old son into my office one day. She explained that his birth had been complicated. He was born with the aid of forceps, which often results in misalignment of the upper bones in the neck. For the first year of his life, he had constant ear infections and was on one antibiotic after another, to no avail.

Around his first birthday he started wheezing and having difficulty breathing and was diagnosed with asthma. He was prescribed various medications for the next two years, one asthma medication after another, and when she brought him in to see me, he was using two inhalers and taking two oral medications. This was a very sick little boy.

What I found was that he simply had a misalignment at the third thoracic vertebra in the upper back, creating interference between his brain and his lungs. I only had to adjust him three times before the asthma symptoms completely disappeared. I can't recall having a patient with asthma that I was not able to help simply by correcting misalignments like this, and I know many other chiropractic physicians who have had the same experience.

If misalignment and nerve interference can contribute to asthma, what about all the other organs and glands and tissues?

It's impossible to overstate the importance of having good communications between your brain and the organs of your body. But it's something that most people give little if any thought to.

When finding and balancing the underlying cause for the misalignment, miraculous things sometimes happen, as Susanne found in the following story.

I Can Breathe Again

A patient in her sixties had had chronic obstructive pulmonary disease (COPD) for many years and rated her difficulty breathing at a 7 out of 10. We found a misalignment of the T3 vertebra, with an associated imbalance (one inherited trapped emotion), which we released. After that we were able to realign the misaligned T3 vertebra energetically. I asked her to get up and walk around a bit and tell me if she was able to breathe any better. After a couple of minutes, she was able to breathe in freely and deeply while walking, which she had been unable to do for many years! She felt like something had opened up inside her chest as if a load of bricks were taken from her. She immediately rated her difficulty breathing at a 0! She was as happy as can be! What a miracle! Thank you, Dr. Brad, for creating this amazing modality!

—Dr. Susanne H., Bayern, Germany

If trapped emotions and other imbalances such as physical trauma energies are not discovered and cleared, you may find yourself needing more frequent chiropractic adjustments, because the underlying causes have not been addressed. In the following story, Antonio shares his experience using the Body Code to keep his spine in proper alignment.

Fixing the Causes

I was told I'd have scoliosis my whole life. With clearing trapped emotions, all the misalignments and subluxations in my spine in different locations went back into alignment and there are no more subluxations. I realized that the trapped emotions were causing inflammation in the nerves, and the nerves connected to the vertebrae were sending bad signals to the different organs of the body. Clearing out all trapped emotions now has my spine, for the first time in my life, fully aligned, with no tightness or subluxations.

—Antonio S., Texas, United States

All of the components that make up the body are made of pure energy, whether they are muscles, tendons, ligaments, nerves, organs, soft tissues, or bones, and they are therefore capable of being corrected energetically, even at a distance. In my experience, some misalignments are more common than others, starting with the bones of the body.

VERTEBRAL COLUMN

EXPLANATION

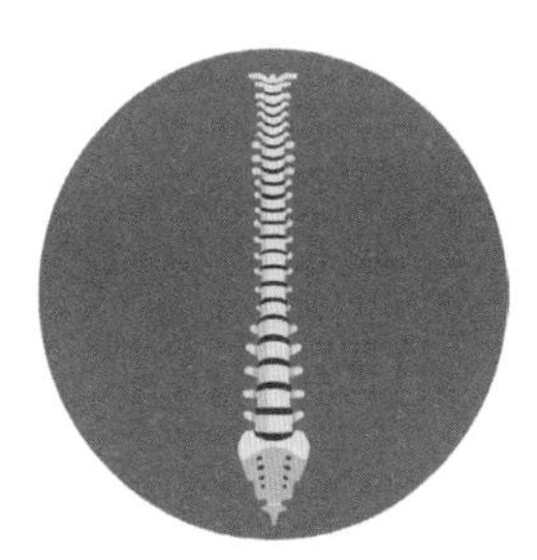

Misalignments that occur anywhere in the spinal column are potentially dangerous because of the interference that results from nerve impingement. As we discussed earlier, nerve interference that occurs from misaligned spinal vertebrae results in diminished or garbled communications between the brain and the organs and glands and other tissues of the body.

Misalignment of the first cervical vertebra, the uppermost vertebra in the neck, is the most dangerous misalignment of all. The reason for this is that it can create interference in the spinal cord itself, at a point where all the communications from the brain to the rest of the body are passing through it. C1, or the atlas vertebra as it is commonly referred to, is uniquely positioned as well as being anatomically different from all other vertebrae. Unique to the atlas vertebra are tiny hairlike ligaments that extend from the inside of the ring of this bone to the spinal cord itself. This is a reason misalignment of this bone can create so many varied kinds of problems, because of the direct interference that can occur in the spinal cord.

Remember that if you find a misalignment of any bone or any tissue, there will most often be an underlying cause or causes, and those will usually be trapped emotions. Clearing the underlying causes will usually result in an immediate correction of the misalignment. If not, simply swipe a few times with a magnet or your hand over the governing meridian with an intention to correct that misalignment and then ask if you have accomplished your goal.

CRANIAL BONES

EXPLANATION

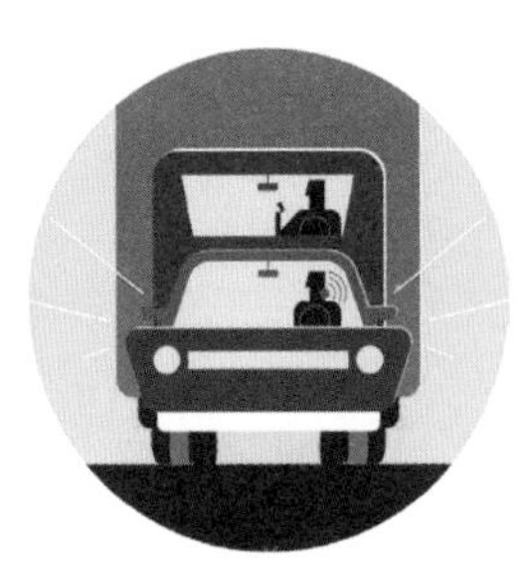

I had a fascinating experience when I was being treated by the holistic doctors that saved me from kidney disease.

I was lying on their treatment table one day when one of them began probing the roof of my mouth with a gloved hand. They said that I had a misalignment of one of the bones in my skull. They began applying gentle pressure to the roof of my mouth, when suddenly something moved. I felt no pain whatsoever, but I suddenly realized that the roof of my mouth had assumed a dome shape that had not been there before. It felt like I suddenly had twice as much room inside my mouth.

I filed this experience away in my mind but never forgot it. Many years later, when I went to chiropractic school, the first book I checked out of the library was a book about the bones of the skull, a book on craniopathy.

After I was in practice for a few years, I attended seminars taught by a renowned craniopath named Dr. David Denton. I learned that the bones of the skull move very slightly as a person breathes in and out. I learned how it is possible to manipulate and realign the bones of the skull and "unlock" the bones to restore their normal motion and function.

Sometimes bones can become misaligned, or blocked in their ability to expand or contract along the joint lines, or "suture lines" as they are commonly called.

It's funny to me how the skull has become a symbol of death and destruction. To me, the skull is a most wonderful and intricate creation. It is actually an incredibly complex three-dimensional jigsaw puzzle of the highest order, and yet it is far more malleable than most people think.

REARRANGING HER FACE

One day we worked on a lovely young woman with an unusual problem. Her face was a bit like a painting by Picasso. Her eyes were not symmetrical, as her left eye was approximately an inch lower on her face than her right eye. It gave her a striking appearance, but it was clear to me that this was not a normal and healthy situation. She told us that her vision had been growing progressively worse over the last few years in her left eye, and that her doctors had told her to expect total loss of sight in that eye within two years.

My wife, Jean, would often work with me as my assistant when I had cranial work to do. This young woman came into the office, and I began muscle-testing her, checking the different bones in her skull. We found a misalignment in both of her temporal bones, the bones that house the ear canals. They were twisted, and that was causing a disruption throughout her entire skull, interfering with the normal function of nearly every other bone.

Following Dr. Denton's procedures, with my wife applying gentle pressure at a certain point with a gloved hand inside this woman's mouth in order to "unlock" her temporal bones, I applied gentle pressure to the temporal bones themselves as she breathed deeply.

In this way, over several treatments we were able to realign her temporal bones. The result was astonishing. Her left eye was now nearly aligned with the other eye. To most physicians and biologists this would seem impossible, for the bones of the skull seem stagnant. When you look at a dried skull from a once-living human being, it seems that no movement could possibly take place.

The result for this young woman was that the deterioration of the vision in her left eye suddenly stopped and began to improve, and the change in her appearance was immediately obvious to everyone who knew her.

TEETH

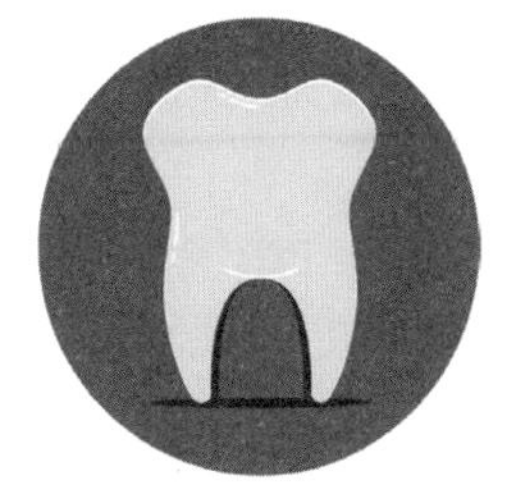

EXPLANATION

Any bone in the body can become misaligned, especially as a result of some sort of accident or physical trauma. This was the case with my son, Joseph, when he was five years old.

ALL I WANT FOR CHRISTMAS . . .

When Joseph was five, he was playing with his older brother, and his front upper teeth violently collided with his brother's head. His right front tooth was visibly bent backward. I gently moved it back into a more normal position, but wondered what was going to happen.

As you might guess, that tooth turned gray. I called our family dentist and explained what had happened. He assured me that the tooth was dead and there was nothing that could be done, but since it was a baby tooth, it didn't matter.

A couple of weeks went by, and I kept having a nagging feeling that something might be done to help Joseph's tooth. I decided to do some more detailed checking. Muscle-testing myself as a surrogate for him, I found that the tooth was still showing that it was out of alignment, but not to the naked eye. I found that the tooth had been rotated a tiny amount in one direction. Using just a fingernail, I made a small correction by flicking his tooth in the opposite direction. The next misalignment that manifested through proxy testing was that the tooth was pushed up into the upper jaw a bit too far. I grasped the tooth and gave it a gentle tug downward. Next, I discovered that the tooth was still misaligned slightly backward, and a small flick of a fingernail in the opposite direction seemed to correct that misalignment as well. There were two other tiny misalignments that I was able to find and correct. This was done in the evening.

The next morning I was shocked to see that Joseph's once-gray tooth was back to its normal color. It apparently wasn't dead after all, but it certainly hadn't been getting any circulation. If you think about the tiny capillaries through which blood flows into our teeth, it is easy to see how a misaligned tooth might disrupt that blood flow.

Today, if I were faced with the same situation, I would simply roll a magnet or my fingertips down the governing meridian three times (the subject's governing meridian, or my own if I am acting as surrogate or proxy), with the intention to the misalignment. In a complex case like this, I might have to do that a number of times, to correct each specific component of the misalignment, but it would work just as well as the physical adjustments that I made in this story.

APPENDICULAR SKELETON

EXPLANATION

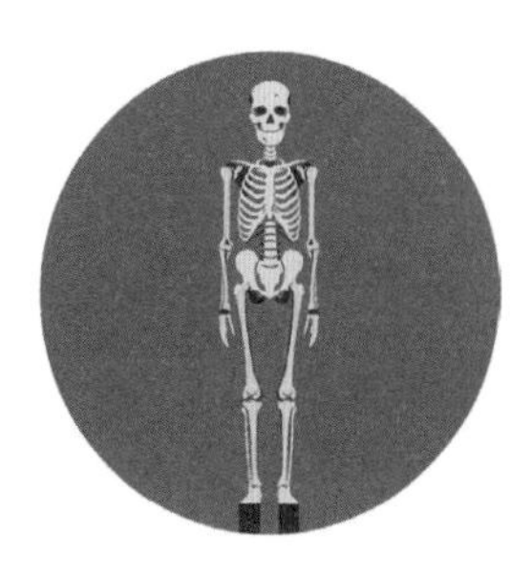

The appendicular skeleton includes 126 bones that make up the pelvis, legs, and feet, as well as the shoulder girdle and the bones of the arms, wrists, and hands, all of which are included in the Body Code System app. If you have not already downloaded it, visit discoverhealing.com/app for more information.

Doreen found that she was able to realign a scapula energetically from a distance as she describes in the following story.

The Sheep Shearer

At 8:00 P.M. one night I had a distress call from a shearer who had four hundred sheep to shear the following day. He was unable to raise his right arm, as it was extremely painful. There was no way he was going to be able to work. Rain was forecast, so time was of the essence to get the sheep shorn. If the sheep are wet, the shearers are unable to shear them until they're dry again.

I immediately checked him using the Body Code and found he had trapped emotions to release and also a misalignment in his scapula, which I promptly corrected energetically. I rang him back about eight minutes later and he was totally astounded that he could raise his arm without any pain. Needless to say, the shearing was carried out.

He booked an appointment for a full Body Code assessment the following week and sent his fellow workmates along to see me also. Many of them had back and neck problems and other health issues that the Body Code was able to remove for them.

—Doreen M., Waikato, New Zealand

For instructions on how to correct a misalignment of any tissue energetically, go to the end of the next chapter. With the Body Code, anything can be corrected from anywhere on the planet. Isn't that amazing?

17

SOFT TISSUE MISALIGNMENTS

Have you more faith in a spoonful of medicine than in the power that animates the living world?

—B. J. PALMER

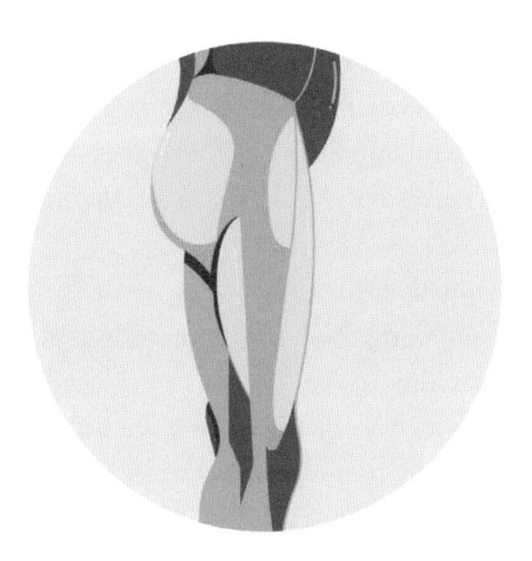

SOFT TISSUE MISALIGNMENTS

Any tissue can become misaligned due to emotional or physical stress or trapped emotions. Although the Body Code System app includes all possible misalignments, in this chapter, I will highlight two of the more common soft tissues that are prone to misalignment, the body's fascial tissues and the kidneys. You can test some of the other tissues of the body using chapter 12, "The Organs"; chapter 13, "The Glands"; and chapter 14, "Systems."

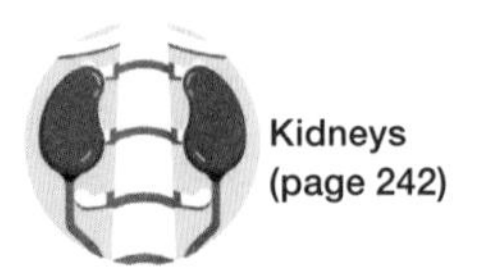

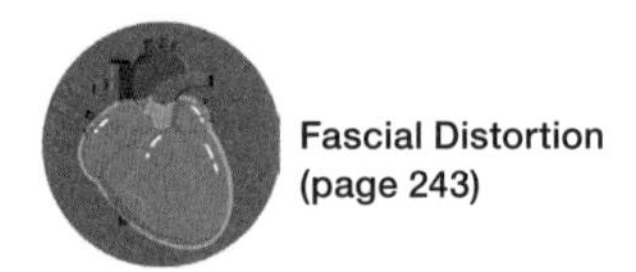

KIDNEYS

EXPLANATION

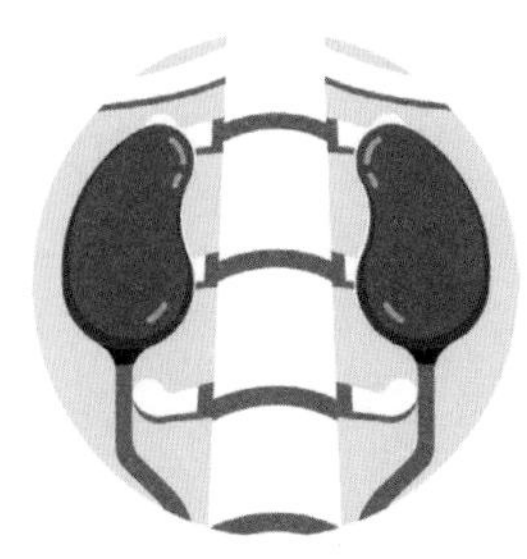

I found out during my years in practice that the kidneys are the most commonly misaligned organs. Many things can cause a kidney to become misaligned, including exposure to sudden trauma, prolonged stress, and dehydration. Caffeinated drinks, energy drinks, black tea, and other toxins ultimately end up in the kidneys as they are being filtered out of the blood, but they may toxify and imbalance the kidneys, often misaligning them slightly.

When a kidney becomes imbalanced it will most often "drop" out of its normal position slightly. The most commonly misaligned organ in the body is actually the left kidney, because again, left-sided paired organs are the first to become imbalanced, with the right-side organs being held in reserve as backups. If you take a look at the kidney information on page 183, you'll see that the kidneys connect energetically to muscles in the lower back. This is the reason why it is so common for people to have low-back pain when the kidney becomes misaligned or imbalanced. I have observed that these are quite often the very same people that are consuming caffeine on a regular basis or that have a problem drinking water.

When either or both kidneys become imbalanced or misaligned, low-back pain is not far behind, and the discs in the lumbar spine are placed at great risk of being damaged or bulging. The discs are like shock absorbers in between the vertebrae that transmit the body's weight through the spine.

In all the years that I was in practice, I treated many patients suffering from low-back disc problems, and I only had to refer two of them for surgical intervention. Why? Because the secret to the low back is actually the kidneys. I never saw a disc problem in the lower back that did not have a kidney imbalance as a major underlying cause.

KIDNEY MAN

I remember at the end of one day when I was finished seeing patients, a man walked in off the street. He was hunched over forward and was also leaning to one side, which is a common position that people will assume if they have nerve impingement in the low back. They are leaning away from the "pinch" to take the pressure off the nerve that is being squeezed. He asked me if I could help him. I replied, "I don't know. How long have you been in this position?" He said, "Two years!"

I brought him back into my treatment room and found that both of his kidneys had actually dropped out of their normal positions slightly. I manually adjusted his kidneys back up into their normal alignment, and then I asked him to stand up. When he stood up, suddenly his posture was perfect. He shouted, "I'm straight! I'm straight! How did you do that!?"

Please realize that if you find a misalignment in one or both kidneys, you can correct them energetically, even from a distance. Find and remove any associated imbalances first, then swipe a few times with a magnet or your hand on the governing meridian with an intention to realign the kidney or kidneys, and voilà. It is that easy.

FASCIAL DISTORTION

EXPLANATION

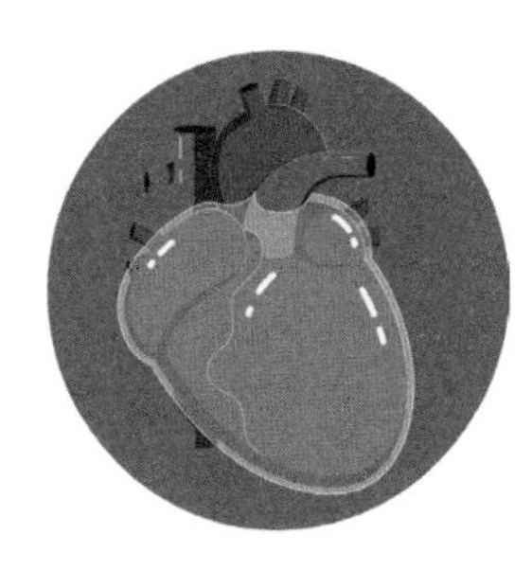

Fascia is a thin layer of connective tissue that can be thought of as the "shrink-wrap" around the various tissues and bones of the body, separating them from each other. Fascia provides a protective coating for every bone, organ, artery, vein, and tissue of the body. For example, the fascial tissue that covers the lungs is called the pleura. When it becomes inflamed, we call that pleurisy. The fascial coating over the brain is called the dura. That's where the word "epidural" comes from. The fascia that surrounds the heart is known as the pericardium, and so on.

The great osteopath Dr. Robert Fulford made tremendous strides in discovering that the fascia can become distorted, or hold abnormal tension. Strong emotions, physical traumas, and other insults that the body may endure can all distort and twist the fascial tissue. The fascia then hold those energies within itself, causing imbalance to occur in the body. If the fascial network in the body is distorted, will the structure of the body be pulled out of alignment? Of course. If the fascia is distorted around the organs in the body, will the chemical processes and reactions taking place in those organs function as efficiently? I don't think so.

Fascia has been found to have a piezoelectric conductive effect, which is believed to be another method of communication used by the body. In his research, Dr. Fulford found that by using a mechanical device called a percussor (essentially a heavy-duty percussing vibrator) he was able to instill motion into the fascial tissues and get them to actually unwind and unravel. The results that Dr. Fulford and others have obtained using percussors to unwind the fascial tissue have been nothing short of miraculous. Long-standing physical problems have immediately resolved themselves upon percussion.

After experimenting with Dr. Fulford's technique in various ways, I began to think that perhaps there might be an additional way to address fascial distortion. At any given time in the body, there is a certain amount of fascial distortion. The subconscious mind, amazing computer that it is, is fully aware of this distortion and comprehends it in the most minute detail. Through intention, and by finding and correcting any associated imbalances, you can help the fascia to return to a balanced state, which can have wonderful effects on health and well-being.

DETERMINING PERCENTAGE OF BRAIN COMMUNICATION

If you're trying to improve the function of a particular organ or gland, you can ask, "What percent of the messages being sent by the brain to this organ are arriving intact, on average?" For example, one of the things that I used to routinely do with people who were suffering from asthma is ask, "What percent of the communications from your brain are actually arriving at your lungs intact, on average?" And then I would muscle-test for the answer to questions like, "Are 50 percent of those messages getting through?" No. "Are 40 percent of those messages getting through?" In this way, it's possible to get a precise number. Determine this percentage before and after structural correction is made to a misaligned vertebra energetically, and I think you will be amazed at the changes you will see.

EXERCISE:
FIND AND CORRECT A MISALIGNMENT

STEP 1.

Ask: "Do I [or you] have a misalignment that can be corrected now?"

- **If yes, continue to Step 2.**
- **If no, you may not have a misalignment at all or you may have one that cannot be corrected now, so you may want to try again later.**

STEP 2.

(Decoding) Ask: "Do we need to know more about this misalignment?"

- **If no, move to Step 3 (Association).**
- **If you have not already determined what tissue is misaligned, use a process of elimination to determine whether this is a misalignment of a bone, an organ, fascia, or some other tissue.**
- **If you have not already done so, feel free to download the Body Code app at discoverhealing.com/app for a complete list and a free trial.**

STEP 3.

(Association) Ask: "Is there an associated imbalance that needs to be decoded?" (Remember that most of the time, misalignments are caused by the distorting effect of trapped emotions.)

- If no, move to Step 5 (Intention).
- If yes, return to the Body Code Map on page 101 and decode and address any associated imbalances, then return here and repeat Step 3.

STEP 4.

(Intention) Swipe three times with a magnet or your hand on any length of the governing meridian, while holding the intention to correct the misalignment.

STEP 5.

Ask: "Did we correct that misalignment?"

- If yes, you can start at the beginning on Step 1 and repeat the process to find another misalignment.
- If no, refocus, say a prayer for help, allow your heart to feel love and gratitude that this is going to help, and swipe three times once again with intention.

HELPFUL TIPS FOR CORRECTING MISALIGNMENTS

Get used to the idea that all of the parts of the body are made of pure energy and can be manipulated or corrected energetically.

You'll find that when a misalignment has an associated imbalance, the correction of that associated imbalance will almost always result in an immediate correction of the misalignment.

RECURRING MISALIGNMENT

If a misalignment recurs, the most common reason will be a trapped emotion, a physical trauma energy, or some other kind of imbalance. Be open to all possibilities.

Structural misalignments are common problems. I would recommend that you find a chiropractor in your local area and follow his or her recommendations to keep your spine in good alignment. But if the day comes when you can't leave your house to see a chiropractor and you're on your own, remember that corrections like this can also be made simply through the energy of your intention.

SECTION 5

TOXINS

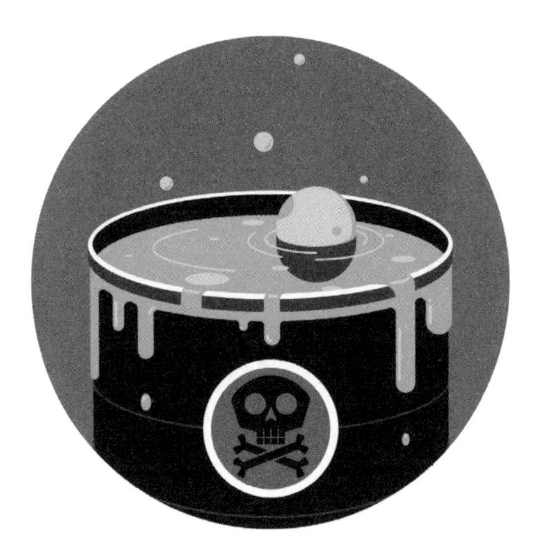

If you don't take care of your body, the most magnificent machine you'll ever be given, where will you live?

—KARYN CALABRESE

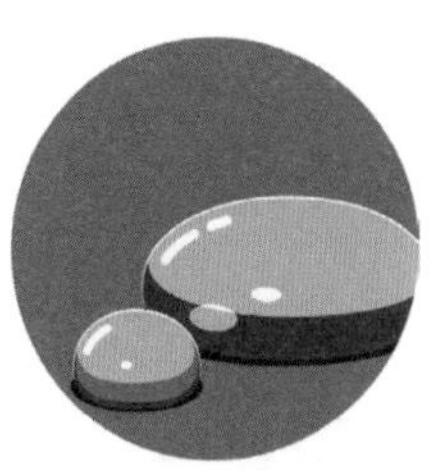

Heavy Metals
(page 252)

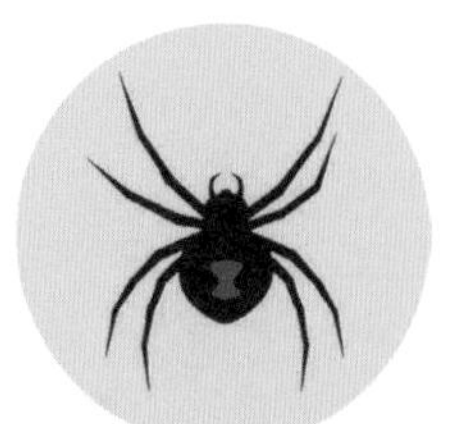

Biological Poisons
(page 259)

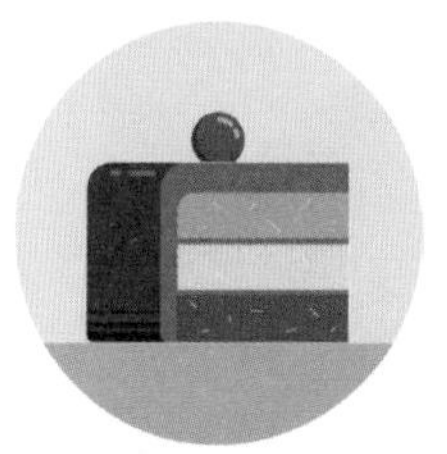

Food Toxins
(page 266)

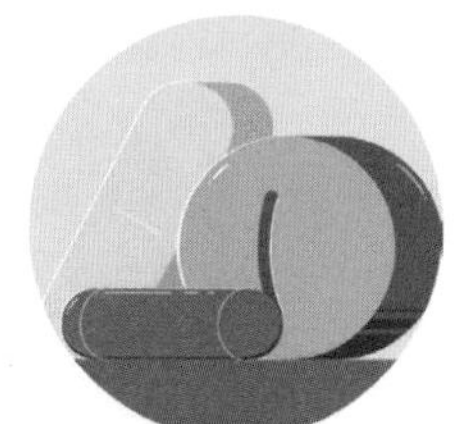

Drug Toxins
(page 274)

There is a veritable universe of toxins that we are faced with on planet Earth. We are exposed to toxins daily through the air we breathe, through the food we eat, and even through the electronics we use.

The purpose of this chapter is to help you understand toxicity, how to detect it, and what to do to correct or eliminate it. There are many different types of toxins that affect our bodies. The types of toxicity discussed in this section include heavy metals like mercury, biological poisons from things such as insect bites, food toxins such as sweeteners and preservatives, and drug toxins, including prescription and recreational drugs.

18

DEALING WITH TOXINS

All things are poison and nothing is without poison; only the dose makes a thing not a poison.

—PARACELSUS

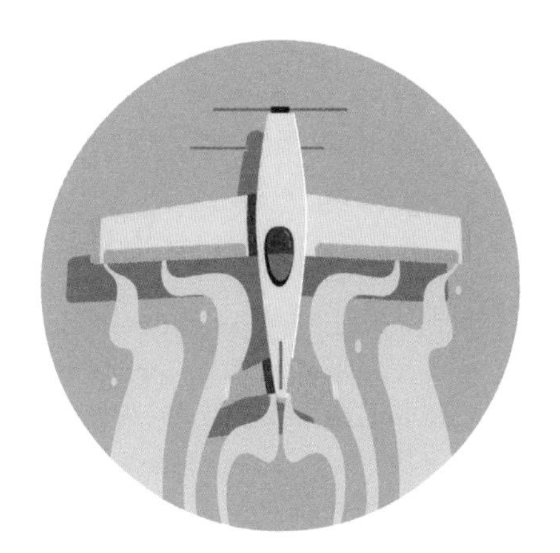

Toxicity refers to the accumulation of toxins, or toxic matter, in the body. For the most part, toxicity is a relatively new phenomenon. Most toxins were introduced into our environment and subsequently into our bodies around the beginning of the Industrial Revolution. This problem continues to increase as the health of planet Earth declines. Toxicity is now a worldwide problem, and unfortunately there's not any place on Earth that's free of toxic pollutants.

A large number of the toxins that we are exposed to comes from the food we eat. The average person in the United States takes in about fourteen pounds of chemicals per year in the form of food additives: humectants, preservatives, food colorings, and so on. The more processed food you eat, the more these toxic food additives will build up in your tissues. These toxins are damaging to the body and interfere with the normal function of the immune system.

The immune system is responsible for the elimination of toxins, a process called detoxification. Not only are the toxins themselves disruptive to the detoxification process, but many other types of imbalances can also interfere. Finding and clearing these associated imbalances can greatly enable the detoxification process, as Melissa experienced when she used the Body Code to detoxify a family pet after it had overdosed on medication.

Cat Overdosed

My sister called me frantically last month. Her beloved cat, Champ, knocked over a whole bottle of her other cat's medication. The pills spilled out onto the floor and must have been flavored, because Champ ate them all! The vet told her to prepare for him to die. I worked feverishly on him for an hour by proxy from my home many miles away. I detoxed that cat every hour that day and several times a day every day after that. The cat is just fine now with no signs of any problems. This is a miracle! My sister has had a lot of traumatic stress lately in her life, and her cat's death may have put her over the edge. I am so thankful for this tool we have!

—Melissa M., Utah, United States

An important thing to remember is that if trapped emotions and other energetic imbalances are present in the body, they will tend to make detoxing more difficult. For example, if you have trapped emotions or traumas that are lodged in the liver—a major organ of detoxification—every chemical reaction now taking place in the liver is going to suffer some degree of interference. The liver function will not be at 100 percent by any means, and getting rid of harmful toxins is going to be more difficult. Similarly, if you have imbalances like this that are lodged in the small intestine, which houses a large part of your immune system, you'll also have a hard time getting rid of toxins.

TOXINS AS ENERGY

All toxins consist of nothing but pure energy, so you can treat them as such with the Body Code. Think of toxins as clouds of energy in the body, just like trapped emotions or other energies. When you find a toxin, you can identify the type of toxin and any other necessary information, including any imbalances that may be associated, as well as the location of the toxin in the body, if desired.

In some cases, treating toxins energetically may be enough, and the body may be able to handle any remaining detoxification on its own with no other help. This will usually be the case if the toxic load is relatively minor and the body's organs are functioning well. At other times however, the body may need some extra help, and a detoxification product or cleanse may be needed.

EXERCISE: IDENTIFYING A TOXIN

STEP 1.

Ask: "Do I [or you] have a toxin that can be found and eliminated now?"

- **If yes, continue to Step 2.**
- **If no, you may want to try again later.**

STEP 2.

If you have not already done so, identify the toxin type. Ask: "Is the toxin on the left side of this chart?" (referencing the toxins chart at the beginning of this section)

- **If yes, it is on the left side.**
- **If no, it is on the right side.**

STEP 3.

Starting at the top of the side identified, ask, "Is this a ____ toxin?" For example, let's say it is on the right side. You would ask, "Is this a biological toxin?" If no, you'd continue down that side and ask, "Is this a drug toxin?" where you should receive a yes answer.

Once the toxin type has been identified, turn to that chapter to learn more about the toxin and follow the exercise instructions to eliminate it.

19

HEAVY METALS

Watching what you eat ought to include knowing what what you eat ate.

—MOKOKOMA MOKHONOANA

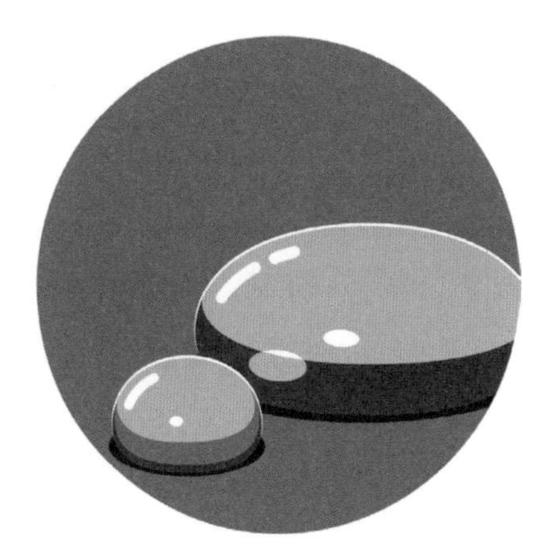

Heavy metals can enter the body through contaminated food, vaccines, polluted air, water, cosmetics, and more. Although trace amounts of some metals are necessary to support life, most heavy metals have no benefit to the human body. When heavy metals accumulate, they can be extremely damaging to the tissues and create interference with metabolic processes.

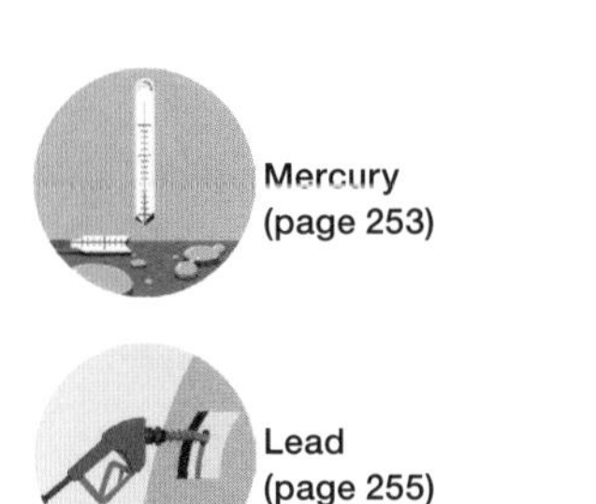

Mercury
(page 253)

Lead
(page 255)

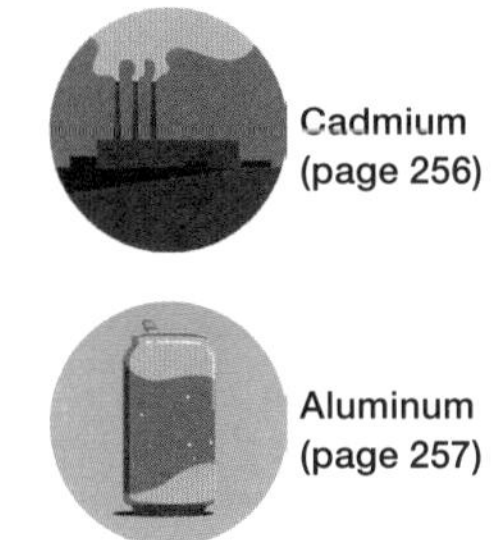

Cadmium
(page 256)

Aluminum
(page 257)

MERCURY

EXPLANATION

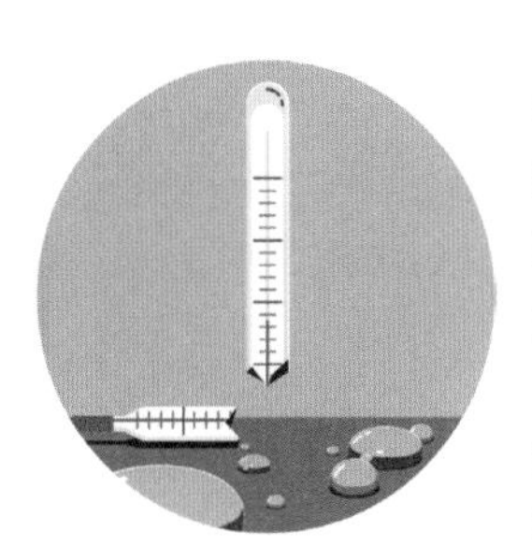

One of the most toxic and commonly found heavy metals is mercury. It is said that only radioactive plutonium is more poisonous than mercury. Mercury can be found in many things, but the largest sources include air pollution, vaccines, and dental fillings.

Coal-fired plants put toxic smoke into the atmosphere, which is absorbed into ocean water and consumed by fish. Larger ocean fish can contain enormous levels of mercury because they eat smaller fish that contain mercury and it builds up in their bodies. The larger the fish, generally speaking, the higher the level of mercury.

In the following story, Sandra discovered she could clear the toxic energy left behind from polluted shellfish.

It's All Energy

In my first year or so of using the Body Code, my husband and I ordered Thai food takeout one night, and my dish was a stir-fry with noodles, shrimp, and vegetables. While I was eating the meal, there was this nagging feeling in the back of my mind about the shrimp, like maybe it wasn't the best. However, I have never had a shellfish problem or any problems from eating shrimp, and the restaurant serves high-quality food, so I ignored my strange thought.

A short time after finishing dinner I decided to change into something else to wear, and as I pulled my shirt over my head, I saw that I was covered in a red stippled rash all over my stomach and up my chest. I did not feel any irritation from it, but it was very noticeable. I showed it to my husband, then I got the idea to see what the Body Code said about it.

I muscle-tested and found only one imbalance causing it—toxins, specifically heavy metals. I used the Body Code to clear the toxin energetically. Curious about if it would work and how long it would take, I checked my torso again after about ten to fifteen minutes and the redness was largely gone; just a mild hint of it remained. I showed the change to my husband and told him all I did was release heavy-metal toxin energy with the Body Code, and he was amazed. He said that was the best proof he had seen yet of how effective the Body Code can be.

—Sandra D., Ontario, Canada

For many years vaccines contained mercury, and it is still found in some vaccines today. According to the FDA, thimerosal, which is approximately 50 percent mercury by weight, has been one of the most widely used preservatives in vaccines since the 1930s.

The largest source of mercury exposure is amalgam fillings. I have seen several cases in which people were diagnosed with a major disease, but by simply removing their amalgam fillings, their health recovered dramatically. Amalgam fillings should always be removed by a dentist with the right equipment and expertise, because when a dentist drills out old mercury fillings, clouds of mercury vapor are released and can be inhaled back into the body.

Great caution needs to be taken if you are considering having amalgam fillings removed. Do your research and find an experienced dental expert that uses every possible precaution during the procedure. Ask if they have the right equipment for the procedure, including a dental dam, nasal breathing system, and air purifier. The dental dam is a rubber barrier that protects you from swallowing any bits of mercury. The nasal breathing system prevents you from breathing toxic mercury vapor. I have first-hand experience of the dangers of not removing an amalgam filling properly.

MY MERCURY STORY

Many years ago, before I knew how dangerous mercury is, I went to a dentist and asked him about getting an amalgam filling removed. He thought the filling wasn't a big problem, but I wanted it replaced anyway. So he went ahead and drilled out just one mercury filling and replaced it with a white composite filling. I felt fine after the procedure, drove home, walked through my front door, climbed the stairs to go to my bedroom, but when I reached the top of the stairs, I collapsed with sudden exhaustion.

The next day, a black growth appeared on my right forefinger and grew very quickly. It was a malignancy that ultimately had to be surgically removed. It was a strange thing to experience, and later muscle testing revealed that it was directly caused by my exposure to mercury vapor.

Mercury can remain in the body and will interfere with the formation of protein molecules, making it difficult to create the enzymes and other proteins that are needed for normal health. There is no safe level of mercury.

LEAD

EXPLANATION

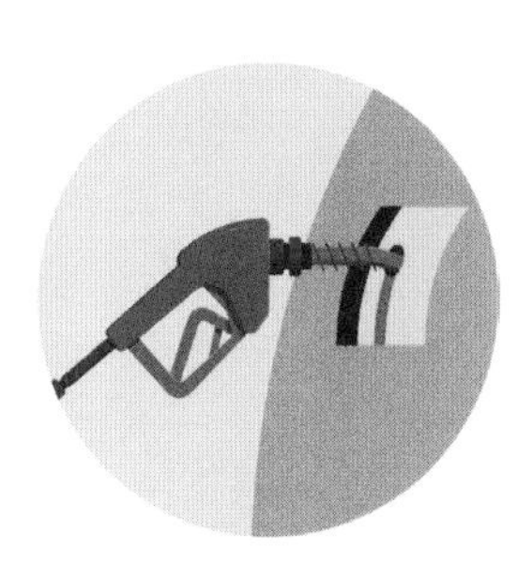

If you were born in the 1970s or earlier, you may remember that at every gasoline pump at every gas station, there was a sign that read: FOR USE AS MOTOR FUEL ONLY—CONTAINS LEAD.

Leaded gasoline was common from the 1920s until the 1980s. Lead was considered an important compound to mix in with gasoline because it helped the engine run more smoothly. Leaded gasoline is still used in certain countries, and on a limited basis for people who drive and maintain historic cars, and low-lead gasoline is used in general aviation. When leaded gasoline was being heavily used, millions of tons of lead were put into the atmosphere in the form of exhaust. As a result, many people in the industrialized world now have high lead content in their bodies.

Lead has also been an ingredient in paint for thousands of years, even though making and using lead-based paint was a known danger. In fact, the paint makers and painters often came down with paralysis and nervous system disorders. Although banned in the United States in 1978, much of the world still produces and sells lead-based paint. Even though many places don't use lead-based paint anymore, old paint chips and dust from buildings and toys pose a threat. Children are at the most risk because old paint chips have a sweet taste, and children are often on the floor where dust resides.

Between 1900 and 1950, a majority of America's largest cities installed lead water pipes—with some cities even mandating them for their durability. And because lead pipes can last seventy-five to one hundred years, the legacy of lead pipes lives on today. Unfortunately, you can't see, smell, or taste lead, so even water that runs clear can contain it. In the following story, a Body Code practitioner found that her client's shoulder pain was due to a buildup of lead from her drinking water.

Shoulder Pain Caused by Lead Toxin

One client has come back to me for more help with the shoulder pain we had addressed previously using the Emotion Code. I used the Body Code app to help navigate this session more smoothly. I loved including the Body Code because it proved just how integral the two systems are at working together. I found not only emotional imbalances that were irritating her shoulder, but physical ones as well. We found out that she was suffering from a toxic heavy-metal buildup of lead from lead piping. I was able to specifically get a time in which this started to affect her body and, lo and behold, it lined up with when she and her family had moved into a new house!

The connections that we made were crazy, and we both learned a lot from the experience. I've checked in on her since, and she says there is definitely more movement in her shoulder since then. . . . She was very thankful for my time and efforts to help her, and it just undoubtedly proved to me that now I know I need to be making this a part of the healing that I use, not only on myself and my loved ones but also so I can officially offer it to my clients to make a real and positive difference.

—Ariel D., Idaho, United States

High levels of lead exposure can be serious and life-threatening. To the cells in our bodies, lead looks a lot like the mineral calcium, which is vital to healthy development and function, strong bones and teeth, and a healthy cardiovascular system. As a result, lead that has been absorbed or ingested can travel through our bodies and cause problems in our bones, teeth, blood, liver, kidneys, and brain, disrupting normal biological function.

CADMIUM

EXPLANATION

Cadmium has been in industrial use for a long time and can be found in mining and smelting activities, phosphate fertilizers, batteries, and contaminated food and beverages. Tobacco smoking is a huge source for cadmium exposure, and tobacco smokers have been found to have four to five times the blood cadmium concentrations of nonsmokers. Cadmium is a known carcinogen that is also used in artist's paints.

Cadmium is not eliminated by the body very well, and it tends to accumulate in the kidneys, liver, and testicles. Even small amounts of cadmium can damage the kidney, liver, and heart, weaken the bones, and in severe cases may cause death.

Vitamins A, C, E, and selenium can prevent or reduce many toxic effects of cadmium.

ALUMINUM

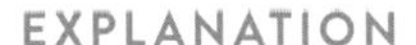

EXPLANATION

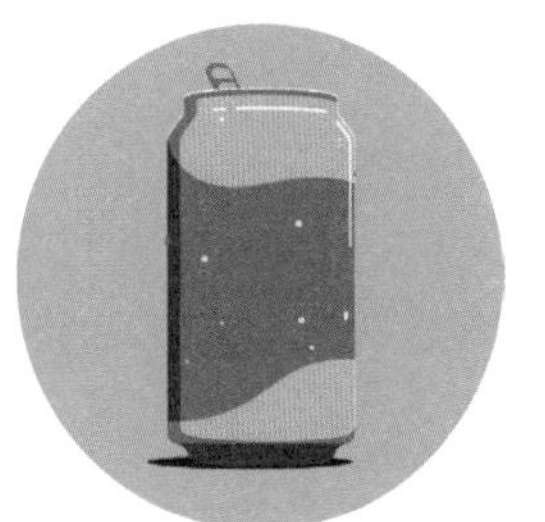

Aluminum is the most plentiful metal in the earth's crust. Aluminum toxicity occurs when a person, usually someone living in an environment contaminated by industrial wastes, ingests or breathes high levels of aluminum into the body. It can also enter the body through the food we eat and the water we drink. Aluminum is used to help purify our drinking water and can be an additive to processed foods.

Packaged table salt often contains sodium silicoaluminate, which contains aluminum, and is used in many baking mixes and baking powders as an anticaking agent as well. If you start reading labels, you will be amazed at how many sources of aluminum there are in seemingly harmless everyday products.

Aluminum is present in many other products, such as deodorants, antacids, cosmetics, and baking tools. Prolonged use of aluminum cookware is not recommended.

Overexposure to aluminum may cause brain damage, Alzheimer's disease, Crohn's disease, and anemia, just to name a few. If you want to keep your brain young, try to eliminate as many sources of aluminum as possible.

IT'S STILL JUST ENERGY

Keeping in mind that everything in the universe is ultimately made of energy, it's possible to address even heavy metals as an energy. Please realize that the efficacy of addressing heavy metals as an energy is dependent upon your own belief as well as the belief of your subject. Remember that subatomic particles change their behavior based on the expectation of the observer. Heavy metals are made of subatomic particles. Your intention, entangled and combined with the intention of whomever it is you are working with, can be a powerful way to detoxify the body of heavy metals.

EXERCISE: FIND AND ELIMINATE A HEAVY-METAL TOXIN

STEP 1.

Ask: "Do I [or you] have a heavy-metal toxin that we can find and eliminate now?"

- If yes, continue to Step 2.
- If no, you may not have heavy-metal toxicity at all, or you may need to try again later.

STEP 2.

(Decoding) Ask: "Do we need to know more about this toxin?"

- If no, move to Step 3 (Association).
- If yes, muscle-test to see which of the following details need to be identified. Sometimes, all that is needed is to identify the heavy metal. Some common heavy metals you can test for are listed in the table at the beginning of this chapter.
- If you don't find the toxin in that table, here is a more expansive list you can use:

Titanium	Manganese	Nickel	Molybdenum	Gold
Vanadium	Iron	Copper	Silver	Arsenic
Chromium	Cobalt	Zinc	Tin	

- Once you have identified a specific heavy metal, return to Step 2 (Decoding) and ask if there is more you need to know. If you do not need to know more about the heavy metal, go to Step 3 (Association), otherwise, you might ask the following questions:
    - Ask: "Do we need to know the source of exposure?"
    - Ask: "Do we need to know the age of occurrence?"

STEP 3.

(Association) Ask: "Is there an associated imbalance that needs to be decoded?"

- If no, skip to Step 4 (Intention).
- If yes, return to the Body Code Map and decode and address any associated imbalances, then return here and repeat the Step 3 (Association) question.

STEP 4.

(Intention) Swipe three times with a magnet or your hand on any length of the governing meridian, while holding an intention to release the energy of this toxin from the body, while at the same time directing the body to remove the toxin through its normal elimination channels.

STEP 5.

Ask: "Did we release that heavy-metal toxin?"

- If yes, you can start at the beginning on Step 1 and repeat the process to find another heavy-metal toxin.
- If no, refocus, say a prayer for help, allow your heart to feel love and gratitude that this is going to help, and swipe three times once again with intention.

HELPFUL TIPS FOR DEALING WITH TOXINS

It is important to note that physical support may be necessary to complete the detoxification process. I recommended seeing a health-care provider for more information about detoxifying heavy metals from the body.

Using good judgment and common sense, avoid this toxin in the future if possible.

20

BIOLOGICAL POISONS

There are moments when the human body can overcome things you would never expect.

—ANDRES INIESTA

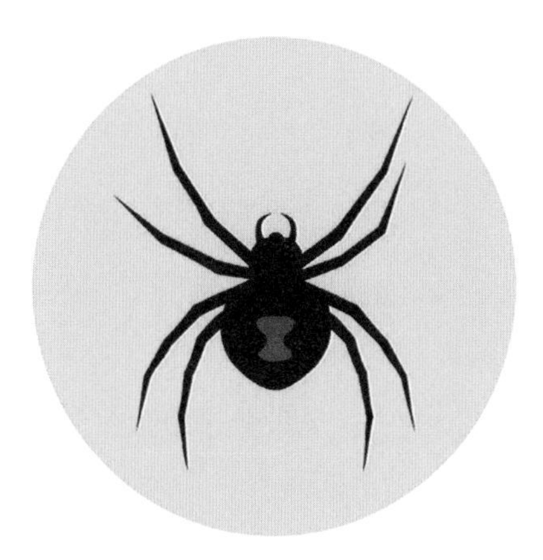

Biological poisons are substances that can cause injury, harm, or even death to organs, tissues, cells, and DNA and are produced by single-celled organisms such as bacteria and fungi as well as plants, animals, and insects.

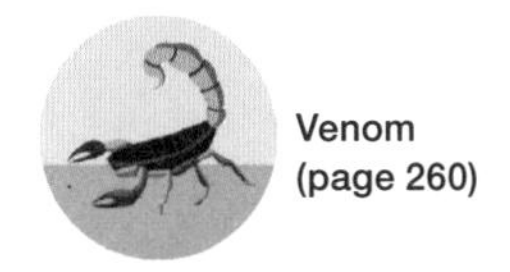

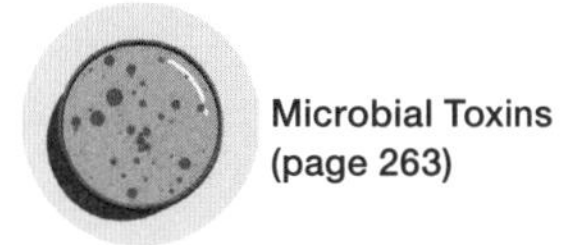

VENOM

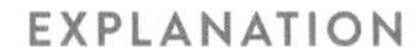

EXPLANATION

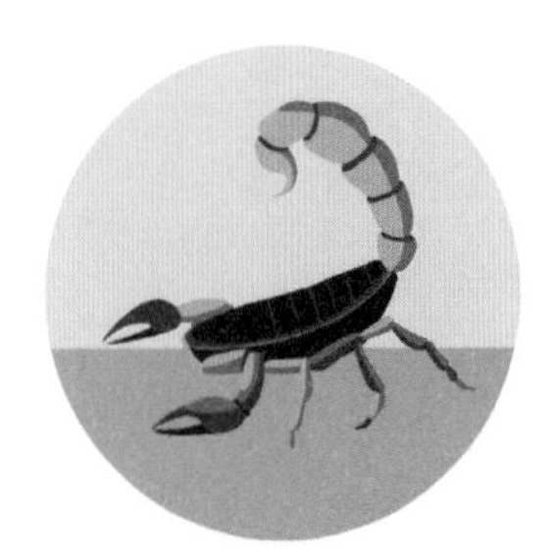

Venom is a toxic secretion that is distinguished from poisons in that venoms are injected by a bite or sting, while poisons are ingested or absorbed.

Venoms are usually comprised of different protein molecules that are responsible for their biological effects. For example, it was recently discovered that king cobra venom contains 113 different proteins.

SICK FROM A SPIDER BITE

After I graduated from chiropractic college in 1988, we moved to Montana to work in Kalispell with Dr. Stan Flagg, a holistic chiropractor.

Dr. Flagg was a very gifted healer, and I felt blessed to be able to learn from him. I spent my workdays following him around the office, taking notes, and trying to comprehend everything that he was doing to help his patients.

One Friday afternoon a woman came into the office with several family members. She was in a wheelchair and was obviously very ill. She told us that she had been sick for about three weeks and had been in the wheelchair since then because she didn't have the energy to walk or move about.

She had been to the emergency room and had seen another medical doctor for her condition as well, but no one seemed to know what was wrong with her. It was a bit mysterious, but her condition seemed grave to me. She looked like she was dying. Her face was very pale, her skin was clammy, her eyes were sunken, and she told us that the only time she wasn't racked with pain was when she was in a tub of very hot water. She said the only problem with that was that it took multiple members of her family to help her out of the tub because she had absolutely no ability to get out on her own.

I took notes as Dr. Flagg examined her and then used muscle testing in an attempt to determine what was wrong with her. Since she was far too weak to be tested directly, he had me act as a surrogate. I put one hand on her shoulder and held my other arm straight out in front of me, parallel to the floor. Her body's responses to his questions would result in my arm being weak for the no answers and strong for the yes answers. It didn't take long before Dr. Flagg got an answer. He asked, "Have you been bitten by a spider, that you can recall?" She had to think about it for a moment, but suddenly said, "Yes, I was bitten by a spider about five weeks ago. It swelled up for a while, but then it went away."

According to the answers that her subconscious mind was giving through my arm in response to Dr. Flagg's questions, the spider venom was the source of the problem. He released the venom using the energetic methods that he used at the time, and at the end of this session her subconscious mind indicated that there wasn't anything else for us to do. Her family members wheeled her out of the office, and I was left wondering what would become of her.

She was our last patient that Friday afternoon long ago. The following Monday morning I came into the office at my usual time and noticed a woman sitting in the waiting room. I started a conversation with her and suddenly was thunderstruck. This was the same woman that was in the wheelchair a few days before, the woman who had appeared to have one foot in the grave. She no longer needed a wheelchair, and she looked wonderful. She had completely recovered and was so grateful that as we talked, her tears flowed freely, and so did mine.

Always be open to other imbalances that may show up to be corrected while you are using the Body Code, as Annelle found in the following story.

Cross-Eyed from a Bee Sting

I recently worked with a twenty-two-month-old little girl who had gotten a bee sting near her eye. Shortly after, her eye turned inward, creating a cross-eyed problem. Her mother said they were working with an eye doctor, but she also asked me to use the Body Code. She told me there have been eye problems on both sides of the family.

So, I began clearing imbalances from this sweet little girl and I found a miasm inherited from her father that went back five generations, and another miasm inherited from her mother that went back seven generations. Both were somehow related to the eyes. Within a week's time, her mother let me know that she was seeing improvement in the eye's position.

—Annelle D., Virginia, United States

People are not always aware that they have been bitten or stung. Sometimes the bite or sting is painless and may go unnoticed by the victim, making it difficult to connect symptoms from it that appear later, sometimes weeks or months later.

EXERCISE:
FIND AND ADDRESS A TOXIC VENOM

STEP 1.

Ask: "Do I [or you] have venom that we can find and eliminate now?"

- **If yes, continue to Step 2.**
- **If no, you may not have a venom toxin at all or one that cannot be removed now, so you may want to try again later.**

STEP 2.

(Decoding) Ask: "Do we need to know more about this venom?"

- If no, move to Step 3 (Association).
- If yes, muscle-test to see which of the following details need to be identified. Sometimes, all that is needed is to identify the venom source. Some common venom sources are listed in this table:

REPTILES AND AMPHIBIANS	ARACHNIDS	INSECTS
Snakes	Spiders	Bees
Frogs	Ticks	Wasps
	Scorpions	Ants

- Once you have identified a specific venom source, return to Step 2 (Decoding) and ask if there is more you need to know. If you do not need to know more about the venom, go to Step 3 (Association), otherwise, you might ask the following questions. Return to Step 2 (Decoding) once the answer to any of these questions is determined.
  - Ask: "Do we need to know the age of occurrence?"
  - Ask: "Do we need to know the location of this energy in the body?"

If yes, using a process of elimination to locate this may be helpful. For example, divide the body in half, and ask if the energy is lodged in the lower half of the body or upper half. Divide the body from left to right and ask if the energy is lodged in the left half of the body or the right half. Continue dividing in this fashion and asking until you've determined the location in the body where the venom is lodged, then return to Step 2 (Decoding).

STEP 3.

(Association) Ask: "Is there an associated imbalance that needs to be decoded?"

- If no, skip to Step 4 (Intention).
- If yes, return to the Body Code Map and decode and address any associated imbalances, then return here and repeat the Step 3 (Association) question.

STEP 4.

(Intention) Swipe three times with a magnet or your hand on any length of the governing meridian, while holding an intention to release the energy of this venom from the body, while at the same time directing the body to remove the toxin through its normal elimination channels.

STEP 5.

Ask: "Did we release that venom toxin?"

- If yes, you can start at the beginning on Step 1 and repeat the process to find another venom toxin.

- **If no, refocus, say a prayer for help, allow your heart to feel love and gratitude that this is going to help, and swipe three times once again with intention.**

HELPFUL TIPS FOR DEALING WITH VENOM TOXINS

Toxins can exist in physical form as well as in an invisible, energetic form. Energetic toxins are vibrational frequencies that were simply unable to be processed, likely because the energy body was imbalanced. A venom toxin energy may be found lodged in your body from any time or point in your life.

Again, physical support may be necessary to complete the detoxification process depending on the severity of the venom. When in doubt, see a health-care provider for more information about detoxifying venom from the body.

MICROBIAL TOXINS

EXPLANATION

Some pathogens create toxins as by-products of their own metabolism and existence in the body. For example, parasites produce uric acid, which often causes joint and muscle discomfort. Also, when pathogens die they release additional toxins that create die-off symptoms and sickness. Microbial toxins promote infection and disease by directly damaging host tissues and by disabling the immune system.

FOOD POISONING

Another unforgettable experience I had when I was working with Dr. Flagg was with food poisoning—my own.

One day, just after lunch, I started feeling ill. I had experienced food poisoning a couple of times before in my life, and this felt familiar. I was feeling feverish, slightly dizzy, and an ominous sense of nausea and abdominal discomfort was rapidly increasing. I was in trouble and I knew it. I told Dr. Flagg that I was going to have to go home and take the rest of the day off and maybe the next day or two as well.

I knew the reason for this sudden sickness. For lunch, I had foolishly eaten a fish sandwich that had been in my car. When I ate it, I thought I could get away with it. I knew it had been in the car a little too long, but it tasted okay, and I thought it would be all right. But I was now regretting my decision.

Dr. Flagg looked at me and asked me what was wrong. After I explained what I had eaten for lunch and how I was feeling, getting worse by the moment, he brightened up and said, "Well, let's treat it!"

As he was working on me I suddenly felt energy surge from my feet up through my body. In that moment, the sickness was gone. The shift was so dramatic that I actually burst out laughing and said to Dr. Flagg, "Okay! Let's get back to work!"

Years later, I realized what a great example this was to me of how even microbial toxins produced by food poisoning can be treated as an energy and released immediately.

EXERCISE: FIND AND ELIMINATE A MICROBIAL TOXIN

STEP 1.

Ask: "Is there a microbial toxin that we can find and eliminate now?"

- If yes, continue to Step 2.
- If no, you may not have a microbial toxin at all or one that cannot be removed now, so you may want to try again later.

STEP 2.

Ask: "Do we need to know more about this toxin?"

- If no, move to Step 3 (Association).
- If yes, muscle-test to see which of the following details need to be identified. Sometimes, all that is needed is to identify the source of the toxin. Some common sources are listed in this table:

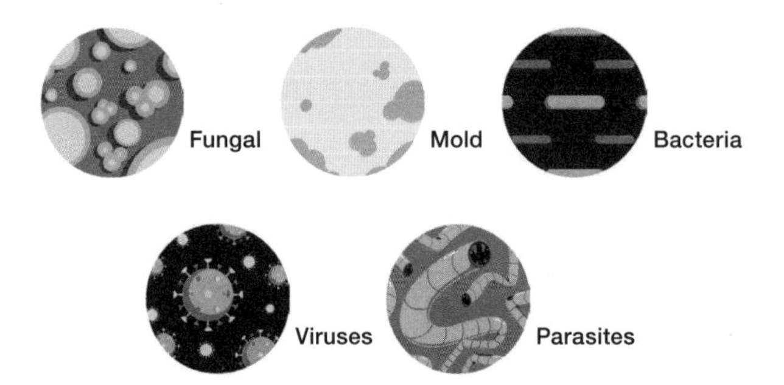

- Once you have identified a specific source of the microbial toxin, return to Step 2 (Decoding) and ask if there is more you need to know. If you do not need to know more about the toxin, go to Step 3 (Association), otherwise, you might ask the following questions:
  - Ask: "Do we need to know the age of occurrence?"
  - Ask: "Do we need to know the location of this energy in the body?"

If yes, using a process of elimination to locate this may be helpful. For example, divide the body in half, and ask if the toxin is lodged in the lower half of the body or upper half. Divide the body from left to right and ask if the toxin is lodged in the left half of the body or the right half. Continue dividing in this fashion and asking until you've determined the location in the body where the toxin is lodged, then return to Step 2 (Decoding).

STEP 3.

(Association) Ask: "Is there an associated imbalance that needs to be decoded?"

- If no, skip to Step 4 (Intention).
- If yes, return to the Body Code Map and decode and address any associated imbalances, then return here and repeat the Step 3 question.

STEP 4.

(Intention) Swipe three times with a magnet or your hand on any length of the governing meridian, while holding an intention to release the energy of this toxin from the body, while at the same time directing the body to remove the toxin through its normal elimination channels.

STEP 5.

Ask: "Did we release that microbial toxin?"

- If yes, you can start at the beginning on Step 1 and repeat the process to find another microbial toxin.
- If no, refocus, say a prayer for help, allow your heart to feel love and gratitude that this is going to help, and swipe three times once again with intention.

HELPFUL TIPS FOR DEALING WITH MICROBIAL TOXINS

Microbial toxins can create all sorts of symptoms, including fatigue, inflammation, hormonal imbalance, and mood swings, just to name a few. You can be exposed to them through your digestive system, lungs, and the skin. We can reduce these toxins by learning how to avoid them as much as possible.

You can build a strong immune system to better resist microbial toxins by reducing stress, having good hygiene, and using the Body Code to find and eliminate pathogens before they are able to become entrenched in the body.

21

FOOD TOXINS

Food, one assumes, provides nourishment; but Americans eat it fully aware that small amounts of poison have been added to improve its appearance and delay its putrefaction.

—JOHN CAGE

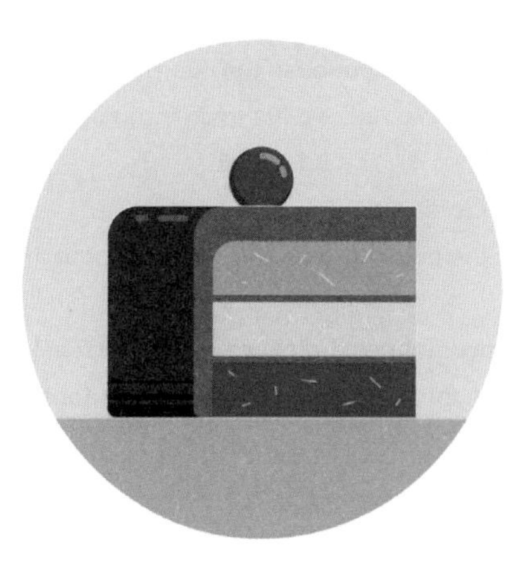

Much of the food that is consumed in the industrialized countries is modified in any number of ways. It's a good thing, in a sense. Without the addition of artificial flavorings and coloring, many things that people eat would be unappetizing and would appear in various shades of gray. Unfortunately, food itself has become industrialized with the addition of all sorts of food toxins, including flavor enhancers like MSG, artificial sweeteners, preservatives, humectants, pesticides, herbicides, and more.

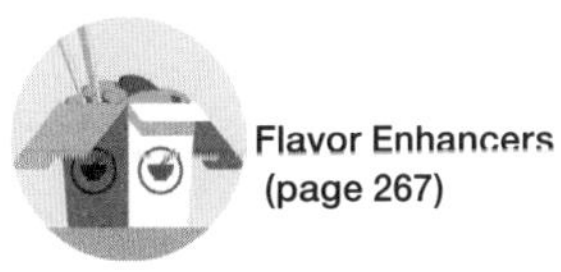

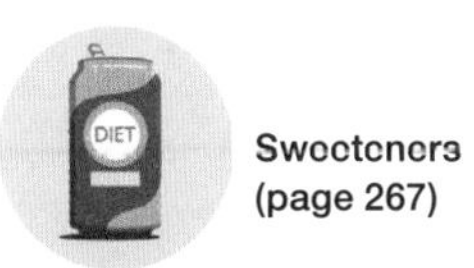

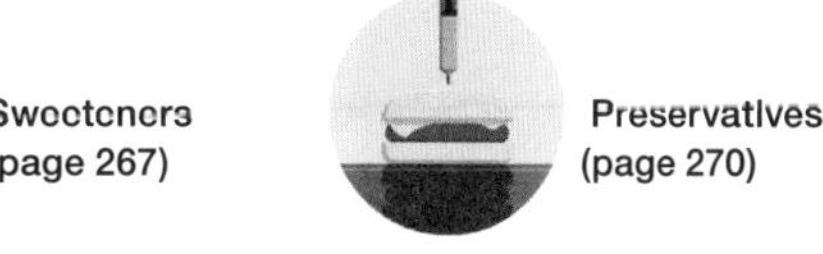

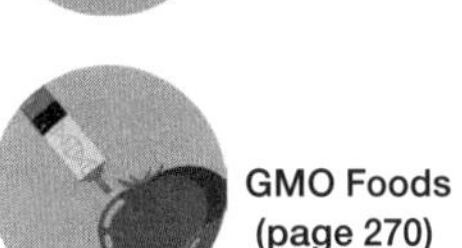

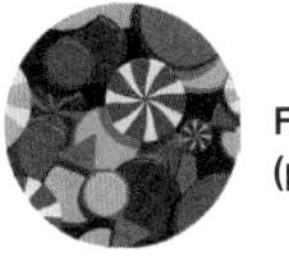

Food Coloring
(page 271)

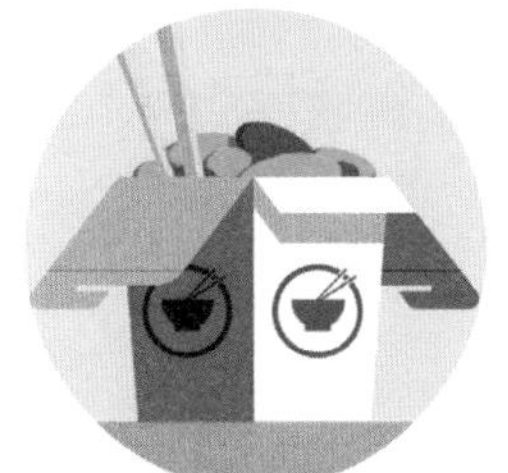

FLAVOR ENHANCERS

EXPLANATION

Flavor enhancers improve the flavor of food and are a major source of toxicity for people.

MSG

Monosodium glutamate, or MSG, was the first flavor enhancer to be developed commercially and is present in a wide variety of different foods, disguised under a slew of different names. The most common code words to watch for are "glutamate," "hydrolyzed," "autolyzed," and "modified." These are all names for MSG compounds that are uniformly toxic and produce the same physical reactions in those who are sensitive to MSG.

You may have heard of "Chinese restaurant syndrome," which includes symptoms such as headache, muscle tightness, fatigue, and nausea following a meal laced with MSG. Most people don't even realize they are sensitive to MSG. The reason for these symptoms is that MSG is classified as an excitotoxin, which means that it can excite nerves to the point of exhaustion. MSG tends to be addictive, is mood influencing, and causes weight gain. In fact, scientists who study obesity in the laboratory create obese rats by giving them MSG. These animals are called "MSG-treated rodents." MSG should be avoided as much as possible.

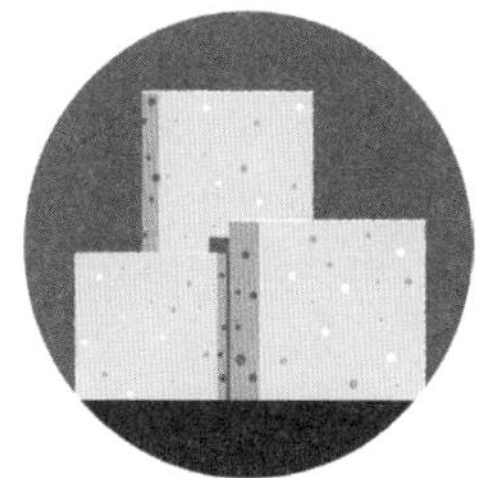

SWEETENERS

EXPLANATION

The subject of sweeteners can be confusing mainly because the terminology is often open to interpretation. Some manufacturers will market their sweeteners as "natural" even though they're entirely synthetic in nature.

The two most common sweeteners used in foods and drinks are aspartame and sugar.

ARTIFICIAL SWEETENERS

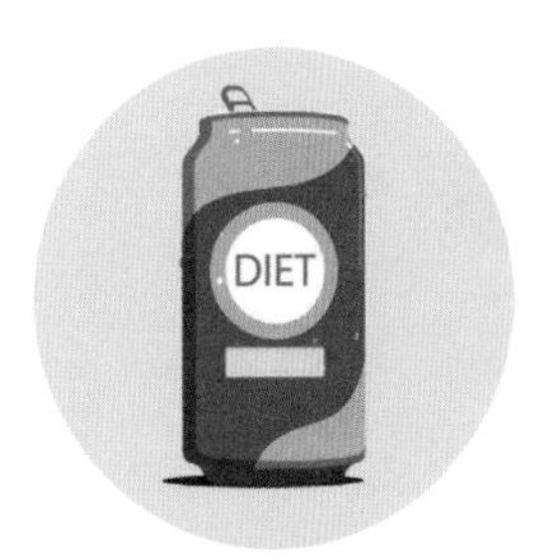

Artificial sweeteners are synthetic sugar substitutes. There are many different names for artificial sweeteners, including acesulfame potassium, aspartame, maltitol, saccharin, sucralose, and sorbitol, to name a few. While a number of them may be on the more natural side, such as stevia and erythritol, even these have their side effects. Of all the artificial sweeteners, the most dangerous is aspartame.

ASPARTAME

Aspartame is a very toxic substance that can be found in chewing gum and in diet foods and drinks. It is marketed as a sugar substitute under the brands Equal and NutraSweet. Aspartame is an excitotoxin, and when ingested can cause headaches, stomachaches, and a long list of other problems, including mental disorders and cognitive dysfunction. It works well as a pesticide to kill ants, likely a sign that you should avoid it. Aspartame can be found in over nine thousand different products now, and that number is climbing. It's less expensive than sugar, and two hundred times sweeter than sugar. However, aspartame breaks down in the body into formaldehyde and methanol, two very toxic compounds indeed.

Lauren was thirty-eight years old when she came to my office for treatment. She had the most severe case of chronic fatigue syndrome that I had ever seen. She was too exhausted even to drive herself to my office. Instead, her father would drive her, and my staff would immediately usher them through our waiting room into a spare room that had a table on which she could lie down.

She brought a brain scan with her that showed dark patches on the surface of her brain. I began to work with her, and before long her subconscious mind, through the Body Code, led us to a very important finding. A reason for the dark patches on her brain was somehow connected to formaldehyde. She was suffering from formaldehyde poisoning. I asked her, "Can you remember a time in your life when you were exposed to formaldehyde?" She thought about it for a bit and replied, "No, not really." She said that she had never done any dissection on cadavers, which are usually preserved in formaldehyde. We exhausted a few other possible sources as well. Having heard that Styrofoam cups can emit trace amounts of formaldehyde, I asked her if she had used them very much in her life. She said, "Well, yes. For quite a number of years I was a traveling salesperson and was on the road a lot. I drank out of a lot of Styrofoam cups, for sure. You think that's the source of this formaldehyde toxin?" I really didn't think that was very likely.

I next asked her, "Do you use any artificial sweeteners, at all?" She replied, "Well, I was addicted to NutraSweet back in those days. I drank a lot of coffee, and I used to use about a tablespoon of it in every cup, sometimes even more. I love the sweet taste of it." A little bit more testing revealed that this was the source of her formaldehyde poisoning. NutraSweet is a trade name for aspartame, and research studies have confirmed that aspartame breaks down into formaldehyde as it is metabolized.

Lauren immediately stopped using aspartame, and it was the beginning of a long, slow period of recovery for her.

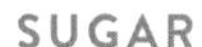

SUGAR

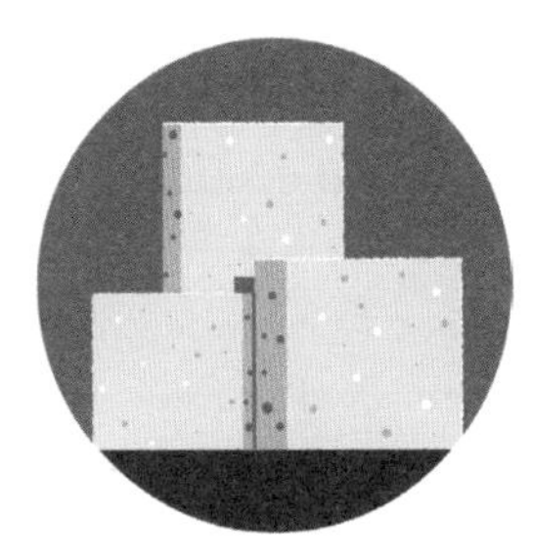

Sugar is highly addictive, making it the most used food additive there is, and the most commonly ingested toxin. In its natural and unrefined form, in fruits, grains, and dairy, sugar is able to be metabolized fairly well. The problem is that nowadays refined sugar is everywhere and in nearly every processed food. Most people eat far too much sugar for the body to process, causing weight gain, mood disturbances, and an overload on the pancreas, which can eventually lead to diabetes.

Excess sugar also weakens connective tissue (think stretch marks), accelerates the aging process, and helps in the formation of damaging free radicals. Overconsumption of processed sugars is a big contributor to many chronic diseases. If you want an in-depth analysis of sugar and its effects on the body, *Sugar Shock!* by Connie Bennett and *Sugar Blues* by William Duffy will both open your eyes to how damaging sugar really is. One of our Body Code practitioners shares a client story of just how addicting sugar can be.

Sugar Addiction Gone

I used to have a serious sweet addiction. For many years, my breakfast was a bar of chocolate or a piece of cheesecake. On good days, when I wanted to have a healthy diet, I would make toast with lots of Nutella added to it. I would add fifteen spoonfuls of sugar in my tea. I was so ashamed of this addiction to the point that I would go buy my tea from the cafeteria, then go to my office and add sugar from the bag that I used to hide there.

While working with Kal, my Body Code practitioner, to clear my Heart-Wall, all of a sudden I didn't crave sugar anymore. I am now enjoying a healthy breakfast (fruits, cheese, egg, etc.). I just don't understand how I was able to drink fifteen spoonfuls of sugar in one cup of tea! If I did this now, I'd throw up. Now, instead of sugar, I add one spoon of honey to my tea, and it tastes amazing! Not only that, when I eat more than a small piece of chocolate I feel like throwing up. So my body really does not need it anymore. I never imagined or thought that one day I'd heal from my chocolate/sugar/sweet addiction. I am so grateful for my practitioner, Kal, for helping me heal using the Emotion Code. And thank you, Dr. Nelson, for your discovery.

—Submitted by Khalid Y., New York, United States

PRESERVATIVES

EXPLANATION

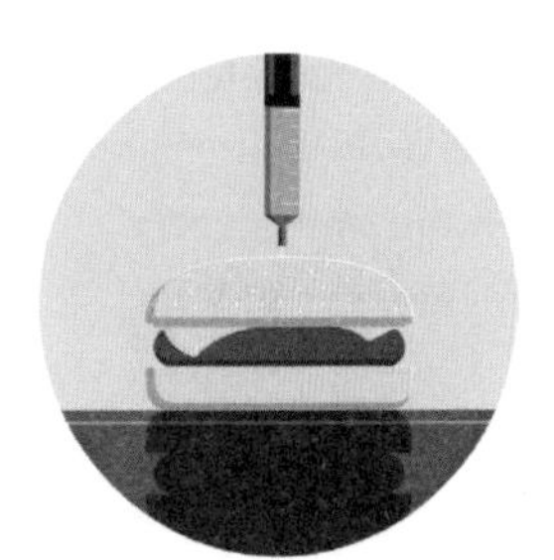

Preservatives are used to extend the shelf life of foods and prevent spoilage. They are toxic and can interfere with normal metabolic processes, leading to the creation of abnormal cells.

An example of a food preservative is sodium benzoate, used in processed foods and beverages to extend shelf life. While it is "generally recognized as safe" (GRAS) by the Food and Drug Administration in the United States, in the presence of vitamin C, sodium benzoate can form benzene, a cancer-causing chemical linked particularly with leukemia and other blood cancers.

GMO FOODS

EXPLANATION

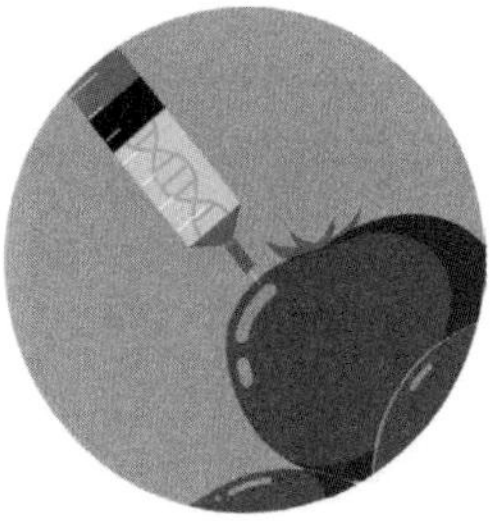

GMO stands for "genetically modified organism." As you are probably aware, modern scientists are combining the DNA of foods like tomatoes, corn, wheat, and so on with all kinds of other DNA, including DNA from insects, poisonous plants, etc. One of the best documentaries about this topic is called *Genetic Roulette*; see GeneticRouletteMovie.com for more information.

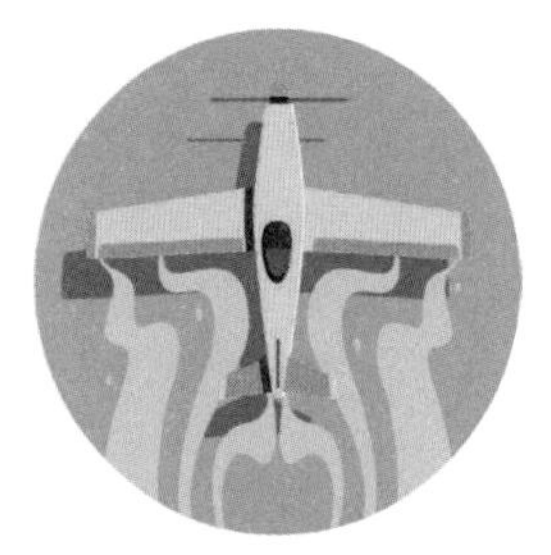

About 90 percent of the soybeans and 70 percent of the corn that is grown in the United States is genetically modified under the label Roundup Ready, 1.8 million tons of which is consumed in the United States annually.* Some studies suggest that Roundup as well as genetically modified Roundup Ready plants are toxic and may lead to birth defects and other serious problems, including loss of energy, autoimmune disease, and more.

*https://www.carlsonattorneys.com/news-and-update/banning-roundup

Pesticides are chemicals that are sprayed on fruits and vegetables to keep insects from damaging produce before it is sold. These chemicals are very harmful to the body. Over 850 million pounds of pesticides are used in the industrial farming industry in the United States alone every year.

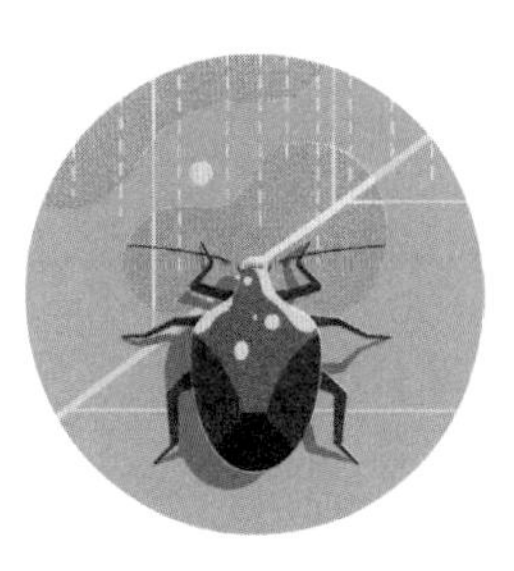

FOOD COLORING

EXPLANATION

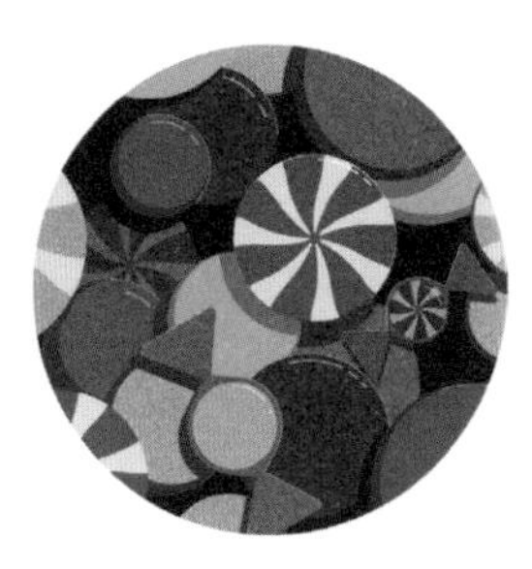

Many common foods such as oranges and salmon are actually dyed so they will look more "palatable." This is done because food's natural variation in color can be unappetizing. Food colorings are generally toxic and have long been implicated in the aggravation of behavioral disorders such as Attention Deficit Disorder (ADD), Attention Deficit Hyperactivity Disorder (ADHD), and autism spectrum disorder. They can also cause typical toxin-related issues such as headaches, stomachaches, irritability, and more.

ADD AND FRUIT SNACKS

I was working on a client whose son had severe behavioral disorders, including attention deficit hyperactivity disorder, or ADHD, and symptoms of autism. She asked if I would test her son to see if we could find any underlying causes for his symptoms. Using the Body Code, I was taken by his subconscious mind to food coloring toxicity. I asked her if she gave him any snacks that might contain food coloring. She told me she really keeps the sugar to a minimum because it upsets him if he gets too much. But she did tell me that she routinely gave him what she thought were healthy fruit snacks. I asked her to go home and check the package for food coloring. Sure enough, there were multiple artificial colors used in that small pack of fruit snacks. She was amazed and began to look at everything else she was feeding him; she found most of it contained food coloring.

After a few months I asked her how her son was doing. She said that after a few weeks of very little food-colored snacks, he was able to concentrate on reading a book and he could hold still long enough to watch a short television show. After about a month, he was not throwing fits anymore and really didn't show any signs of autism or ADHD. It is amazing how food coloring can affect the brain!

EXERCISE:
FIND AND ELIMINATE A FOOD TOXIN

STEP 1.

Ask: "Do I [or you] have a food toxin that we can find and eliminate now?"

- If yes, continue to Step 2.
- If no, you may not have a food toxin at all or you may have one that cannot be removed now, so you may want to try again later.

STEP 2.

(Decoding) Ask: "Do we need to know more about this toxin?"

- If no, move to Step 3 (Association).
- If yes, muscle-test to see which of the following details need to be identified. Sometimes, all that is needed is to identify the source of the toxin. Some common sources are listed in the table at the beginning of this chapter.
- Once you have identified a specific source of the toxin, return to Step 2 (Decoding) and ask if there is more you need to know. If you do not need to know more about the toxin, go to Step 3 (Association), otherwise, you might ask the following questions:
    - Ask: "Do we need to know the age of occurrence?"
    - Ask: "Do we need to know the location of this energy in the body?"

If yes, using a process of elimination to locate this may be helpful. For example, divide the body in half, and ask if the toxin is lodged in the lower half of the body or upper half. Divide the body from left to right and ask if the toxin is lodged in the left half of the body or the right half. Continue dividing in this fashion and asking until you've determined the location in the body where the toxin is lodged, then return to Step 2 (Decoding).

STEP 3.

(Association) Ask: "Is there an associated imbalance that needs to be decoded?"

- If no, skip to Step 4 (Intention).
- If yes, return to the Body Code Map and decode and address any associated imbalances, then return here and repeat the Step 3 (Association) question.

STEP 4.

(Intention) Swipe three times with a magnet or your hand on any length of the governing meridian, while holding an intention to release the energy of this toxin from the body, while at the same time directing the body to remove the toxin through its normal elimination channels.

STEP 5.

Ask: "Did we release that food toxin?"

- If yes, you can start at the beginning on Step 1 and repeat the process to find another food toxin.
- If no, refocus, say a prayer for help, allow your heart to feel love and gratitude that this is going to help, and swipe three times once again with intention.

HELPFUL TIPS FOR DEALING WITH FOOD TOXINS

Sometimes toxin energies will have associated imbalances such as trapped emotions that will need to be released.

Try to eat organic foods when possible, and do your best to keep your sugar intake low, avoiding artificial sweeteners such as sucralose and aspartame, etc. Use good judgment and common sense to avoid food toxins in the future when possible.

22

DRUG TOXINS

The human body is a self-regulating organism. Meaning, it's programmed to heal itself. Pills only mask and suppress the symptoms. The cure lies within you.

—THE MINDS JOURNAL

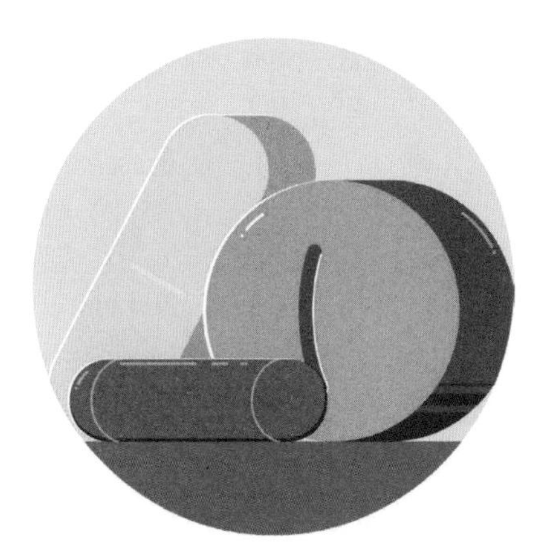

Medications are used to suppress symptoms or to achieve a certain effect, but there are often unintended or unwanted side effects. Side effects are simply the result of toxicity in the body and range from skin irritation to headaches to nausea and even death.

The liver and kidneys are especially vulnerable to medical toxins because they are the organs of detoxification. Some drugs are so toxic that people have to see their doctors every week or sometimes even daily so they can test the liver and kidneys to see if they are starting to fail.

Millions of people, particularly the elderly, are using dangerous combinations of medications that are untested, yet they are still being prescribed every day without full knowledge of the possible complications that could take place. A colleague of mine had a patient who was taking a certain medication that was so powerful, one of the side effects was a syndrome known as "furry tongue." The medication actually created fur or hair growing all over this person's tongue.

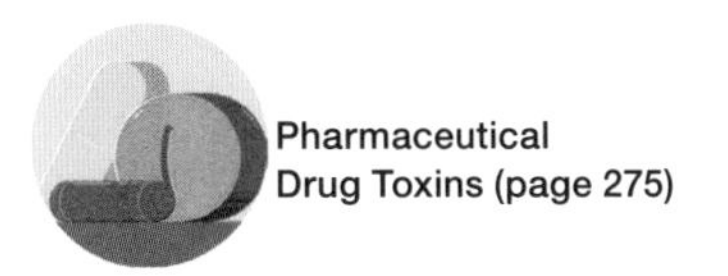

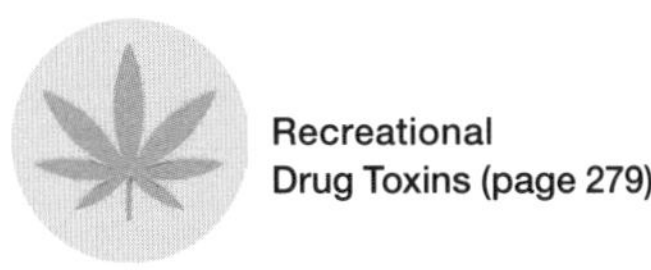

PHARMACEUTICAL DRUG TOXINS

EXPLANATION

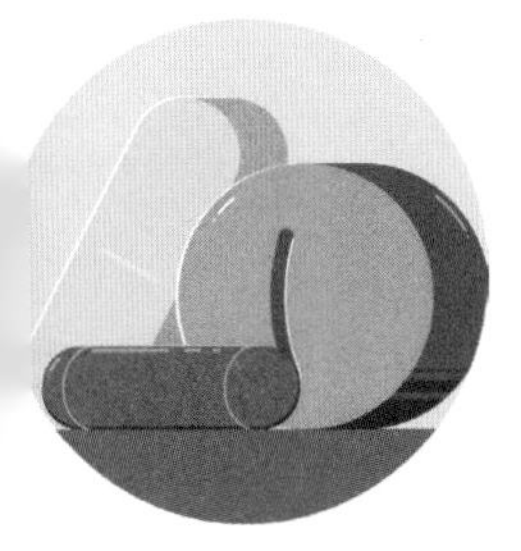

Medications may be necessary and appropriate at times. Always talk to your doctor about any questions or concerns or before changing or stopping any medication. Using muscle testing to determine whether a person should stop taking a medication or to adjust medication dosage is not advised unless you are a prescribing physician. On the other hand, if you muscle-test to see which prescription you are using is causing a particular side effect for you, and you find something, then you could visit with your doctor about it so he or she can help you determine what to do about it. In the next story, a registered nurse suffered neurological symptoms from all the medicine she was taking.

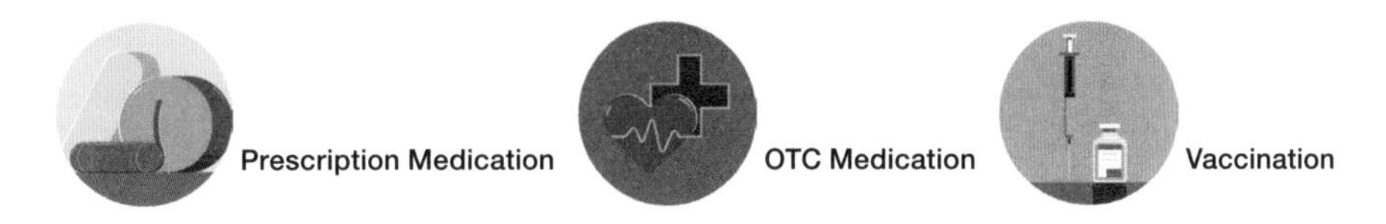

A Nurse's Mental-Illness Journey

I spent the last eight years of my life looking for answers to my struggles with mental health. I had been diagnosed with bipolar, agoraphobia, top 1 percent ADD, major depressive disorder, and panic disorder. My prescriptions included Celexa, which caused serotonin syndrome, and Lexapro, which caused me to be hospitalized. I was prescribed Latuda, Seroquel, trazodone, Lamictal, clonazepam, Prozac, lithium, hydroxyzine, Abilify, Adderall, and lastly Geodon, which caused me to have significant neurological symptoms. Later I spent five days in a mental hospital.

I could not leave my home by myself, could no longer think well enough to pump gas in my car, and had to use Google maps to find my way home. Eventually, I found out about EMDR and the Amen Clinics. With much research, I realized I was in fact suffering from extreme emotional trauma. When I would ask primary doctors, psychiatrists, and neuropsychologists if the anxiety and depression could have anything to do with three members of my family dying, they all said, "You are bipolar. You will have to learn how to manage the symptoms."

At the Amen Clinic, a SPECT scan of my brain showed I had significant PTSD. I later learned that was from my father dying by suicide, my sister dying in a car wreck, and my brother dying in a car wreck. When I started processing those events, my childhood memory started coming back, and I realized I had suffered from extensive sexual abuse as a child, as well as physical and emotional abuse from my mentally ill father. After leaving the Amen Clinic, I started processing the emotional trauma with a therapist who used the Brainspotting modality, but my body could not handle the emotional release, as my blood pressure would shoot up to 210/110 and I would have seizurelike activity. I also tried acupuncture for PTSD, and it helped some. I did a twenty-session round of Neurofeedback after having a brain map, and it helped minimally. My body was out of balance from all the stress and medications, so I started replenishing it with the help of a local practitioner that does bioenergy scans.

I thought I had exhausted all of my options for healing. But then I found out about the Emotion Code. I bought the book and went to a local practitioner. It took a lot of sessions to work through all of my life trauma, but I now no longer have anxiety or depression. We worked together for approximately ninety sessions in seventeen months, which included the Emotion Code, the Body Code, and the Belief Code. It changed my life. I can honestly say I am truly happy for the first time in my life. My recovery has been tested by new difficult situations in my family, and I'm happy to report that I have been able to respond reasonably without excessive worry, panic, and catastrophizing.

I am extremely grateful for this natural healing method that gives so much hope to people who are hurting. I am currently working with about fifty people to help them for free as I complete my certifications in the Body Code System and establish a coaching business. The ripple effects I see happening to all the people that have so graciously been willing to work with me are amazing! I never gave up or lost all hope. I have a purpose and a story to share. I was told by all my medical practitioners that I would never be well and functioning. I'm not 100 percent yet but probably 97 percent. My area has significantly poor ACE (adverse childhood experience) scores, a lot of serious mental-health statistics, and a lot of poverty. My goal is to plant as many seeds as possible of growth, positivity, grace, and love and to watch the ripple effect of the Body Code System, one person and one heart at a time. Thank you for this opportunity!

—Karla D., Oklahoma, United States

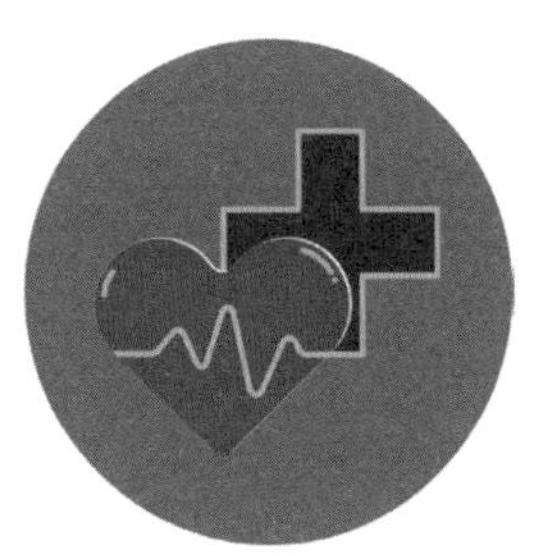

OVER-THE-COUNTER MEDICINES

Over-the-counter medicines (OTC) are medicines that can be purchased without a prescription. All drugs, including OTC medications, are toxic to the body to some degree and require the body to process them both physically and energetically.

THE CAMPHO-PHENIQUE CULPRIT

Julie came to my office for treatment and told me that her problem was a chronic cough that had been going on for about two years. She said that she coughed all night long and throughout the day as well.

She looked at me in a very serious way and said, "Dr. Nelson, I'm afraid that if I can't get rid of this cough, I may actually end up getting divorced. My husband now sleeps every night as far away from me as he can, in another bedroom. I've seen a couple of doctors for this, but they can't find anything serious going on. I've been taking their medications and over-the-counter remedies as well, but nothing is really working. I don't know what to do. You are my last resort. I hope that you can help me."

I took comfort in the knowledge that her subconscious mind would know why she had this chronic cough. A cough like this is a symptom, and symptoms are caused by imbalances, and the Body Code helps find imbalances.

When I used muscle testing to ask her subconscious mind for an underlying reason for her cough, the very first thing that showed up was chemical toxicity. When I used a list of common household products, I was taken to Campho-Phenique, a commonly used pain-relieving antiseptic liquid.

I said, "Julie, do you use Campho-Phenique?" Startled, she said, "Yes! I use it every day! I have an elderly friend that I check in on every night. She's very old, in her nineties, and every night while I'm visiting with her she loves me to rub her feet with Campho-Phenique!"

Campho-Phenique contains phenol, which can be irritating to the eyes and nose, mucous membranes, and nervous system. My patient Julie and I hit this one out of the park. All Julie had to do was stop using Campho-Phenique, and her coughing problem was solved.

This is just another great example of how the Body Code can enable you to find the root cause of problems that you might otherwise miss if you are taking medications to suppress symptoms.

VACCINATION

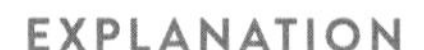

EXPLANATION

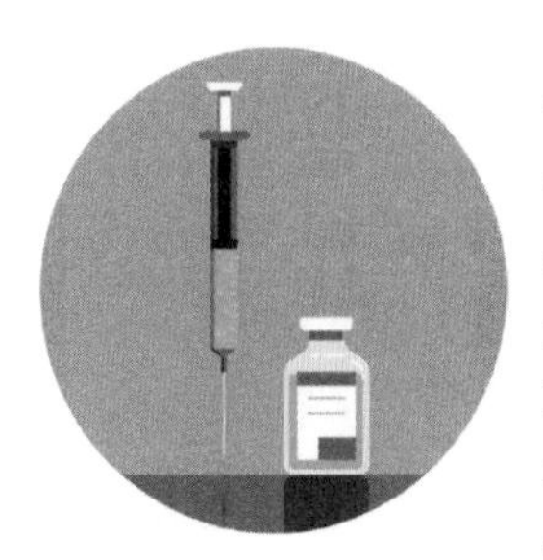

The debate about vaccines has been ongoing for years. Parents are faced with the troubling question of whether they should vaccinate their children or not. There is so much data available from many sources, pros and cons, that it is hard to get the essential proven facts. I recommend checking out the National Vaccine Information Center (NVIC.org) for a source of unbiased information. I encourage you to make your own health-care decisions based on your judgment and research and in partnership with your health-care professional. There have been known side effects from vaccines, as Ingrid illustrates in this next story.

Shingles Vaccine Reaction

I am seventy-three and had a shingles vaccine to prevent getting the virus. I had a horrible reaction, ending up with all the shingles symptoms—the rash, lots of pain, and tiredness. It was really bad. My niece is a Body Code practitioner and she immediately started working on my symptoms. With each Body Code session, there was a reduction in my symptoms, and after eleven sessions or so, it was completely gone, never to return. I don't know what I would have done without her help.

We have worked on many things, such as the grief and heartache on the passing of my husband, and my heart condition. I have nine stents. I feel so blessed to have a niece who does this amazing thing called the Body Code.

—Ingrid G., Ontario, Canada

RECREATIONAL DRUG TOXINS

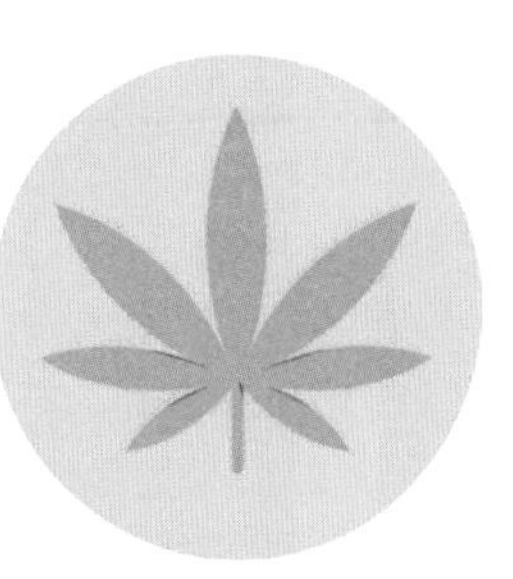

EXPLANATION

Recreational drugs are a scourge of the world in our day, destroying countless lives. Some are extremely toxic and damaging to the body quickly and sometimes permanently. I believe that drugs (excluding caffeine and tobacco) open the body to invasion by entities as well. Marianne Williamson stated it eloquently when she said,

Trying to suppress or eradicate symptoms on the physical level can be extremely important, but there's more to healing than that; dealing with psychological, emotional, and spiritual issues involved in treating sickness is equally important.

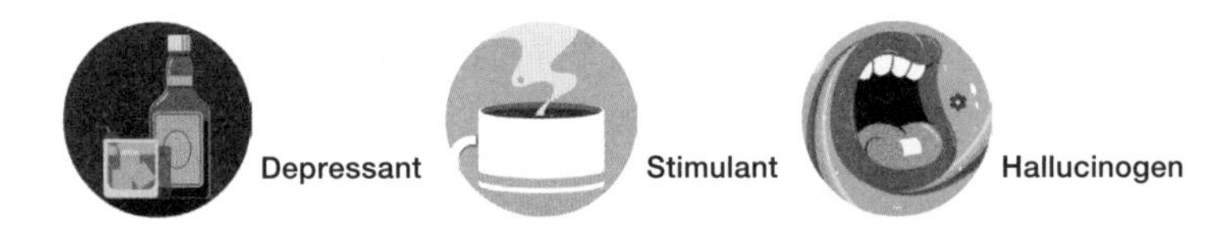

Many people will turn to drugs to suppress symptoms, when the Body Code provides a better way. The following are descriptions of some common recreational drugs and what they can do to your body.

CAFFEINE

Caffeine is one of the most common toxins people ingest. I'm classifying it as a recreational drug because it's addictive, toxic, and so many people rely on it for its druglike effects on the body.

Because caffeine creates imbalance in the kidneys, it will also tend to create low-back pain. In fact, I believe it is the largest single factor that causes low-back pain today. Caffeine is more dangerous than just this, however. It causes fibrocystic breast disease as well as benign prostatic hypertrophy—a condition in which the prostate becomes enlarged, creating difficult urination.

Caffeine can raise blood pressure for hours, stimulate the intensity of the heart's contractions, and actually exaggerate the effects of stress on the body. Faye tells the story of how caffeine has affected her mother.

Too Much Caffeine

My mother woke up one morning with her heart racing and feeling very unwell, which was subsequently diagnosed as fast atrial fibrillation (A-fib), and while on hold to the doctor I did some work to see if we could get to the bottom of it. The Body Code showed "sleep" as a need, a requirement for magnesium, and to avoid coffee. We had to go into hospital to get it under control, where we found out the top three triggers for A-fib are . . . exhaustion, low magnesium, and too much caffeine!!

—FAYE C., HERTFORDSHIRE, UNITED KINGDOM

ALCOHOL

Taken sparingly, alcohol is metabolized fairly well. Too much alcohol can overwhelm the liver, which has to work overtime to process it. Alcoholism over time leads to a diseased liver, a condition known as cirrhosis, which can ultimately result in liver failure and death. In this story, Eva tells how the Body Code was able to help her overcome a painful past linked to alcohol abuse and find a better and happier life.

Rising Above Childhood Trauma

I was born in Zimbabwe (then Rhodesia) in 1972 to alcoholic parents who sank further into alcoholism after my thirteen-year-old sister committed suicide when I was a baby. My mother took her rage out on me. Drunk at night, she would charge into my room while I was sleeping to beat me up. I was called stupid, good for nothing, and everything else under the sun. My father was too weak and frightened of my mother to protect me.

When I was finally able to leave home, I turned to alcohol, drugs, and sex, looking for love with the most awful men. I was overweight and a total mess. Eventually, I hit rock bottom with thoughts of suicide and of taking my four-year-old daughter with me. I was guided to get help from Jane, a practitioner of Dr. Nelson's work. We released absolutely everything, from conception energies, entities, curses, negative beliefs, abundance blocks, and relationship blocks. I threw my antidepressants away, and the light started to enter my life!

My life is now happy, abundant, joyful, and I am basically a new me. I would dread to think where I would be now if this amazing healing modality hadn't been discovered. After participating in the Emotion Code seminar in London, it is my mission to help others as I have been helped. It was an honor to meet Dr. Bradley Nelson and his lovely wife, Jean, and I was so grateful that I was able to thank him personally for saving my life through the grace of God. Thank you, thank you, thank you!

—Eva T., Hertfordshire, Great Britain

TOBACCO

Tobacco is one of the top three most popular toxins out there, along with alcohol and caffeine. Tobacco is a recreational drug in and of itself, but processed cigarettes also contain thousands of different toxic chemicals. One of these chemicals is actually an insecticide called hydrogen cyanide—the same drug that was used in Nazi Germany in the gas chambers. If you have a smoking addiction, use of the Body Code may help, as Kay found in the following story.

Cigarette Addiction Resolved

After a session with a practitioner, we found and released a trapped emotion that kept me in a habit of smoking cigarettes. Since then, I have stopped smoking!

—Kay H., California, United States

MARIJUANA

Marijuana is widely thought of as being fairly harmless, but studies are beginning to show that adolescents who smoke marijuana at least once are more than twice as likely to develop schizophrenia as those who have never smoked. In addition, those who have smoked it fifty times or more are six times more likely to develop schizophrenia. So beside the more widely recognized lack of motivation and paranoia issues, smoking marijuana may not be as safe as people think. My belief is that marijuana use leads to joint problems and eventual arthritis, but there are no studies I have found to support this beyond my own observations in practice.

AMPHETAMINES

Amphetamines are chemically engineered psychostimulant drugs that act to speed up the nervous system, causing euphoria, increased concentration, hyperactivity, and other more agitating symptoms. Speeding up the natural rhythms of the body is harmful to the adrenal glands, the kidneys, and the liver.

Amphetamines include pharmaceutical drugs such as Adderall, but also methamphetamine, an illegal street drug commonly called meth or speed. Amphetamines in any form are toxic, and when introduced to the body, the liver will attempt to break down the chemicals into hopefully less toxic components. The physical effects of amphetamine use are harmful and include weight loss, insomnia, increased blood pressure, numbness, tachycardia, increased heart attack risk, and many more.

Psychological effects of amphetamine use include anxiety; a false sense of confidence, strength, or well-being (all of these being dangerous to the user's safety); and possible psychosis.

COCAINE

Cocaine is a drug that stimulates the central nervous system and is both harmful and incredibly addictive. Like any other drug, cocaine causes health problems that become worse with prolonged or excessive use, which can result in heart and blood pressure problems, paranoid delusions, seizures, and strokes.

ECSTASY

Ecstasy, also known as MDMA, is a dangerous psychoactive amphetamine street drug that happens to be very toxic. It causes an imbalance in the serotonin transporters in the brain, which unfortunately makes you feel great while you're on the drug, but the side effects can be difficult to devastating. At the lesser end of the spectrum, Ecstasy will cause increased depression and anxiety, even after a user has quit using it. This is because the serotonin levels in the brain have been depleted and they don't automatically go up to normal again. On the other end of the spectrum is disaster.

I had a patient from California who had tried Ecstasy twice. The first time she tried it, she didn't notice much of anything, but the second time she tried it, it destroyed her health completely. When she came to me, she was twenty-three years old and had such terrific fatigue and such terrible fibromyalgia that she couldn't work anymore. It was all she could do to get to the store to buy enough food to survive on each week.

HEROIN

Heroin is an extremely addictive and very damaging drug made from opium poppies. Psychological dependence is what makes heroin so addictive, because of the euphoria experienced when the drug is taken. Like other drugs, it is toxic and destroys the body, causing respiratory problems, which are often what kills the user, as well as decreased liver function and heart problems.

KETAMINE

Ketamine, or Special K, is a drug used medically in anesthesia, but is a street drug as well. It causes impaired senses, hallucinations, and problems with respiration and circulation. It is both addictive and toxic.

LSD

LSD, or lysergic acid diethylamide, is a psychedelic drug invented for medicinal and psychiatric purposes but now more frequently used as a street drug. It causes hallucinations, paranoia, and euphoria. LSD as a substance is considered to be nontoxic, however it will show up through muscle testing as a toxin in the body.

NIGHTSHADES

The most commonly known toxic nightshade is the psychoactive "deadly nightshade" or belladonna. Tobacco is also a nightshade, as are edible plants such as potatoes, tomatoes, eggplants, and peppers. Nightshades are known to cause inflammation and pain due to the alkaloid chemicals they produce. The most common include nicotine in tobacco, the hallucinogenic and deadly tropane alkaloids in belladonna, and the mildly irritating alkaloids in tomatoes, potatoes, and other food nightshades. I often advise sensitive individuals to avoid nightshades altogether, although most people tolerate edible nightshade plants very well.

EXERCISE: FIND AND ADDRESS A TOXIN

STEP 1.

Ask: "Do I [or you] have a drug toxin that can be eliminated now?"

- If yes, continue to Step 2.
- If no, you may not have a drug toxin at all or one that cannot be removed now, so you may want to try again later.

STEP 2.

(Decoding) Ask: "Do we need to know more about this toxin?"

- If no, move to Step 3 (Association).
- If yes, muscle-test to see which of the following details need to be identified. Sometimes, all that is needed is to identify the type of toxin. Some common drug types are listed in this table:

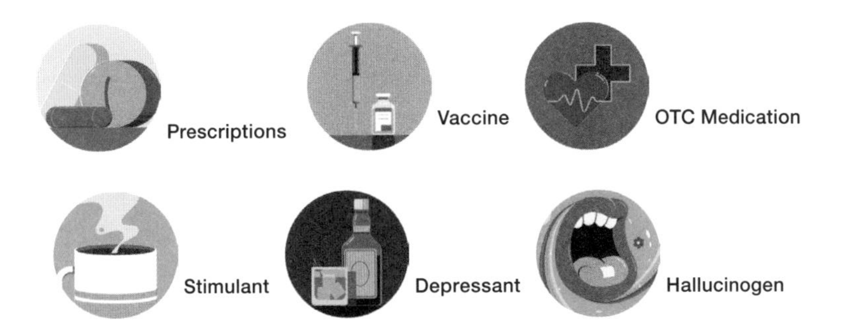

- Once you have identified a specific type of drug toxin, return to Step 2 (Decoding) and ask if there is more you need to know. If you do not need to know more about the toxin, go to Step 3 (Association), otherwise, you might ask the following questions:
  - Ask: "Do we need to know the age of occurrence?"
  - Ask: "Do we need to know the location of this energy in the body?"

If yes, using a process of elimination to locate this may be helpful. For example, divide the body in half, and ask if the toxin is lodged in the lower half of the body or upper half. Divide the body from left to right and ask if the toxin is lodged in the left half of the body or the right half. Continue dividing in this fashion and asking until you've determined the location in the body where the toxin is lodged, then return to Step 2 (Decoding).

STEP 3.

(Association) Ask: "Is there an associated imbalance that needs to be decoded?"

- If no, skip to Step 4 (Intention).
- If yes, return to the Body Code Map and decode and address any associated imbalances, then return here and repeat the Step 3 (Association) question.

STEP 4.

(Intention) Swipe three times with a magnet or your hand on any length of the governing meridian, while holding an intention to release the energy of this toxin from the body, while at the same time directing the body to remove the toxin through its normal elimination channels.

STEP 5.

Ask: "Did we release that drug toxin?"

- If yes, you can start at the beginning on Step 1 and repeat the process to find another drug toxin.
- If no, refocus, say a prayer for help, allow your heart to feel love and gratitude that this is going to help, and swipe three times once again with intention.

HELPFUL TIPS FOR DEALING WITH DRUG TOXINS

Millions of people are using dangerous combinations of medications, over-the-counter drugs, and recreational drugs, overloading and weakening the liver and kidneys. With repeated exposure, toxins often accumulate in the body, causing a multitude of problems.

Physical support may be necessary to complete the detoxification process. It is recommended that one see a health-care provider for more information about detoxifying this substance from the body. Use good judgment and common sense to avoid drug toxins in the future when possible.

SECTION 6

NUTRITION AND LIFESTYLE

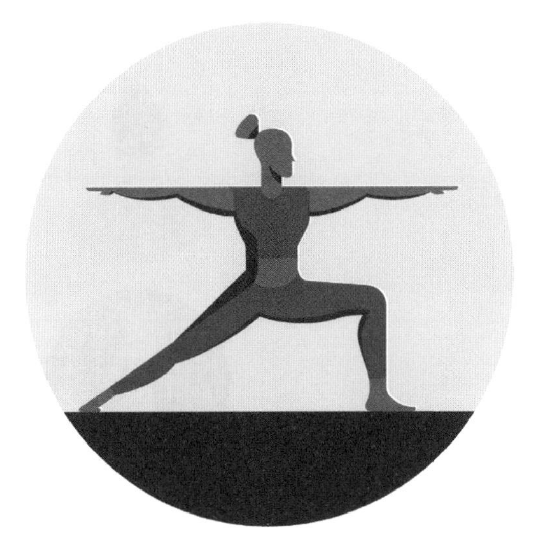

The natural healing force within each one of us is the greatest force in getting well. Our food should be our medicine. Our medicine should be our food.

—HIPPOCRATES

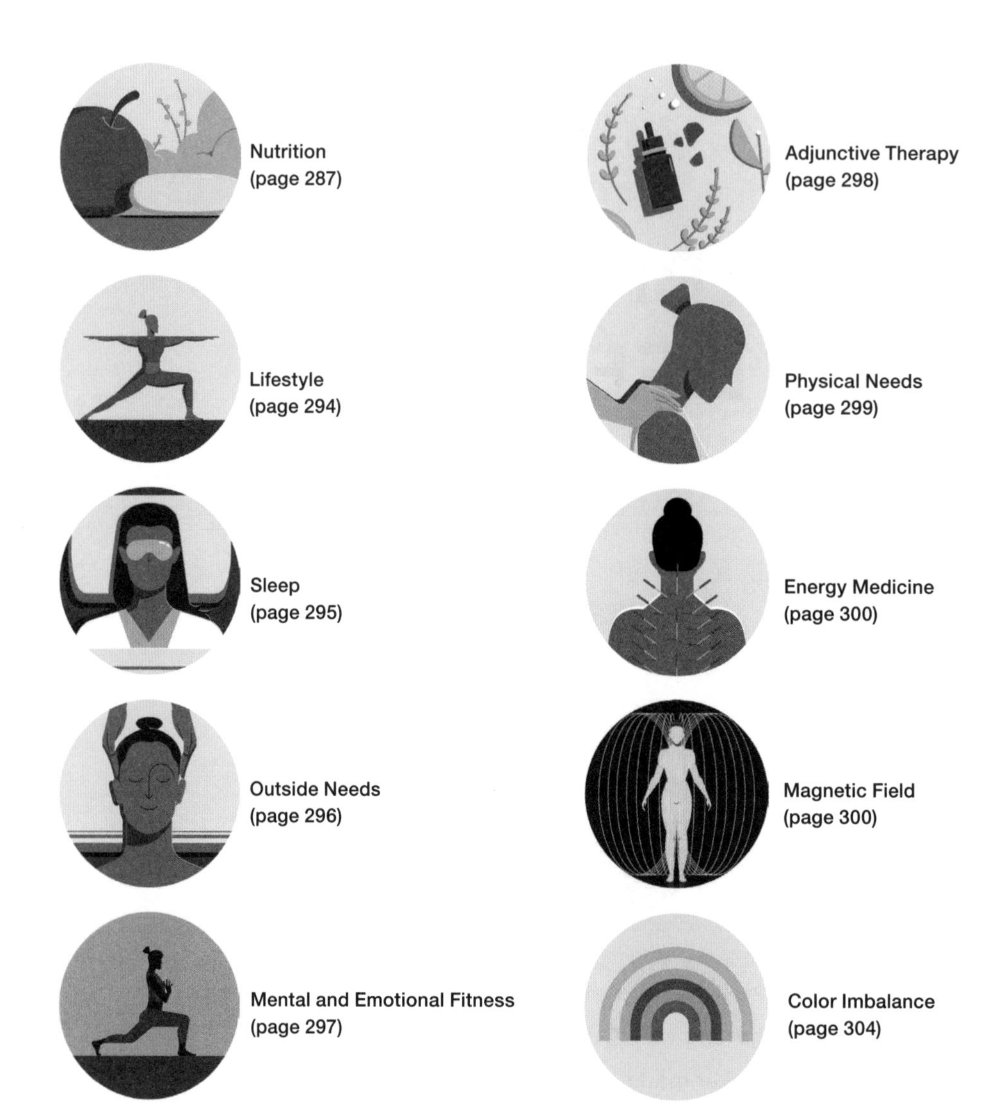

Nutritional imbalances and lifestyle needs can easily be undetected sources of suffering. What are they? How do we detect them? How do we correct them?

In this section we will discuss nutrition, sleep, outside needs, magnetic field imbalances, color deficiency, and more.

23

NUTRITION

The human body is a river of intelligence, energy, and information that is constantly renewing itself in every second of its existence.

—DEEPAK CHOPRA

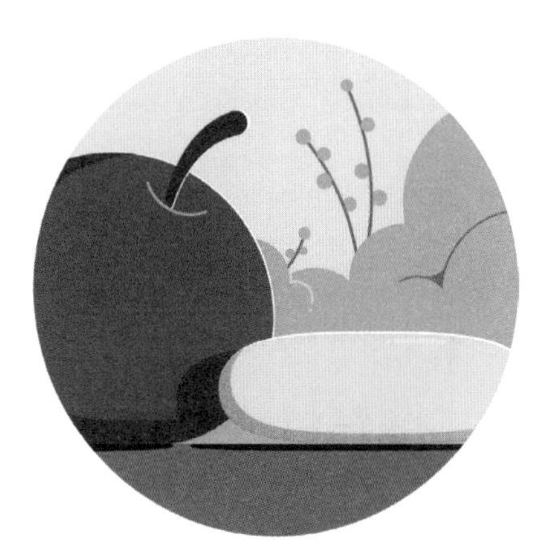

Eating nutrient-dense food is vital to our health and is becoming more and more so as time goes on. While it is often better to eat conventionally grown fruits and vegetables rather than none at all, this is not always the case. For example, commercially grown fruits and vegetables are often sprayed so heavily with toxic pesticides and herbicides that you're better off leaving them on the shelf. Unfortunately, pesticides and herbicides are not the only things you need to watch out for.

Many fruits, vegetables, and grains are also genetically modified organisms (GMOs), meaning their DNA has been altered to achieve certain effects. These organisms are usually seen as toxic by the body, even though they may look the same as their organic counterparts.

In fact, genetically modified foods may even appear more appetizing, fresher, and without the bruising that you sometimes see in other produce. But don't be fooled. This is because their DNA has been specifically changed so the produce will be tougher to survive the often long, rough road from farm to store.

If your fruits and vegetables still seem fresh two weeks after you buy them, you may want to question how healthy they really are for you. Many are genetically modified so they will grow in unnatural conditions, such as a colder or warmer climate. For example, scientists combined the DNA of tomatoes with the DNA of the flounder fish. This allowed them to grow tomatoes in an unnaturally cold climate, where normal tomatoes would not be able to grow. These tomatoes may look normal, but your body knows better.

Avoiding toxins is a good reason to eat organic foods, but it's certainly not the only reason. Organically grown fruits and vegetables have been proven to be many times more nutrient rich than those commercially grown. A study done a number of years ago by Rutgers University found astounding differences in mineral content in organically grown versus commercially grown vegetables.

In simple terms, organically grown snap beans had seven times the amount of boron and twenty-two times the amount of iron, and organic tomatoes had two thousand times the amount of iron than their commercially grown counterparts.

All of the mineral contents were dramatically higher in organically grown vegetables than in commercially grown vegetables.

Eating organic foods is by far the best way to nourish the body and give it all the nutrients it needs. What your body needs is probably a little different than what my body needs, of course, depending on any number of factors. But at the end of the day, organic food is best for all of us.

If you are able to, I highly recommend that you grow some of your own vegetables and fruits. If you've ever grown your own vegetables, you know how much better they taste. If you don't have a garden of your own, I recommend reading a book called *Square Foot Gardening* by Mel Bartholomew. In it you'll learn how you can have a garden, even if you live in an apartment and you don't have much room.

NUTRITIONAL IDEAS CHANGE

If there's one thing that is certain, it is that ideas about nutrition change continually. You may be old enough to remember the great egg scare during the 1990s. Scientists promoted the notion that eggs were causing heart disease because of the cholesterol they contain, recommending that no one should eat more than one egg per week. Of course, a few years later, they discovered that these ideas were actually wrong: it turned out that eggs are not dangerous after all.

Keep an open mind when you hear about what foods you should and shouldn't eat, because you never know what information might be outdated or incorrect. Remember that what is really best for the body is different for everyone, so use muscle testing to determine what you need and what you should avoid.

WHAT'S RIGHT FOR YOUR BODY

The perfect diet does exist, but it will never be a one-size-fits-all type of plan. It is the diet that is specifically for you, the one your subconscious mind already knows all about. Your body knows exactly what it does and does not want, what will nourish you and what will cause problems if you eat it. All you have to do is ask. You can get as specific as you want, even creating complete and extensive meal plans.

Remember that if you have trouble with a certain food, there may be an underlying reason (especially if the food is not inherently toxic), so use the Body Code and clear whatever you find. Keep in mind that your dietary needs will likely change over time, depending on what is going on in your body and in your life. So keep an open line of communication with your body and keep giving it the proper fuel. A great resource that will teach you how to use your body's wisdom to eat what your subconscious mind really wants you to eat is the book *The Food Codes* by Lana Nelson, a certified Body Code practitioner.

As I learned to ask the subconscious mind what a person needed, I often found that there was some sort of nutritional deficiency that needed to be addressed for the person's recovery to take place. Vitamins and minerals are needed for the countless number of chemical reactions taking place in your body every moment. If you are deficient in any vitamin or mineral, it will be essentially impossible for you to attain vibrant health.

One of the most widely known examples of this is the disease known as scurvy. Scurvy is a condition that results in nosebleeds, loss of teeth, anemia, exhaustion, and ultimately death if a severe vitamin C deficiency is allowed to exist. The British navy found that scurvy could be beaten simply by eating fresh fruits and vegetables. They began storing and shipping barrels of limes on voyages, preventing scurvy and giving the British sailors the nickname "limeys."

While it's uncommon in our day to see deficiencies as severe as scurvy, it's not unusual for most people to be deficient in a few minerals or vitamins at any given time. Rather than leading to textbook vitamin-deficiency diseases, these deficiencies instead result in a wide variety of lesser illnesses and loss of energy.

Luckily, the human body knows exactly what it needs. Not only does your subconscious mind know the history of your every cell as well as your entire existence, even prior to conception, it also knows if you need more of a certain vitamin, mineral, essential oil, herb, and more.

THE SUBCONSCIOUS KNOWS

Remind yourself frequently that the healing power is in your own subconscious mind.

—JOSEPH MURPHY

Ginger was an athletic twenty-eight-year-old woman who had been hospitalized for five days because of severe abdominal pain. Her doctors couldn't figure out what was wrong with her, and after five days of exhausting all of their diagnostic tests, they released her from the hospital after telling her that there was nothing they could do to help her.

She showed up at my office on a Monday morning, the day after she had been released from the hospital. Her pain was not any better, and she was distressed that something was seriously wrong with her, as well as being confused that the doctors at the hospital couldn't find a cause for her pain.

Using the Body Code, I began muscle-testing her, asking her subconscious mind what the reasons for her pain were. I found a couple of trapped emotions and released those, as well as a couple of other imbalances. At some point during this session, muscle testing took me to the nutrient section of the Body Code, to a very specific nutrient called chromium. I recommended that she get herself a chromium supplement and gave it no more thought.

I couldn't find anything else to correct, so even though she was still in a lot of pain, I told her to go home and come back the next day.

She was one of my first patients the next morning but she wasn't any better. In fact, her pain was clearly worse than it was the day before. I remember thinking that somehow, something serious must have been missed in the hospital.

Not knowing what else to do, I started again using the Body Code and muscle-testing her to see what her subconscious mind had to say. I was once again taken to the nutrient section of the Body Code to—you guessed it—chromium. I suddenly remembered that chromium had shown up the day before, which I thought was a random finding.

I told her, "You need chromium. I don't know why, but you seem to really need it. I want you to leave my office right now, drive down the street to the health food store, and buy some chromium. Ask them for a glass of water and take some of it right there in the store, then come back here to my office."

Twenty minutes later Ginger was back in my office waiting room literally jumping for joy, exclaiming, "I'm fixed! I'm fixed! The moment I took the chromium, the pain was instantly gone!"

She excitedly asked me, "How did that work? Why did taking chromium make the pain go away?" My reply was, "Honestly, I have no idea. All I know is that your body needed chromium. The pain was a signal to you that you didn't have enough chromium. Luckily, your body was able to communicate its need to me, and I was able to communicate it to you, and for whatever reason, it worked!"

This story is a wonderful illustration of how powerful it can be when the subconscious mind is given a clear way to indicate what it needs.

NUTRIENT DEFICIENCY

EXPLANATION

Most Western diets are deficient in vitamins and minerals. Factory-farming practices have depleted the soil so that the vegetables and fruit growing from it are not rich in nutrients like they once were. In addition to that, most people don't eat enough fruits and vegetables as it is, so it should be no surprise that many people have nutrient deficiencies. The body's organs and tissues need a certain amount of vitamins and minerals in order to function properly. When they don't have the nutrients they need, imbalance and eventual breakdown are the result.

EXERCISE: IDENTIFYING A NUTRIENT DEFICIENCY

To find out if you have a nutrient deficiency, ask, "Is there a nutrient deficiency that needs to be addressed?" If yes, find the nutrient on the following Nutrients chart. If no, you may not have a deficiency and can skip this exercise.

NUTRIENTS CHART		
	A	B
1	Antioxidants Boron Calcium Carbohydrates Carnitine	Methionine Molybdenum Omega-3 Omega-6 Oxygen
2	Carotenoids Chloride Cholesterol Choline Chromium	Phenylalanine Phosphorus Potassium Probiotics/Prebiotics Protein
3	Coenzyme Q10 Cobalt Copper Enzymes Fat, Monounsaturated	Selenium Sodium Sulfur Threonine Tryptophan
4	Fat, Polyunsaturated Fat, Saturated Fiber Flavonoids Histidine	Valine Vitamin A Vitamin B1 (Thiamin) Vitamin B2 (Riboflavin) Vitamin B3 (Niacin)
5	Iodine Iron Isoleucine Lecithin Leucine	Vitamin B5 (Pantothenic Acid) Vitamin B6 (Pyridoxine) Vitamin B7 (Biotin) Vitamin B9 (Folate) Vitamin B12 (Cobalamin)
6	Lutein/Zeaxanthin Lycopene Lysine Magnesium Manganese	Vitamin C Vitamin D Vitamin E Vitamin K Zinc

STEP 1.

(Decoding) Ask: "Is the nutrient in column A?"

- If no, it is in column B.

STEP 2.

Ask: "Is it in an odd row?"

- If no, it is in an even row (2, 4, or 6).

STEP 3.

For odd, ask, "Is it in row 1?" (Name odd rows one by one.)

- For even, ask, "Is it in row 2?" (Name even rows one by one.)

STEP 4.

Ask: "Is it ____?"

- Name each nutrient one by one, and muscle-test for the answer.
- Once the nutrient is identified, continue the decoding process by asking the following questions.
  - Ask: "Am I taking in enough of this nutrient?"

If no, look for information about the recommended daily allowance online or in other resources available. Then continue by asking the next question.

- Ask: "Am I taking in the right quality of this nutrient?"

If no, make an effort to find a different or higher quality source of this nutrient.

STEP 5.

(Association) Absorption/Utilization: Ask, "Is there an associated imbalance that we need to decode in order to help your body absorb or utilize this nutrient?"

- If yes, return to the Body Code Map, decode and address any associated imbalances, then return here and repeat the Step 5 (Association) question.

STEP 6.

(Intention) Using caution and common sense, add the needed nutrient into your diet via food or supplement.

HELPFUL TIPS FOR TESTING FOR NUTRITION

You can also try testing for foods, supplements, proteins, or any other nutritional categories to see what you are missing in your daily diet. As with any change in nutrition, always use common sense and moderation. Consult your health-care provider or a nutritionist with any concerns or questions.

For more information about each nutrient and its recommended daily allowance (RDA), search online.

24

LIFESTYLE

If you restore balance in your own self, you will be contributing immensely to the healing of the world.

–DEEPAK CHOPRA

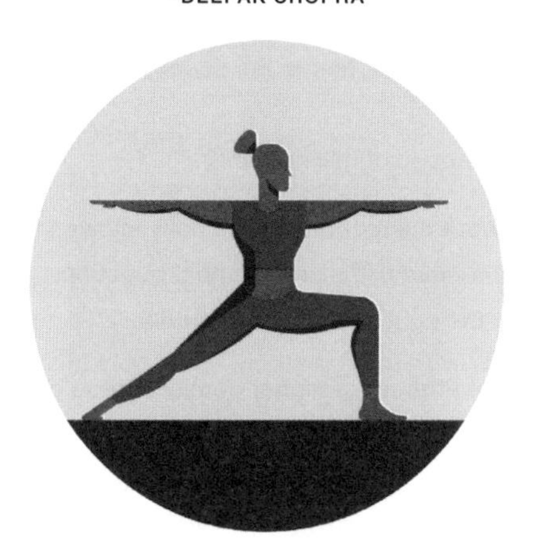

How long you live and how healthy you are depends to a great degree on lifestyle. The purpose of this chapter is to discuss a few lifestyle categories, what they are, and how you can test to see if you need to do something in that category to improve your lifestyle.

SLEEP

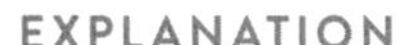

EXPLANATION

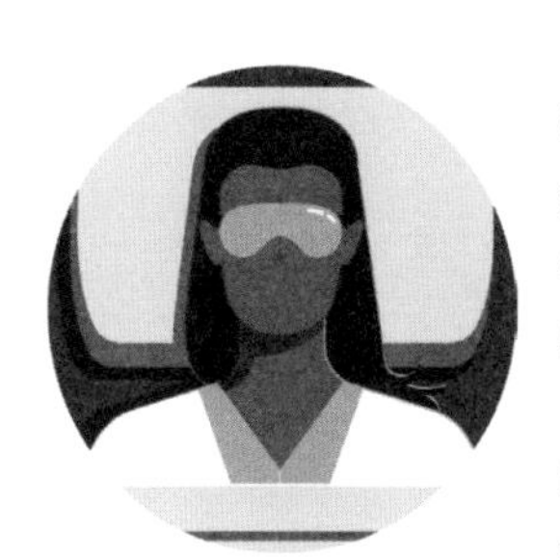

Sleep is a restful state that allows for accelerated healing, growth, and a general rebalancing of the mind, body, and spirit. Many people have a sleep deficit, often spending enough time in bed but still not getting proper restorative sleep.

Sleep is made up of different recurring stages and is influenced by the internal circadian clock that aligns with normal day/night cycles. With the advent of artificial light, sleep patterns have been altered in most modern countries. The human body has been shown to prefer sleeping at night. Working and wakefulness during the normal hours of sleep are highly disruptive to health.

In my first year of practice, I saw a lot of patients who worked at a local factory. The difference between the patients who worked the day shift and those who worked the night shift was quite remarkable. Those patients working the night shift had a much more difficult time recovering their health. In fact, in some cases the disruption to their sleep schedule was the single biggest factor in their inability to get well. Getting these patients back to a normal daytime shift for work often became critical to their recovery.

Beyond working when you should be sleeping, there are many different underlying reasons why sleep may be disturbed. One of the most common areas of imbalance has to do with the autonomic nervous system, the "automatic" portion of the nervous system that runs all the processes of the body, which may become stuck in "fight or flight" mode due to trapped emotions or other traumas. In the following story, Stefanie finds her fatigue was due to trapped emotions.

Difficulty Waking Up

In my first session with an Emotion Code practitioner, I asked her to focus on my issue of having difficulty waking up in the morning. This had plagued me for several years because of various chronic illnesses and emotional traumas, but after healing most of those problems, I still could barely get out of bed each day, making it difficult to take care of my children and get them to school on time. The practitioner found twenty-four trapped emotions contributing to this issue . . . coming from the years that I had suffered from chronic illness and fatigue. The next day, I woke up feeling like a new person! It's been nearly six weeks, and I am able to get out of bed without hitting the snooze button or feeling a sense of dread or exhaustion upon waking. I can clearly tell the difference between feeling tired and needing more sleep, and feeling like I don't want to face my day. This has been a total game changer for my productivity and confidence. I now wake up with a sense of joy and purpose each day without anything holding me back, and I actually look forward to mornings again!

—Stefanie W., Nebraska, United States

EXERCISE: FIND AND RELEASE A SLEEP IMBALANCE

STEP 1.

Ask: "Am I [or are you] getting enough restful sleep?"

- **If yes, great!**
- **If no, continue to Step 2 (Association).**

STEP 2.

(Association) Ask: "Is there anything interfering with my [or your] ability to get enough restful sleep?"

- **If no, move to Step 3 (Intention).**
- **If yes, return to the Body Code Map decode and address any associated imbalances, then return here and repeat the Step 2 (Association) question.**

STEP 3.

(Intention) Swipe three times with a magnet or your hand on any length of the governing meridian, while holding the intention to reset the body's sleep mechanism.

HELPFUL TIPS FOR FINDING SLEEP IMBALANCES

There are many different underlying reasons why sleep may be disturbed. A thorough decoding process using the Body Code Map is recommended to resolve sleep issues fully.

OUTSIDE NEEDS

EXPLANATION

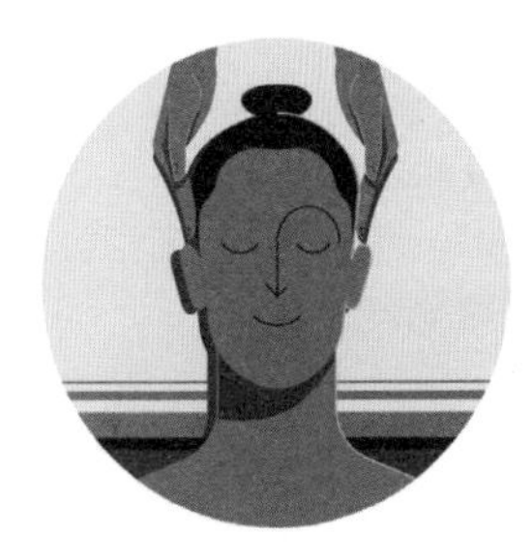

If one's body or lifestyle is lacking in some crucial area, the subconscious can communicate that need to you through the use of the Body Code. "Outside needs" refer to anything else that can help achieve balance and ultimate healing, apart from the imbalances and needs listed elsewhere in the Body Code System. These outside needs can be anything from mental health care to massage to homeopathy. These are grouped into four categories: mental and emotional fitness, adjunctive therapy, physical need, and energy medicine.

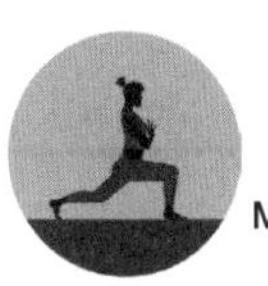
Mental and Emotional Fitness

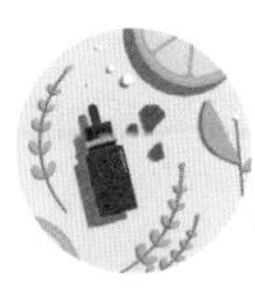
Adjunctive Therapy

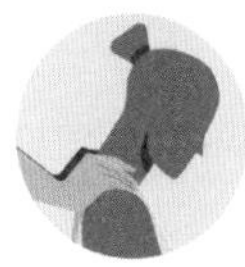
Physical Need

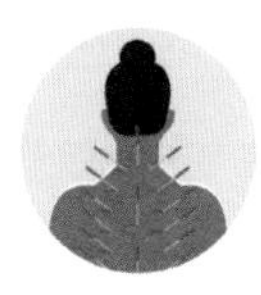
Energy Medicine

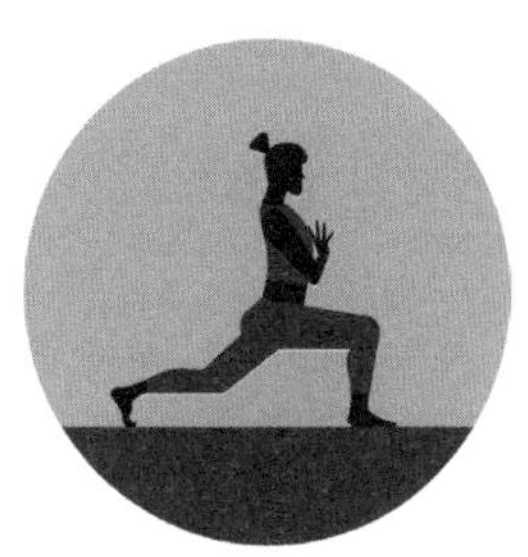

MENTAL AND EMOTIONAL FITNESS

EXPLANATION

Mental and emotional fitness include activities to help creativity as well as balanced thinking and emotions, and may assist in avoidance of the formation of new trapped emotions.

EXERCISE: IDENTIFYING A MENTAL OR EMOTIONAL FITNESS NEED

STEP 1.

(Decoding) Ask: "Would I [or you] benefit from ____?" (Fill in the blank using intuition, creativity, and the following list.) Be creative, ask friends for suggestions, and do research online to help you decide how to proceed. Some ideas for this category are listed in this table:

MENTAL AND EMOTIONAL FITNESS

Acts of service or charity	Counseling or therapy with a licensed professional	Socializing
Reading, watching, or listening to uplifting materials	Meditation	Physical movement (dance, exercise, etc.)
Spending time appreciating nature and/or animals	Journaling	Creating art or pottery
Spending quality time with loved ones	Enjoying music, live or otherwise	Creative writing
Laughter therapy	Hiking	Anything else that helps you feel positive, uplifted, and nourished

STEP 2.

(Association) Ask: "Is there an associated imbalance that needs to be decoded?"

- If no, move to Step 3 (Intention).
- If yes, return to the Body Code Map, decode and address any associated imbalances, then return here and repeat the Step 2 (Association) question.

STEP 3.

(Intention) Try any or all of the activities that tested positive, and see what feels right and nourishing.

HELPFUL TIPS FOR MENTAL AND EMOTIONAL FITNESS

If one of the aforementioned activities is indicated, it's always important to give this subconscious wisdom and communication the importance it deserves, as doing so may facilitate a more complete and efficient recovery process.

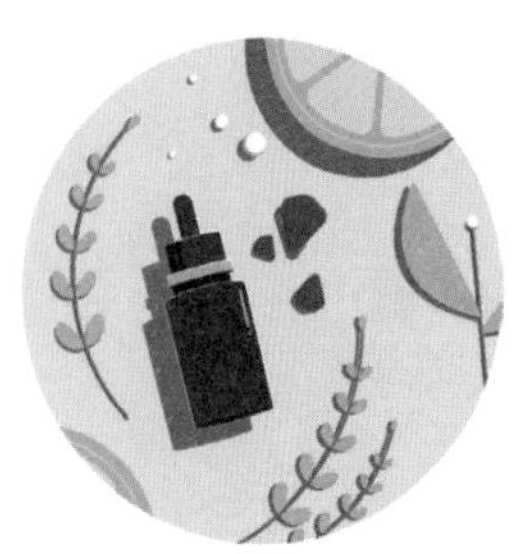

ADJUNCTIVE THERAPY

EXPLANATION

Sometimes the subconscious mind may want outside help or an additional therapy to maximize the effectiveness of healing and recovery. This category includes common therapies such as homeopathy and flower remedies.

EXERCISE: IDENTIFYING AN ADJUNCTIVE THERAPY NEED

STEP 1.

(Decoding) Identify the particular remedy the subconscious mind would like. (A remedy can be selected based on the symptoms present, however, it is suggested that you do some research, as well as muscle-test to see which remedy at your local store or online may benefit you.)

- Ask: "Would I [or you] benefit from a homeopathic remedy?"
- Ask: "Would I [or you] benefit from a flower remedy?"

STEP 2.

(Association) Ask: "Is there an associated imbalance that needs to be decoded?"

- If no, move to Step 3 (Intention).

- If yes, return to the Body Code Map, decode and address any associated imbalances, then return here and repeat the Step 2 (Association) question.

STEP 3.

(Intention) Take any remedies as directed, following manufacturer recommendations, and consult your health-care provider or homeopathic doctor for advice. Remember to use common sense and moderation.

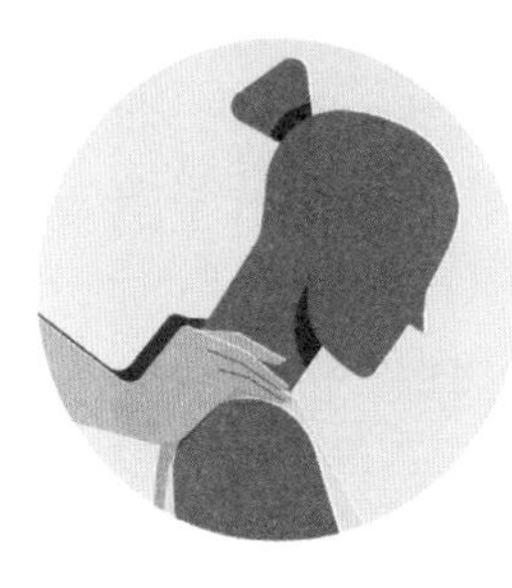

PHYSICAL NEEDS

EXPLANATION

The "Physical Needs" section of the Body Code includes important activities such as body work, detoxification, and exercise.

EXERCISE: IDENTIFYING A PHYSICAL NEED

STEP 1.

(Decoding) Ask: "Would I [or you] benefit from ____?" (Fill in the blank using intuition, creativity, and the following list.) Be creative, ask friends for suggestions, and do research online to help you decide how to proceed. Some ideas for this category include:

Walking	Chiropractic care	Yoga	Acupressure
Swimming	Resistance training	Craniosacral therapy	Sports
Hiking	Massage	Dance	Reflexology

STEP 2.

(Association) Ask: "Is there an associated imbalance that needs to be decoded?"

- If no, move to Step 3 (Intention).
- If yes, return to the Body Code Map, decode and address any associated imbalances, then return here and repeat the Step 2 question.

STEP 3.

(Intention) Depending on what your answer was, try any or all of the activities that tested positive, and see what feels right.

HELPFUL TIPS FOR PHYSICAL NEEDS

A wealth of information about each of these methods is available on the internet, or you can learn more by visiting a provider of the method you want to learn about.

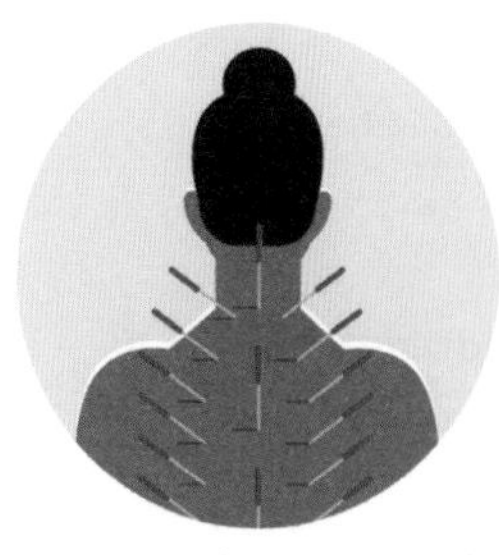

ENERGY MEDICINE

EXPLANATION

Energy medicine includes additional kinds of energy healing techniques and practices found around the world, apart from the Emotion Code and the Body Code.

The items in these categories do not constitute an exhaustive list, and you may add your own pieces to this puzzle of complete health. If you have a technique or modality not listed here, add it as part of your tool kit. The subconscious knows exactly what the body and spirit need—you just need to ask!

EXERCISE: IDENTIFYING AN ENERGY MEDICINE NEED

STEP 1.

(Decoding) Ask: "Would I [or you] benefit from ____?" (Fill in the blank using the categories above.) Here are additional energy methods that may be beneficial and essential for complete healing and recovery:

- Traditional Chinese medicine
- Ayurveda
- Reiki
- Acupuncture

STEP 2.

(Association) Ask: "Is there an associated imbalance that needs to be decoded?"

- **If no, move to Step 3 (Intention).**
- **If yes, return to the Body Code Map, decode and address any associated imbalances, then return here and repeat the Step 2 (Association) question.**

STEP 3.

(Intention) It is suggested to continue using the Body Code in conjunction with whatever protocol your energy medicine practitioner recommends.

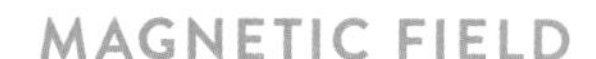

MAGNETIC FIELD

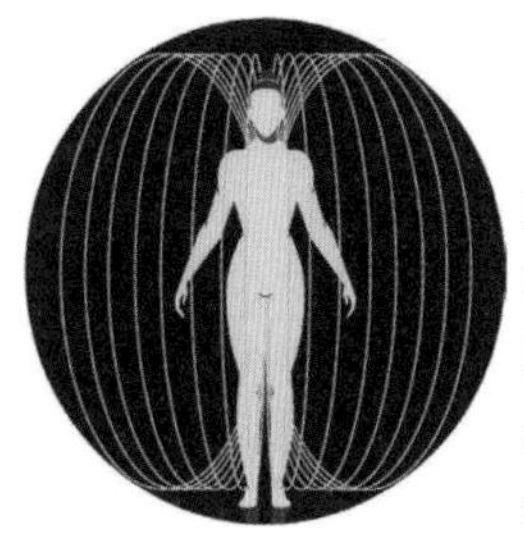

EXPLANATION

It's possible to have a deficiency of magnetic energy, which is often caused by a lack of connection with the earth's magnetic field. It's also possible to have a distortion of the body's magnetic field, usually resulting from some associated imbalance, such as a trapped emotion, a trauma energy, a miasm, and so on.

Magnetic-field imbalances or deficiencies will tend to cause mild to acute discomfort, fatigue, and insomnia and often contribute to other chronic issues. In the following story, Weston found that pain in his friend's elbow was from a magnetic-field imbalance.

Elbow Pain Relieved

I had a friend who was experiencing severe elbow pain. He was headed out of town and really wanted this elbow pain to go away. In real time, over the phone, we discovered a magnetic field imbalance due to trapped emotions. As the emotions were released, so was all of his pain in his elbow. A big "wow" was expressed from him. This elbow pain went away after being corrected and has never come back.

—Weston M., Arizona, United States

My first experience with the healing power of magnets occurred many years ago when I was in practice. I had just purchased a magnet from Nikken, a Japanese company that manufactures magnetic products of all kinds. The particular magnet that I had purchased was called a Magboy, consisting of a blue plastic case containing two silver magnetic balls that could be rolled over areas of discomfort.

Lying facedown on the chiropractic adjusting table directly in front of me was a patient that had come to me for treatment of her fibromyalgia, a debilitating condition primarily characterized by widespread muscular pain of unknown origin.

I had been treating her for about a month, and we were just barely beginning to make some headway in her constant unremitting pain. In her particular case, all of the pain was in her upper body. Her shoulders were particularly affected, to a point where her ability to move her arms in the various ranges of motion was very limited, and it was impossible for her to raise either arm past the horizontal.

Seeing her lying there on the table gave me the thought, "Here is a perfect opportunity to put these magnets to the test." I chose her left arm for my experiment, and for the next five minutes I engaged her in conversation while I rolled the magnet continuously back and forth on her arm.

I had no expectation that it would actually work, but I was curious, having heard stories about these magnets from my brother, Greg, who was a practicing chiropractor as well. The five minutes were soon up. I had her sit up on the edge of the adjusting table and I said, "Okay, I want to check the range of motion in your arms now. First, see if you can raise your right arm for me."

She raised her right arm until it was almost parallel to the floor, and I could see that she was in a good deal of pain, so I had her stop. This was what we had seen on her last visit, without any change.

Now I said, "Okay, go ahead and raise your left arm now." She smoothly raised her left arm past the point of being parallel to the floor and continued on up over her head without any obvious discomfort.

This was totally unexpected. She exclaimed, "What *is* that thing?! I don't have any pain at all where you were rolling it!" I was amazed at this result. I went on to test her arm further, and to my amazement, her left arm seemed to have made a complete and sudden improvement. All of her ranges of motion in her left arm were now normal! We looked at each other for a moment, and I looked down at the magnetic device in my hand and replied, "Well, I'm not really sure. It's a magnet that I got from my brother." She said, "Can I buy it from you? How much does it cost?" I replied, "Well, I don't really know, but let's find out."

Within a few minutes, she paid for the Magboy (now called the MagDuo) and took it with her. I didn't see her again for nearly six months. When she finally returned, I said, "Hey! Where have you been? I haven't seen you for quite a while. How are your fibromyalgia symptoms?" She said, "I'm doing great! Whenever my fibro flares up, I just rub the magnets on the area, and it seems to go away!"

As it turned out, this was just the first of many amazing things that I saw over the next few years using Nikken products in my practice. It was easy to put these products to the test, as I had a never-ending supply of people who were in pain.

One patient, for example, had a long-term shoulder problem that immediately went away when she put the Nikken magnetic insoles in her shoes. I saw four different patients in the midst of acute asthmatic attacks get immediate relief by simply placing a large magnet on their chests. I saw allergies suddenly improve dramatically by simply placing a magnet on the surface of the body. I saw terrible bruises go away literally overnight. I saw broken bones heal from their fractures in half the time. I saw disc bulges, which had been candidates for surgery, reduce and disappear, to the bewilderment of radiologists. I saw all of these things and more.

Magnetic field deficiency is like any other deficiency. If you don't get enough magnetism, then you need to supplement that need somehow. Interestingly enough, the earth's magnetic field is now about 10 percent weaker than it was when the German mathematician Carl Friedrich Gauss started keeping tabs on it in 1845. Because of the nature of our lives and our loss of contact with the soil, as well as our constant exposure to negative electromagnetic fields, magnetic field deficiency syndrome, or MFDS, is a very common problem.

A randomized, double-blind study done at Tufts University in Boston on fibromyalgia patients using magnetic mattress pads concluded that "Sleeping on a magnetic mattress pad with a magnetic surface field strength of 1100, plus or minus 50 gauss, delivering 200 to 600 gauss at the skin surface, provides statistically significant and clinically relevant pain relief and sleep improvement in subjects with fibromyalgia. No adverse reactions were noted during this 16-week trial period." All that, simply from sleeping on a magnetic mattress pad.

Another study using magnetic mattress pads was carried out over a one-year period in three of Japan's foremost hospitals, using 431 patients. The conclusion was that sleeping on magnetic mattress pads proved effective in helping relieve neck pain, shoulder pain, back pain, lower limb pain, insomnia, and fatigue, an average 83 percent improvement in all those ailments. There were no harmful side effects either, because these patients were simply getting what their bodies needed in order to return to a state of balance.

Of course, refrigerator magnets are widely available and work just fine for releasing trapped emotions and correcting energetic imbalances of all sorts, but the Nikken magnets seem to work best for treatment of MFDS and for a lot of other problems as well, as I confirmed in my own practice. Their magnets are of the highest quality, will last a very long time, and are professional strength, so they are well worth the investment.

Note that it's best to not expose pregnant women or anyone with a medical device or electronic implant, such as a pacemaker, to strong magnets.

If you are interested in more information about Nikken magnetic products, please visit discoverhealing.com/magnets.

EXERCISE: IDENTIFYING A MAGNETIC DEFICIENCY

STEP 1.

(Decoding) Ask: "Do I [or you] have a magnetic field deficiency?"

- **If no, great!**
- **If yes, continue to Step 2 (Association).**

STEP 2.

(Association) Ask: "Is there an associated imbalance that needs to be decoded?"

- **If no, skip to Step 3 (Intention).**
- **If yes, return to the Body Code Map, decode and address any associated imbalances, then return here and repeat the Step 2 question.**

STEP 3.

(Intention) You can supplement your magnetic field with the following:

Grounding or "earthing" by spending time outdoors with bare feet, or using earthing products (available on the internet)

Therapeutic-grade magnetic products, such as magnetic insoles (available on the internet)

COLOR IMBALANCE

Color is simply energy, energy made visible. Colors stimulate or inhibit the functioning of different parts of our body. Treatment with the appropriate color can restore balance and normal functioning.

—LAURIE BUCHANAN, PHD

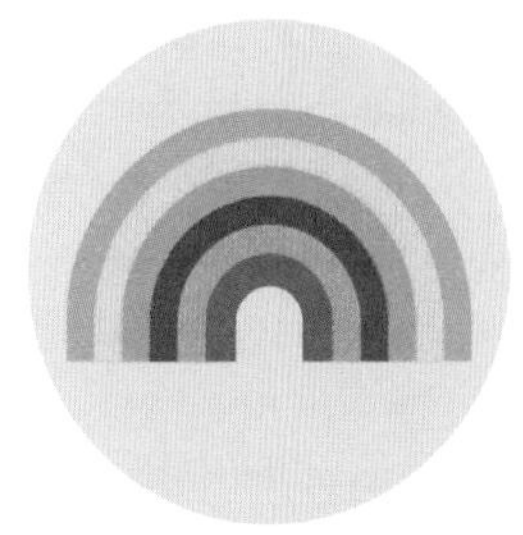

EXPLANATION

Occasionally, you may become deficient in a certain color. Keep in mind that colors are just frequencies that can affect the overall energy field and therefore the body. In some situations, the vibration of a color can be the perfect remedy for restoring balance.

Color deficiency can be corrected in various ways. Most often, the best way is to start wearing clothing of that color, but looking at things that are that color could also work. In some cases, using colored light therapy is the best method.

It's also possible to develop a "color excess," usually if we are exposed to too much of a certain color on a continual basis and are not balanced by exposure to other colors, or if there is an associated imbalance causing the problem.

EXERCISE: IDENTIFYING A COLOR DEFICIENCY

Here is a list of basic colors, with some variations of each listed in parentheses to help you narrow it down even more, if desired:

Pink (ballet pink, fuchsia)
Blue (baby blue, cyan, electric blue, turquoise, royal, navy)
Red (salmon, maroon)
Indigo (cornflower, midnight)
Orange (peach, brown)
Violet (lavender, purple, plum)
Yellow (cream, goldenrod)
White
Green (lime, mint, forest, emerald, olive)
Black (gray)

STEP 1.

(Decoding) Ask: "Do I [or you] have a color deficiency?"

- If yes, use the list to determine the specific color.
- Once you've identified the color, find out why the deficiency exists.
    - Ask: "Do I have this color deficiency simply due to a lack of exposure?"

If yes, move to Step 3 (Intention).

If no, this indicates an associated imbalance. Continue to Step 2 (Association).

STEP 2.

(Association) Return to the Body Code Map and ask, "What associated imbalance needs to be decoded and released in order to be okay with this color?"

- Decode and release any associated imbalances, then go to Step 3 (Intention).

STEP 3.

(Intention) The subject should receive more exposure to this color in any way desired. This can be through wearing clothing of that color family, looking at pictures of that color, wearing sunglasses of that tint, finding that color in nature, etc.

HELPFUL TIP FOR A HEALTHY LIFESTYLE

When you find and release imbalances in the categories mentioned, there are other things you can do beyond that to improve your health. Did you know that feeling gratitude can improve your health? If you choose to be grateful for whatever is going on in your life, you will find your vibration rising. Is it possible to be grateful even for the difficult things in your life? It is (although it can be challenging), and it's a secret to living a happy life.

PART IV

CHANGING THE WORLD

You don't have to get it perfect, you just have to get it going. Babies don't walk the first time they try, but eventually, they get it right.

—JACK CANFIELD

25

THINGS TO CONSIDER

A healer's power stems not from any special ability, but from maintaining the courage and awareness to embody and express the universal healing power that every human being naturally possesses.

—ERIC MICHA'EL LEVENTHAL

Is it possible that you might have imbalances that are unknown to you that have not caused any sort of symptoms yet? Finding and correcting imbalances before they actually start to cause symptoms and sickness is practicing true preventive medicine.

Think about this for a moment. Do you have some sort of mental, emotional, or physical symptom? Are you in pain right now? Do you have a headache or neck pain? Is your low back bothering you, or do you have knee pain? Have you been struggling with depression or anxiety lately? If you can't identify any kind of symptom or issue in your life, that's okay, too. You can still find and release imbalances you didn't even know were there.

PROCESSING

Generally, we find that we can address and correct from one to twelve imbalances in an individual session before a person's body needs time to process the work that has been done. Once your muscle testing isn't giving you any more answers, it's probably because you are done with this particular session. The body needs to do its healing work and needs to adjust to the new state of things before more corrections can be made. When a session is over, "processing" begins.

Processing is the healing period after an emotional or energetic release. Generally, processing lasts for one or two days but can be longer if the energies released were from a particularly intense emotional episode. During that time a person may or may not experience some symptoms, such as emotional ups and downs, crying, sleeplessness, a need for extra sleep, vivid dreams, and, in rare cases, nausea or headache.

Most often, people feel immediate improvement from having a Body Code session. But sometimes people tend to be slightly more emotionally sensitive than normal, if anything. If you find yourself experiencing any of these symptoms, try holding the intention to process with grace and ease.

It's important to note that people will always go through this processing period when emotions and other energies are released, but only about 20 percent of the time will they experience these negative symptoms.

I recommend that when you work on someone you let them know that they may experience some of these processing symptoms. Let them know that it is all part of the healing process. If you don't advise them of the possibility, and they have any processing symptoms, they may think your work made them worse. If you have advised them of the possibility of some symptoms like these, and they do experience them, their minds will be more at ease.

Also, holding an intention for your subject to have a gentle and easy processing experience often helps.

Processing time is often the reason results are not seen immediately. Kati, a chiropractor, was surprised to discover that her sugar addiction actually did dissipate, but not until several days after her Body Code session.

Sugar Addiction

My sugar addiction is now *gone*! I was eating sugar left and right and sneaking it whenever I could. Because gluten-free baked goods and treats are not easily or readily available, I would specifically seek them out on a daily basis.

I would get candy bars on my way home from work to eat before I got home. I would get cookies and brownies every time I went to the grocery store and would eat them before I got home. I would guiltily hide chocolaty treats from my husband so he wouldn't steal them. Ice cream, cookies, cupcakes, candy bars, chocolates, fruit snacks—anything—I would eat daily.

I used the Body Code on myself, and the next day at work I had two snack-size fruit snacks, three chocolate pieces, and a peppermint milkshake. I thought maybe it didn't work, or there may have been more imbalances to remove. Well, about five days later it occurred to me that sometimes issues can take extra time to go away because of required processing time.

That's when I realized I had not craved, itched, twitched, or sought out *any* sugar after that! It has been a week and a half at this point, and I still have *zero* urge for sugar. It's completely out of my mind.

—Dr. Kati O., Washington, DC, United States

CHOICE

Choice is the foundation of all progress. If your subject is reluctant or skeptical, you are not as likely to see great results. A person who wants to be his or her best self and who chooses to do whatever it takes is much more likely to see results in any endeavor. Choice and agency are paramount in this work. You can make a conscious choice to do something, but you also need the capacity and power to make your choice become reality.

For most of us, part of our power to act has been taken over by our subconscious mind and its baggage. It's important to desire to be well, healthy, and prosperous, both consciously and subconsciously. For instance, you may consciously want to lose the extra fifty pounds you are carrying, but if your subconscious mind wants you to keep that weight on because of the trapped emotions and beliefs it has formed, no amount of dieting will bring lasting results. Aligning your subconscious desires with your conscious commitment can make you unstoppable in reaching your goals.

Here is a story about a woman who released trapped emotions to get her subconscious and her conscious mind more aligned to lose weight.

Feeling Amazing

I have been working with my mother to heal my own personal issues through the Emotion Code. One clear difference in my life has been my ability to stick to a diet. I have struggled with my weight and emotional eating my entire life. I would start a diet and then constantly think about the foods that I was not "allowed" to have. The pattern has been that it would always get the better of me and I would fall off my diet.

I have been on many diets, but never for longer than twelve weeks. After working through some emotional barriers, I have now successfully been on my diet for sixteen weeks without faltering. I have lost nearly seventy pounds and am feeling amazing! I still have a long way to go, but I feel like I can complete this lifelong goal of health. Finally!

—Clarissa C., Utah, United States

DON'T PLAY DOCTOR

The Body Code is designed to find imbalances of any and all types. For example, muscle testing may indicate that your subject has an infection of some kind. You would want to say something like, "Your body is suggesting that you may have an infection." You can follow the instructions to clear this imbalance energetically, noting that some imbalances may need medical attention.

Let your subject know if this is the case, and let the person make his or her own decision regarding making a doctor visit. Make it clear that you're not diagnosing anything. Instead, you are letting the subject know what the subconscious mind is indicating. If you think that somebody may need to see a doctor, tell them so. Don't be the reason that somebody delays treatment for something. Doctors are there for a reason, but sometimes you may find imbalances that have doctors puzzled, as Bonnie found in the next story.

The Mystery Cough

I was asked to find out what a woman with a cough had because her doctors couldn't find the reason for her cough and fatigue. They just kept giving her asthma treatments and antibiotics. When she came to me for a Body Code session, her body said that she had a fungal infection in her lungs. Her doctor confirmed the condition and gave the right medication for it, and she has now recovered.

—Bonnie L., California, United States

MEDICAL EMERGENCIES

Always seek medical help in an emergency. If you feel the severity of a symptom needs medical care immediately, let the person you are working on know that. Seeking medical help and using the Body Code can be a synergistic as well as life-saving. Colleen found in this next story.

Severe Pain Vanished

My daughter-in-law was in severe pain—rolling and crawling around, feeling like she would throw up. She couldn't sit up or stand up. My daughter was talking to a medical person who thought it was appendicitis. While they prepared to go to the emergency room, I started using the Body Code to help us find answers.

I tested and found that it was not the appendix, but the spleen. With so much going on around me, I had to talk to myself to just trust the results I was getting. I continued testing and cleared two trapped emotions in the spleen, then I found a physical/physical disconnection at 72 percent, then prions.* That brought the disconnection down to 22 percent. Next, I found a memory field (hard memories about a son in the marines), a trapped emotion of low self-esteem, and then a "no will to live" energy. I cleared all of these energies, and all of a sudden, the pain was gone . . . gone completely!

—Colleen B., Utah, United States

CANCER

The Body Code is not intended to be used to diagnose diseases. Rather, it is used to find the imbalances that stand in the way of the body's natural healing abilities. Even if you are asked to do so by a well-meaning subject, do not use muscle testing to diagnose cancer or any other disease. Let me tell you a story that will illustrate why.

I had a patient who came to me who had been diagnosed with cancer. She had had a sigmoidoscopy and the doctor had found a cancer in her colon that was about the size of a golf ball. Her doctor had taken photographs of this cancer, and she brought those with her when she came to see me. There were color photographs of this ugly, bloody mass in her colon, which had been biopsied and found to definitely be cancerous. I decided to ask her body some questions about the cancer to determine what imbalances might be contributing to it.

The first thing I thought to do was to ask her body if she had a cancer. We already knew that she did, but I just wanted to see what response I got from her body on muscle testing. At the time, it seemed like a good way to start the session so that we could find any imbalances that were contributing to the cancer.

After establishing a baseline muscle test to make sure she was testable, I said, "Do you have a cancer in your colon?" As I pressed down on her arm, she was unable to resist my downward pressure, signaling a no answer. I was surprised, so I then took the pictures of the cancer and held

*Included in the Body Code System app, available at discoverhealing.com/app

them up for her to see, thumbing through the pages, thinking that would help. I put the binder down, had her hold her arm out, and said, "Do you have a cancer in your colon?" and muscle-tested her again. No was the clear answer.

I had her make the statement "I have a cancer." We got the same answer: no. I tried phrasing the question in different ways, but her body would always reply with no. It took me two weeks of work before her body would admit that she actually did have a cancer. What does that tell us? Sometimes the subject doesn't want to recognize or admit that they have cancer. Sometimes the body is disconnected from the cancer, for whatever reason. So you can see how it's best to steer clear of that subject, unless of course you are a doctor and diagnosing cancer is your expertise.

If your friend comes over and says, "Hey, test me to see if I have cancer," what should you do? Let's say that the person does have cancer and it's a case, like that patient of mine, of the body not recognizing the cancer. What happens if the person you test really does have cancer, you get a no answer, and you say, "No, you don't have cancer." Then what happens if the person dies a few months later? At the funeral, the family is going to be grieving, and they're going to be talking about you, saying, "Mom would still be alive if only that neighbor hadn't told her she didn't have cancer." You could find yourself in legal trouble, not to mention the guilt you'd feel for making that kind of mistake. This is not a situation you want to find yourself in.

Using the Body Code allows us to find and remove imbalances that may interfere with healing, but you should never make any claims or promises that by using the Body Code any condition or ailment can be diagnosed or "cured."

When I was in practice, I made it a habit not to make an issue of whatever steps people were already taking regarding their recovery. If people were undergoing chemotherapy or having radiation treatments, my policy was not to interfere. I would simply work to help balance their bodies and release whatever might be in the way of their getting well.

Anything you can do to help the body function better is a good thing if you are battling a disease process. But you don't ever want to guarantee anything. You can and probably will see amazing results from your sessions; just be careful about what you say and what expectations you set.

You might say to your subject, "Let's see what we can do," or "Let's see what happens," or "What have you noticed?" In this way, you're not making promises. Meanwhile, you should always expect a miracle yourself. That is what faith, belief, love, and gratitude are all about, as Cate reveals in the following story.

Cancer-Free Diagnosis

I used the Body/Emotion Code to provide me with a tool to access God's grace to remove my breast cancer naturally. Faith, grace, proper food, and two years later, I was given a cancer-free diagnosis by my MD, who uses muscle testing and homeopathy as well. I had done it!!!

—Cate C., Utah, United States

Far better than dealing with disease is to find and remove imbalances before they create suffering. "May you never know what you have prevented" is a popular saying in the preventive medicine community. With a little bit of education and the Body Code System, you can practice preventive health in the privacy of your own home, on your own loved ones, friends, and family. May you never know what you have ultimately prevented!

ROADBLOCKS

We've all felt stuck at one time or another in helping others find healing. Sometimes a few clues can make all the difference. And sometimes the reason we are not able to help a subject move forward is because we are not using the Body Code System as it was designed to be used.

Consider these principles:

TUNE IN TO THE RIGHT SOURCE

Positive and negative energies swirl around us constantly. The Body Code is well rooted in accessing positive energies, by prayer and by our own choice to hold love and gratitude. If we try to do a session in a space of ego, irritation, impatience, disbelief, judgment, or pride, our sessions may not produce the results we are looking for, and if we do get results, their source may be suspect.

STAY OPEN-MINDED

When we become rigid in our thinking or convinced of our own knowledge, then the truth cannot flow through us. We know by experience that anything can cause anything when using the Body Code System. We must stay curious and open to all possibilities or we will project our own experiences into our sessions and prevent the truth from showing up and true transformation from happening.

ASK THE RIGHT QUESTIONS

Questions are essential to this work. Learning to ask the right questions will help us get to the real issues. If you want to be excellent at the Body Code, you must practice and be open to the guidance you receive from above. Your Higher Power knows what you know and will help you build upon that.

REMEMBER THAT ANYTHING CAN CAUSE ANYTHING

In other words, because every person is unique, and every condition or situation is also unique, you never know what you may be led to find.

It's important to maintain a high vibration while you are using the Body Code. You don't have any power over what the subject's body does, so you just gratefully love your subject and find and remove whatever blockages you can. Your contribution is only to do what you are shown and then let go. After that, what happens is up to the subject's body.

HEALING CAN TAKE TIME

Sometimes healing doesn't come quickly. Many things take time to unravel, just as they took time to get established and embedded. I've given examples of issues that took a long time to resolve, and yet in other cases many issues were resolved in the first few sessions. Sometimes we have to clear away layers before the deepest truth shows up.

During the last ten years of my practice, I saw many patients suffering from chronic and supposedly incurable diseases. The vast majority of them were able to get well using the Body Code principles. Some got well very rapidly. Some got well over weeks, some over months, and a few over many months.

When you're asking the subconscious mind for the true underlying causes of sickness, you are getting to the heart of the matter, but it can take time. The subconscious will reveal what is next on your list as you ask the body using muscle testing. It's like peeling an onion, layer by layer.

Releasing imbalances using the Body Code may not be the only thing needed. Part of a person's healing journey may require lifestyle changes, seeing a doctor, talking with a counselor, taking supplements, physical therapy, changing behavior, and even changing beliefs. These things are known to your subconscious mind and can all be brought to your awareness by the Body Code.

We all would like a magic bullet to fix whatever ails us, but a critical part of our responsibility for our own healing is doing what we know is in our best interest and for the highest good. The Body Code can point you to those things. Examples include eating clean, nutritious foods, exercising, and being kind to yourself and others. A simple practice of gratitude and forgiveness plays a surprisingly significant role in physical and mental health. The body won't cooperate if we keep doing the things that hinder its progress, such as remaining in a toxic environment. The Body Code is not going to make unhealthy behaviors good for you. Some people expect healing without doing their own part. That will rarely work.

The Body Code works very well to find imbalances, but sometimes there is other work to do. In the following story, Samantha's subconscious mind was giving her a clear message that aspartame was not good for her, but it took her months to get over her addiction.

COLLAPSED LUNG

My wife, Jean, and I stopped in to visit a neighbor one day. As we spoke with Samantha, she told us that she had just been released from the hospital. When we asked her what was going on, she said, "Well, suddenly I couldn't breathe very well and I had sharp pain on my left side. I went to the ER with my daughter, and when the doctor examined me, he found that my left lung had spontaneously collapsed. He asked me if I had fallen or had any kind of traumatic thing happen, and I told him that I hadn't. It just came totally out of the blue. I've never had this happen before, and it was pretty scary."

We told her about the Body Code and asked her if she would like us to check and see if there was anything that we could find that might help. She was very open to it, so after saying a short prayer and asking for help from above, we opened the Body Code System app on my iPad and started asking questions.

My first question was, "Is there an underlying reason why you had this lung problem?" The muscle test was strong, indicating a yes answer. Looking at the Body Code Map I asked, "Is this imbalance on the left side of this chart?" Yes. "Is it in the energy area?" No. "Is it in a circuit or system?" No.

At this point, the only choice left was "toxin." I touched that icon on my iPad and the toxin page appeared, with eight new icons representing different categories of possible toxins.

I tested the subcategories, asking, "Is it a heavy-metal toxin?" No. "Is it a biological poison?" No. "Is it a food toxin?" Yes.

So I asked about the various possibilities one by one.

"Is it a flavor enhancer?" No. "Is it a processing agent?" No. "Is it a sweetener?" Yes.

I knew the two most common sweeteners in foods are aspartame and sugar, so I asked, "Is it artificial sweetener?" Yes.

I noticed that mother and daughter were looking at each other rather intensely at this point, and I could tell that the daughter had something to say, so I paused.

She said, "I've been trying to get my mom off her diet drinks for a long time now. I've been telling her how bad they are, and she knows it, but she won't quit. She drinks them constantly, all day long!"

Samantha said, "Do you think that the diet drinks have something to do with my collapsed lung?"

"Well, let's dig a little bit deeper. There are different kinds of artificial sweeteners, and none of them are good for you, although I've never heard of this particular situation happening from the use of an artificial sweetener. On the other hand, anything can cause anything."

I pulled up the list of sweeteners and said, "Let's see what your subconscious mind says about the sweeteners on this list, okay?"

I said, "Is saccharin the issue for you?" No.

"Is aspartame the issue?" Yes.

"Is aspartame an underlying reason why your lung collapsed spontaneously?" Yes.

Checking further, I found that we didn't need to know any more details about this toxin, and there was nothing associated that we needed to decode.

So I swiped three times down the middle of her back with my hand, holding an intention to release the energy of the aspartame from her body.

Her lung healed, and, while she was not able to get off her diet drinks right away, she did cut back significantly, and within a few months she was able to get off of them completely.

She's never had another problem with her lung to this day. I think the moral of this story is that the subconscious mind will usually try to let us know that there is something wrong, or that we are doing something that is negatively affecting our body. If you eat something and notice a sudden twinge of pain, it may be a message. If we are listening to our bodies instead of ignoring them, we can often avoid dramatic hospital visits.

There is always a choice when it comes to change. When you choose to make a change, patience is important because we are human and have weaknesses. Sometimes it takes time and effort to fully recover your health or achieve your goal.

WHEN NOTHING IS WORKING

Do you feel as if you have tried every remedy known to man and you are still suffering? This can be heartbreaking, and frustrating, and create moments of wanting to give up. One factor to consider is that people's bodies are not perfect. There is often purpose in the weaknesses we have, something to be gained in the experience. If you are open and willing to see, there may be a silver lining or a blessing in it.

I used to tell my patients, "If you have learned what you need to learn from this condition, and if God is willing, there is no reason you cannot get well." One of the purposes of life is to learn. If this is a possibility for you, that you or your subject hasn't yet learned a certain lesson, ponder this question: "Is this problem here to teach me something?"

It is also important to know that you may be able to fix or clear up to about 90 percent of your own imbalances. But you'll most likely never get to 100 percent by yourself. Someone else may need to help you. Some things you simply may not be able to find on your own. Besides, working regularly with another practitioner is an ongoing education in itself, as you learn from each other.

26

WORKING WITH ALL AGES

For me, spiritual means love in action. So if you are working for love, then you are a spiritual person.

—PATCH ADAMS

If you feel drawn to help others when they are suffering, you are likely a healer! There are many different ways to support others and contribute your offerings to the world.

Some of the most important talents and skills we can develop are those that enable us to help others. We want to assist, encourage, make a difference, and relieve suffering. We all know the frustration of feeling helpless as a loved one hurts, mentally or physically. Learning how to use the Body Code System will empower you to make a difference in others' lives. You will also discover that as you serve others, you will find healing for yourself. Bringing the energy of love and light to others will change you. This is the law of reciprocity. A friend of mine put it this way: "Cast your bread upon the waters, and it will come back toasted and buttered."

As good as that sounds, helping others lead happier, healthier lives and finding more peace for yourself does take some effort on your part. First, it takes courage to believe you can really make a difference. Second, you have to muster up gratitude and joy for healing that has not yet taken place, especially if you are suffering with the one you want to help.

Perhaps the biggest challenge of this work is doing so with faith. Instead of feeling pity for those suffering and empathizing so deeply that you feel awful for them, you get to bring the joy of hope and possibility. As you hold the feelings and energy of vibrant health and perfect alignment for others, seeing them as whole and complete, you are helping them transform with energy they may not yet have for themselves.

Know that all things are possible and that you are simply the conduit for a power much greater than you—a power that also wants peace and health for your loved ones. Begin your work in a space of trust, love, and gratitude.

You don't need to be "good" at this. Many great plans never unfold because someone was not willing to begin. Everyone who does this work of love started with only a measure of belief and a humble first step of doing it. If you were doing this all on your own power, by your own gifts and abilities, then you should be self-conscious and worried. But you are not. Instead, know that you are not alone.

This method is based on first asking your Higher Power for help and then acting in faith that it will work. You have every reason to believe it will work and can be grateful that you are fortunate enough to be the vehicle through which healing is taking place.

With practice, your abilities will increase and you will become a great gift to all those you serve.

A woman in the United Kingdom wanted to serve others using the Body Code, but self-doubt had kept her from starting other worthy endeavors in the past, and she was sure her depression would keep her from doing this. She did her own work by releasing her Heart-Wall and afterward said she felt like she had a new lease on life. "I feel better every day and more positive about life. I not only believe, but I know I am going to make a huge success of being an Emotion Code practitioner."

Later, she related the following examples of the differences she is making on a daily basis, helping others live happy, fulfilling lives.

Making a Difference in the United Kingdom

I have had so many success stories, it amazes me. My mother-in-law had arthritis in her middle finger; she could hardly bend it. She described it as being like a claw. After one session with me, she could close her fist fully. She was blown away.

I went to the hairdressers, and my stylist was in pain with her tailbone. She explained that it had hurt ever since giving birth to her son a year and a half before. While my color was on my head, I gave her a session, and her pain completely disappeared. She was so excited, she gave me half off my bill.

I did a session online by proxy with a lovely lady who has no cartilage in one knee. It had escalated to the point where she was in pain just walking down the stairs and was really struggling at the gym. She had run marathons before and was desperate to get back to running. Thirty minutes after our session, she was running up and down the stairs!

—Sol C., Kent, United Kingdom

No matter where people are located physically around the world, you can assist them from your own home by using the Body Code. You can also work with someone who is physically next to you, as well. I don't think it could be any more accessible or any easier to bring healing to another.

The most important thing we can do for the success of another is to remove the obstacles hindering their progress. We don't make decisions for them. They still have to do what they need to do, and we simply remove what we can that's in the way.

Not every need is about a specific illness or difficulty. Sometimes we just feel stuck or we lack joy. Marianne shared her first experience with the Body Code, which helped her find true connection with her family.

Getting Unstuck

In my first Body Code session we released some inherited trapped emotions, but the biggest change came from releasing my broadcast message of "I am stuck" and putting "love" back in. We also released an allergy to the idea of "being rejected" that was associated with my right kidney.

I called my mom after my session. For the first time, I didn't feel a wall or blockage toward her. I feel more openness and love for my husband. I couldn't stop smiling after my session. Now I am more open toward people I don't know. But maybe my biggest overall change is about my attitude toward the Higher Power. I knew it was there, but I couldn't feel it. Now I can feel it. There is so much love on this earth.

—Marianne S., South Dakota, United States

One of life's greatest treasures is feeling the joy of love for others and for the Divine. Often, imbalances are all that's in the way.

The Body Code can help us at any point of our life, even when we are in the womb, a very special time indeed. When we have the love and intention to help others, we are sometimes delighted and surprised at what we can do to influence an outcome, as in this next story.

Preparing for Birth

My friend was due to deliver her baby, but she had a concern. The baby was posterior (faceup) and needed to flip over so she could go into labor. She had tried to get the baby to turn, but it wasn't working, and she was already having painful contractions, signaling that her labor was beginning. I asked if she wanted me to try to get the baby to flip over by doing a Body Code session.

With her permission, I worked on her and the baby by proxy that evening. I discovered that the baby was afraid to face labor, so I removed some trapped energy and energetically told the baby it was now safe to turn. The next day my friend texted me that just after a nap, her baby flipped. Eight days later she had a great delivery of a very healthy baby. What an incredible blessing and way to use the Body Code!

—Kristi D., Alaska, United States

You can be that special person in the lives of others that brings healing and relief in ways they could not find on their own. Getting rid of imbalancing energies has helped many people achieve their goals, return to full health, finally lose the excess weight, find love, and create more abundant lives. Doing this work may just bring you and your loved ones a new sense of clarity, a new inner calm, and profound healing where nothing else has before.

HOW TO EXPLAIN THE BODY CODE TO OTHERS

If you aren't sure what to tell people when you're describing the Body Code, here's a description that might help:

"I am learning a fast and easy way of helping people to function better and feel better. It helps the body return to a state where it can heal itself. The Body Code works for both physical and emotional issues. Do you have a few minutes when we can try it out together?"

Often, that simple introduction and invitation is all it takes for a person to be willing to give it a go. For someone who wants more information than that, you could continue with something along these lines:

"Your body is self-healing. It knows perfectly what's wrong with you and what you really need to function optimally. The Body Code is how we 'decode' those needs. We can use it to identify underlying causes of your issues and use our combined intention to clear them or find out what else you may need. This technique is not meant to replace any medical treatment, but by correcting underlying imbalances, we help the body's innate self-healing ability to take over. And many appreciate that this healing process does not require you to share intimate details of past traumas or upsets."

If someone wants to learn more before or after a session, you can suggest that they read the book or listen to the audiobook of either *The Emotion Code* or *The Body Code* or both. They are easy to read or listen to and are filled with fascinating true stories and explanations of the methods. This helps people overcome their concerns and gives them a mental framework to understand how this works, and even to try it on themselves.

If you're talking with someone who is not familiar with "energy work," you could share something like this basic explanation:

"Quantum physicists have been telling us now for over a century that the human body is actually a very complex energy field. Not only current science, but also the major healing methods of the ancient world all revolve around restoring balance to this energy field. The Body Code is a system that allows us to harness the power of quantum physics to create balance in the body's energy field."

NEVER MAKE CLAIMS

When discussing the Body Code with others, especially during a session, be sure to choose your words carefully. You don't want to be misunderstood as practicing medicine without a license. Don't make any claims that you or the Body Code System can heal or cure anything or that it relieves pain. Definitely do not diagnose, unless you are a certified medical professional that has a license to do so. Instead, try saying something like, "The Body Code may help you feel better and relieve your discomfort." Don't make any guarantees. Instead, do it together as a "let's give it a try" approach.

WHERE TO START

When you are ready to start working on someone, remember to be open-minded, patient, and positive. Ask for permission and what the person's issues or goals may be for the session.

Remember to have a moment of silence to ask for help from above, hold love in your heart for the person that you are working on, and hold an intention of gratitude that this is going to work for them.

You can work on anyone, with permission, from the elderly to adults and children. In the following sections you will read true stories of how people used the Body Code to help others of all ages.

CARING FOR ANCESTORS

Imbalances do not always start within ourselves. Sometimes we inherit imbalances, especially trapped emotions from our parents or grandparents or from any ancestor. A field of science called epigenetics proves that trauma can be passed from one generation to another but cannot explain fully how it happens.

The popular "mice and cherry blossom experiment" demonstrates the link between ancestors and inherited trauma. A set of mice was given a slight shock every time a cherry blossom scent was pumped into their cage. Over time, they developed a fear response to the same scent, even when no shock was given. The sperm of those traumatized mice were artificially inseminated into female mice who had no exposure to the scent nor the shock and had no fear of the scent. However, the baby mice who were born from those mothers had an instinctual fear of the cherry blossom scent, even though those baby mice never met their fathers.

Sometimes the roots of our problems are inherited. When these are discovered, a special opportunity is set before us.

In this story, Izabela explains how identifying and removing her inherited emotional blocks changed her life.

Taking on Grandpa's Issues

I've been stuck for a long time. Or maybe a better word is held back. I needed to make some brave decisions in my occupational and personal life. During a Body Code session, we found a Heart-Wall made of three negative emotions, all of which I inherited from my grandfather. He died before I was born, so I had never met him. But in doing this work, I felt like I finally connected with him—not his body, but his spirit. It was the first time I felt him in such a close and personal way. Removing those difficult energies was like opening the door to my own courage and decision-making. Finally, all by myself, I created my business website. And I improved my relationships with my kids and my husband.

—Izabela C., Warsaw, Poland

In *The Emotion Code* book, I describe in detail how to work with inherited trapped emotions. While the most common type of imbalance that is inherited or passed down from an ancestor is trapped emotions, it's possible for other energies to be inherited as well. In this story, Vickie found the answer to her question in an unexpected way.

Speechless

I had been working like crazy to figure out my dad's high blood pressure, or hypertension. We cleared many things from him with the Body Code, and he was using natural remedies, but it still was not enough. So I prayed, and the answer came to me in my sleep. I needed to check him for and remove an inherited trapped emotion that was a cause of his hypertension. It worked! I am happy to say he now does not have hypertension, and his doctor is speechless. I love how all of this works and everything comes together. Thank you for your wonderful gift.

—Vickie B., Missouri, United States

Not only can we remove these imbalances from ourselves, but by doing this work, we remove them from our ancestors as well, and even our children if they, too, inherited the same disruptive energy.

We are connected to our ancestors. Sometimes their imbalances and traumas are passed down to us. When these types of blocks are discovered, we have an unprecedented and sacred opportunity to help deceased family progress. Their trapped emotions are often shared with us and affect both us and them. In this next story, ancestors shared their thanks for the work that was done on their behalf, something they could not do for themselves.

Releasing Trapped Emotions from All Relatives

One client I had struggled with anger issues and serious allergies. Among other imbalances, we released an inherited trapped emotion of "lost." Well, that's where the interesting story began. It turns out that this inherited energy went back to the time period when people were brought over in slave ships from Africa. Her male ancestor trapped the emotion of "lost" as a result of being torn from his family and brought to the New World.

I released this from my client and from all her relatives who had also inherited it. It was wild! My office was crowded with these beings. My client felt the same thing in her home some thirty minutes away from me. It was so powerful. She was in tears! She later told me from that point on, she had received numerous "gifts" that happened in her life that she had no reason to expect. She said that she knew these gifts were from all these people saying thank you to her for the release of this trapped emotion of "lost." I will forever remember the power and healing of that experience! I am so grateful to have been a part of that restoration to so many beautiful people caught up in a dark time of our civilization.

—Deborah P. M., Florida, United States

I believe our ancestors know about this work, and they may be waiting for us to do this work for them. Over the years, when an inherited emotion comes up for someone I'm working on, sometimes I'll ask if the direct-line ancestors are in the room waiting for this to be released from them as well. The answer is always yes! Once the trapped emotion is released, I'll ask if the ancestors are still in the room, and I usually get a no answer, unless there is more that we are about to find and release from them. They came for the release of their baggage and left when it was completed. Others are finding this to be the case as well, as Patti explains in the next story.

Ancestors Wanting Help

By clearing my own aches and pains with the Body Code, I gained important experience in working with ancestral issues. Often, when I would find an inherited trapped emotion, I would feel tingles over my whole body, and an intense emotion of gratitude, often to the point of tears. I became convinced my deceased grandmother or whomever I was working with was present and grateful for the help. What started out as discomfort and an annoyance that I needed to "waste" time on myself became a great blessing for my ancestors and for me, as well as a meaningful connection to them.

For example, my left thumb started aching. I've wondered about eventually having arthritis myself since my grandmother suffered terribly with rheumatoid arthritis that fused joints and deformed bones. My grandma's hands were gnarled and claw-like. Most of her life was remarkably difficult. As I started working on my thumb, inherited emotions kept coming up to be cleared, and I had remarkable experiences feeling the presence of deceased grandparents.

It didn't take long for me to realize that my ancestors were lining up for help. Word must have gotten out that I had the skills to help all of us let go and progress. Each difficulty in my own body was an opportunity to not only clear imbalances in myself, but also help out my ancestors.

Now I no longer see my discomforts or pain as worrisome. Instead, I just smile and know I have work to do, and hopefully ancestors to help. I would never do this work for my family if I felt perfectly well all the time. I wouldn't know where to start. Now I see purpose and meaning to my aches and pains that I never before imagined, and a way to release them, not just from myself, but from my ancestors, too.

—Patti R., Utah, United States

Anytime we find inherited imbalances and release them, we are serving our ancestors. Even if we don't feel a connection to them while doing this work, imagine what relief they are experiencing as you release the inherited trapped energies that are in your way. Your ancestors were real people who lived real lives and had real struggles at times. In the following story, a young couple in love were prevented from marrying a long time ago.

Heartbroken Ancestor

For most of my life I struggled with ongoing sadness. I couldn't afford to pay for professional help. So I started watching Dr. Nelson, read his book, and worked on myself. I didn't know what I was doing, but the more I tried and practiced, the more I was able to help myself.

One day I found an inherited trapped emotion from my father. He inherited it from his father, and so on, for twenty generations, traced back through the paternal line. I discovered that this man had fallen in love with a woman but couldn't marry her because of his social status. I released it and went to bed.

The next day, when I told my sister, June, she said, "No way! Yesterday I found an inherited emotion, jealousy, trapped in a man twenty generations back, all on the fathers' side. He and a woman had fallen in love with each other and were unable to marry because her parents wanted her to marry a man with a higher social status!" We were amazed! When June released that trapped emotion of jealousy, she sobbed for a minute until the feeling subsided, then she sat in wonder. If there was any doubt that this work is inspired, it vanished that day.

I am now free of this sadness for the first time in many years, and I have been able to rid myself of a Heart-Wall full of emotional baggage that made me believe that I wasn't smart enough or strong enough to be successful and support my family. I am no longer afraid to try.

—Michelle M., Alberta, Canada

STRENGTHENING THE ELDERLY

Watching our parents age and change is not for the faint of heart. We love them deeply and want to do all we can for them, especially when they are ill or in pain. What we often fail to understand is that, consciously or subconsciously, older people are engaged in an effort to understand their legacy. They are mentally putting together what their lives have meant and the memories that will live on after they die.

This can be a profoundly painful process if they feel their own life doesn't amount to much or wasn't all it could have been, or they keenly feel the mistakes they made that have affected their children adversely. Our connection to our elderly dear ones, our show of love, is vital in their later years. They need our compassion, our attention, and they need to feel honored and loved by us. But there are many reasons why that can sometimes be difficult. One simple way to deepen relationships and find things to share with each other is by doing the Body Code work together.

We can help them release many blocks to their happiness and contentment in their later years. Of course, physical issues can be more frequent. Being the one to help them find relief is often bonding and joyful. Hope is the great motivator of progress, and you can bring that hope. Here are several real stories of bringing hope and joy to our elderly loved ones.

Most of us have met or loved someone with some form of dementia. In this story, a doctor shares what may be possible with the Body Code.

Is Alzheimer's Reversible?

When I started working with my elderly client, she couldn't answer any of my questions. She needed twenty-four-hour supervision and couldn't do simple tasks like getting a glass of water for herself. She was paranoid and delusional. She had trouble making friends and was very isolated.

After three and a half months of working together with the Body Code, she now can engage in conversations and get her own water. I'm told she is taking care of herself in other ways, like regularly taking out the trash and even recycling!

Before, she wasn't able to shop without supervision but now can go with a fellow resident. She makes friends easily and participates in all the activities with her retirement community. Her delusions and paranoia have decreased by about 75 percent. I expect and hope they will continue to decrease as we do more work together.

My doctoral research in neuroscience and epidemiology was in Alzheimer's disease. Back then, we believed that the best thing we could do was to halt the progression of the disease. Now I'm beginning to suspect it might be reversible!

—Dr. Tina H., PhD, Washington, United States

So don't believe everything you are told. We don't understand everything there is to know about energy or regeneration, but it seems that healing is often possible when others don't think it is.

Sometimes it's our own parents that we have the opportunity to help. In the next story, Beth helped her father in a big way.

A Major Stroke

I just want to give a huge thank-you to Dr. Bradley Nelson and share this story. My father has gone from "about to die" or "survive as cabbage" after having a major stroke, to "back to normal"! I worked back-to-back along with many other fellow Body Code and Emotion Code practitioners to save my father. I prayed that if he didn't return as a man, then we would let him go. This was the hardest thing to do. Yet he walks, talks, and even wanted to get a train to go to a family funeral.

I am amazed! This happens all the time. . . . I never fail to be amazed. I am eternally grateful and so blessed to have met you and trained with you. This remarkable lifesaving and life-changing energy practice works!

He is not only recovering quickly but has gone from not believing in my work to being a believer, as have the rest of my family. Thank you to you, Dr. Brad, and everyone who supports you and all the fellow practitioners. I do believe in miracles!

—Beth F., Hertfordshire, United Kingdom

Whether the elderly are our parents or grandparents or someone else's, they will benefit from your help.

HELPING CHILDREN

What greater gift can you give a parent or caregiver than the ability to assist a child with his or her emotional and physical issues. Whether this is in-person or at a distance, it is extremely empowering and humbling to have the skills and tools to help a child with larger health issues or something as simple as unhealthy behavior, and it can often be resolved quickly and simply, as we see in this next story.

Separation Anxiety

My six-year-old had his first Emotion Code session, and I asked the practitioner to focus on the separation anxiety and unhealthy "neediness" he experienced with his dad. Whenever they were home together, my son begged for his constant attention and got very upset if his dad even went into another room of the house without him. This behavior was even worse on the weekends, so we were pleasantly surprised to see that the day after his session, a Saturday, he played independently for several hours without needing to be entertained by his dad. He also had a huge burst of creativity and created the most beautiful and imaginative art the entire weekend! He was joyful, generous to his sister, and lovingly affectionate toward his dad without expecting anything in return. This was truly miraculous for our family!

—Stefanie W., Nebraska, United States

Being a parent can be a heavy responsibility, especially when your child is not happy. Many children at one time or another become withdrawn, secretive, and uncommunicative—and it's always for a reason. But it's really hard to help when the child won't share or even connect with you. This can make us feel helpless, frustrated, or even angry. It's important to recognize that it is natural to feel this way, and to keep our emotions under control so we can help our children feel safe.

Kids face some big stressors in addition to homework, grades, and peer pressure. Concerns about bullying, relationships, the future, and general self-worth add more layers of stress.

Neurological disorders are more common in children than ever. Autism, Asperger's, ADHD, ADD, panic disorders, and so many more are stretching families to their limits. I've seen the Body Code improve these issues for many children.

A Sensory-Processing Success

My daughter was two years old when she was diagnosed with sensory processing disorder. Even after two years of therapy, she still had the constant issue of not being able to sleep and of having horrific meltdowns in the middle of the night. By the second Body Code session, the emotions, negative cords, and other issues we released from her were amazing. I could see the change in my daughter's face, the new zest she had for life, and the joyful energy she was radiating in everything she did. The night after the session, she fell asleep within two minutes of lying in bed and slept peacefully the entire night! I know we still have more work to do, but this is the greatest blessing for my daughter and our family.

—Stefanie W., Nebraska, United States

In some cases, we may believe a child is on the autism spectrum, especially if he or she is not speaking by the age of two or three years old. In actuality, it could be something as simple as trapped emotions, as Deborah found in the next story.

Anger and Speech Issues Disappeared

I worked remotely on a two-and-a-half-year-old that did not speak, and he had a serious issue with anger. His parents were very concerned. They had planned to take him to a speech therapist when he was three years old.

I did three sessions on him and identified and released all the trapped emotions and associated imbalances as to why he did not speak. The morning after I finished the third session, this baby didn't just begin speaking, he began singing in the car as his father drove him to day care! The singing and speaking continued to everyone's amazement.

Additionally, within a few days, he toddled up to his mother and wrapped his little arms around her legs so as to say, "I love you!" He had never done anything like that before in his life. His anger was gone! This family was so blessed by this development.

—Deborah P. M., Florida, United States

My wife and I learned many years ago that we could work on our own children very easily when they were sleeping. We saw profound changes, and in this story, so did Lynn.

Working with a Sleeping Child

The mother of a five-year-old boy asked me to do a distance session for her son. He was having behavioral issues of outbursts of anger, hitting other children, and not listening. I did the treatment when the little one was asleep using proxy testing. I emailed the results to his mother the next morning. She told me that at about 11:00 p.m., which is just when the session was over, he got out of his bed and crawled into bed with her. A month later, she called me to say that there had been a pronounced change in his behavior immediately after the session. He was willing to listen, was much gentler with his siblings and other children, and was much more positive. What a wonderful way to help little children, while they are sleeping peacefully and without fear or trauma on their part.

—Lynn G., British Columbia, Canada

Every day, children have bumps and bruises and little crashes. A Band-Aid can do wonders for a crying child. But what if you want to do more, even need to do more? Having a tool that can be used anywhere and at any time is invaluable. This next story shows how normal playing can result in a seemingly insignificant blow but can create real consequences.

A Boy and His Dog

My client's son had a collision with the family's big dog while playing. The boy got a large bump on his forehead. The client asked me for help, so I did a Body Code session by proxy over some distance. There were a couple of imbalances, like a physical trauma, a trapped emotion of shock, an absorbed trapped emotion of anxiety from the mother, misalignment of the frontal bone, and a few others. By the next morning, the bump was totally gone, and her son was fine.

After a week, she wrote to me that their dog was unwell. He wouldn't eat and didn't want to play. She asked me again for help, so I did a Body Code session for the dog. This session was very interesting. There was the physical trauma from the crash, an absorbed trapped emotion of anxiety from the mother, a shared trapped emotion of shock with the boy, a trapped emotion of guilt related to the crash, and a misalignment of the lower jaw from the crash. After clearing all these imbalances, the dog was fine, and he ate and played with the children again.

—Heidi R., Vienna, Austria

It's not surprising to see trauma in animals as Heidi had experienced in her session with her client's dog. Animals can benefit from the Body Code as well, as you will find in the next chapter.

27

WORKING WITH ANIMALS

Clearly, animals know more than we think, and think a great deal more than we know.

—IRENE M. PEPPERBERG

Animals give us love, play, and comfort beyond anything we can return in kind. Their emotional intelligence and complex biology also make them susceptible to trapped emotions and dysfunctional energies, just as we are. Just like people, animals can have trapped emotions and energetic imbalances that affect their health and happiness. These issues can cause animals to behave in negative ways, due to the emotional or physical discomfort they are feeling. Energetic problems in pets often stem from past traumatic experiences that leave residual energies in their bodies, but may include finding toxins, as Sharon did in the following story.

Toxin Nearly Takes a Dog's Life

Last night my daughter called in tears. Her dog was barely walking, more like wobbling in circles, head near the floor, tongue nearly touching the ground, panting, drooling, and disoriented—and had been that way for nearly an hour. They live way out in the desert in Arizona and have no way to get to a vet and no money. She called me and asked, "Can you do anything?"

I had her pet the dog, using me as proxy, and I tested weak as she touched the left ear and all connections to the rib cage. I started yawning until my jaw almost popped, and continued to yawn the entire session. Using the Body Code, the dog's subconscious mind guided me to "toxicity," then I tested for pesticides and herbicides, with ant poison testing strong, but with no underlying causes.

I asked, "Can I release this energy?" Yes, so I did the magnet swipe. I am telling the truth, it wasn't twenty seconds until Vicky started screaming, "MOM, MOM! She walked over and is drinking! Mom, she didn't wobble!"

Toxins tested strong for being cleared, so I continued to "herbicides." Her friend interrupted: "Would biting that toad do it?"

I asked the body. The toad had been exposed to herbicides. Again, no underlying causes, so I did three swipes with the magnet. The rib cage area now tested strong, but I decided to see if there was any reason this dog was determined to get herself into dangerous or unsafe situations (she eats and chews and sticks her nose into *everything* and won't listen to "Get out!" or "No!").

I was taken to "addictive heart energy," which meant I had to release a Heart-Wall also. Was taken to "panic," "shock," and "unworthy."

At that point my daughter related that her neighbor had a yard full of wolf dogs and this was the runt of a litter that had been attacked and abandoned. When she saw the neighbor throw it over the fence to die, she took it home and spent the next two weeks doing all she could to keep it alive.

I was still doing those releases when Vicky interrupted: "*Mom!* She got done drinking and walked over to her bed normally! No panting, drooling, or anything! Her head wasn't dragging on the ground. She curled up and has gone to sleep."

I got a text the next morning: "She slept all night and is up and at 'em this morning."

—Sharon D., Auckland, New Zealand

MUSCLE TESTING WITH ANIMALS

Many energy healing techniques that benefit humans can easily be used with pets! Using the Body Code on animals is exactly the same process as using it on another person. So if you are already doing the Body Code on other people, then you are already an animal whisperer. You can conduct surrogate sessions with a partner for an animal, or you can work by yourself as either surrogate or proxy.

In this image, Jean and I are working on our dog, Max. You can refer back to surrogate muscle testing in chapter 4 if you need a refresher on how to do that. No touching is necessary when working on animals, especially if you feel they may be dangerous.

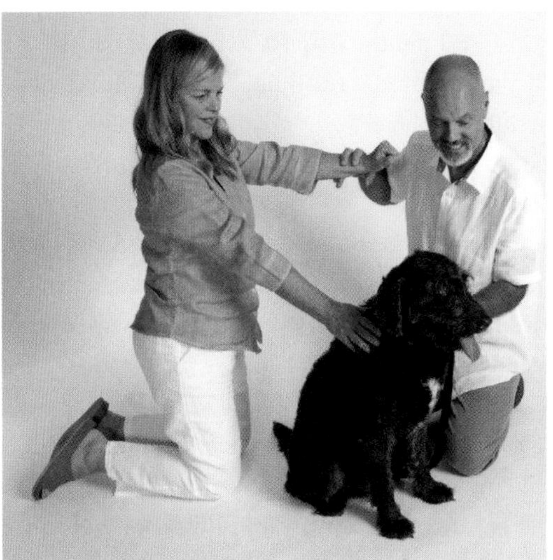

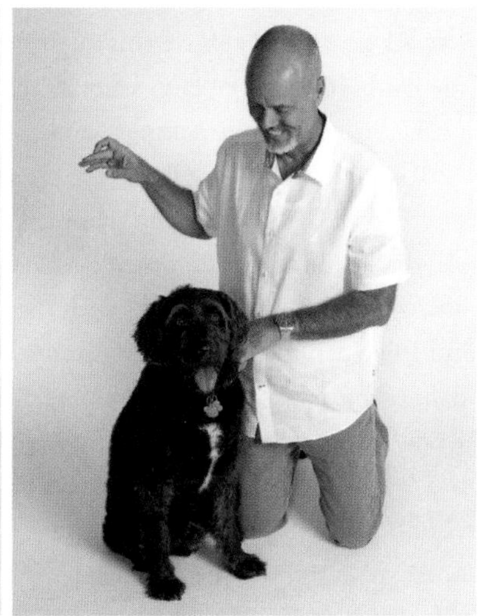

If you don't have a partner with whom you can work on an animal, self-testing works just as well. You can release imbalances on the animal or just release them on yourself. If the animal may not be safe to touch or be close to, or if it feels threatened, you can use proxy testing for it, again with either a partner or by yourself.

As you are preparing to work on an animal, keep in mind that animals are supersensitive and can pick up on your energy. If you are nervous about working on them, they will be nervous as well. Take a moment to relax and focus, then come to the session full of love and intention to help them, and they will be ready to receive the energy work. Fortunately, we can assist our pets with their peace of mind and physical well-being, as Gail tells in the following story of giving peace to her high-anxiety cat.

Shadow's Anxiety

My cat, Shadow, has always been a bit demanding. He would meow incessantly, seeking attention. But after his sibling was taken by a coyote, he became extremely nervous, meowing and crying all the time. It was heartbreaking.

I picked him up one day and set him on the shelf of the cat tree. He was crying and constantly moving, in a very anxious state. I started using the Emotion Code on him, and after the third trapped emotion was cleared, Shadow dropped down onto his side and began batting at the stuffed mouse hanging on the cat tree!

I burst into tears at the sudden change from anxiety-ridden cat to play-mode kitty! It was such a contrast to his prior emotional state. He's had two more sessions since then, and he is now a peaceful kitty. He meows a greeting but is not frantic, like before. The change is phenomenal.

—Gail B., California, United States

LANGUAGE IS NO BARRIER

Ample evidence shows that animals are emotional beings, dating back to Charles Darwin's 1872 book *The Expression of the Emotions in Man and Animals.* We animal lovers know that they establish emotional bonds with each other and with us. In our love for them, we are eager to learn how we can help our pets and even wild animals recover from trauma and difficulties.

Do you remember the 1998 Robert Redford film *The Horse Whisperer*? It's about a girl and her horse who are both injured in a riding accident. The girl's mother takes them to a legendary "horse whisperer" played by Redford, who heals the horse after uncovering the cause of its trauma.

Wouldn't it be incredible if we all could understand what animals are saying and what they need? While we may not speak the same language as animals, still we can reach out to their subconscious minds, just as we do with humans, via muscle testing, as Michele did in the following story.

Diabetic Horse

Joseph is a handsome horse, a sixteen-year-old gelding affectionately known as "The Guardian." He loves his job as the lead horse healer in our equine-assisted psychotherapy program, helping highly traumatized and dissociative children heal from their painful pasts. Laminitis (similar to diabetes in humans) has plagued Joseph over the past few years, and recently, he had a severe laminitis episode that resulted in lameness.

Thanks to the Body Code, I am able to provide extensive care more adequately and address underlying imbalances that cannot be detected through X-ray, blood work, or radiography. The Lord has already healed Joseph through the Body Code for other issues, and I am believing in Him for another miracle healing.

Daily, I begin the session with various horse anatomy charts, asking if there are any imbalances, and I use the Body Code app to address any associated imbalances, then release them as his subconscious directs. I determine precisely the amounts and types of herbs, supplements, feed, and even the length of time the ice boots need to remain on his legs.

I consulted with an expert veterinarian and informed him of my work using the Body Code. Another equine professional validated the presenting imbalances as very typical with laminitis. She was amazed at the combined use of horse anatomy charts and the Body Code. So far, Joseph has not needed outside support, such as my veterinarian, equine chiropractor, specialist, or radiography, other than for consultation.

The Body Code has been invaluable for mental/emotional health as well! Joseph is very sensitive, and I release at least one related imbalance daily. This has greatly improved his spirits and playfulness, even in the midst of his discomfort. Following the sessions, Joseph relaxes, drops his head, and often nuzzles me . . . his way of saying, "Thank you, Mom." Because of the Body Code, we no longer need to guess what is going on internally or how to support recovery.

I may have despaired were it not for this amazing modality and the Lord's goodness. Joseph and our family send the entire Discover Healing team much love and gratitude. I look forward to registering for the Body Code Certification course, next week! Blessings in abundance.

—Michele Y., Colorado, United States

I really believe the animals understand on a heart-to-heart level. In my practice, I found that language really isn't necessary. I had a man come to me once from India for treatment. He didn't speak a word of English and I didn't speak a word of Hindi, and initially I wasn't sure what to do. I went ahead and asked questions in English, and the response from his subconscious mind was able to help us find whatever he needed to help him. I also learned that you don't really need to use language with animals.

When working on an animal, you really don't need to talk out loud, because the animal's subconscious understands implicitly what you are thinking and what your heart is communicating with your intention to help them. You can ask the questions out loud or silently. You can even do this without the animal nearby, as Beate experienced in the following story.

Lilly's Fear of Stairs

Lilly, the dog of a family friend, suddenly no longer wanted to go up the stairs in her home and only managed to do so with a lot of start-up and motivation from her owner. Nothing seemed to be wrong physically. By the time my friend shared this with me, sitting together in a café, it had been going on for a long time. So right there I connected remotely with Lilly, the dog, and released a few of her trapped emotions. When my friend got home that afternoon, Lilly ran up the stairs without any complaints. A few days later, when her "fear of stairs" came back, I was able to solve a few more things. Now Lilly has no more problems walking up the stairs.

—Beate S., Frankfurt, Germany

DEALING WITH PETS AND LOUD NOISES

Fear of loud noises is quite common in dogs and cats, and alleviating it often requires ongoing, patient training to try and get them used to it. It is so much easier to use the Body Code to find the underlying cause as to why they react the way they do when presented with a loud noise.

As many animal lovers know, the noise from fireworks can be a nightmare for our four-legged friends. The sounds of fireworks, especially firecrackers, often send them into a panic. They jump, try to hide, or tremble and salivate, and some of them even escape and run away, leaving their desperate owners searching for them, sometimes for days. Patricia shares her story of how she used the Body Code to release the reaction her dog, Temper, had toward fireworks.

Afraid of Fireworks No More

My older dog, Temper, has grown more and more concerned about really loud bangs over time. This year, on December 30, he reacted to the first occasional firecracker sounds by getting up from his sleeping place and sitting next to me, tense and trembling and panting. I tried to distract his attention with food and play, but he did not show any interest and instead kept sitting in his tense posture, continuously trembling and panting.

I expected to find a few trapped emotions, so at first I intended to go straight to the Emotion Code Chart. But my intuition told me to begin on the Body Code's front page. To my big surprise, I was led to toxins instead of emotions as the underlying reason for my dog's acute symptoms. Testing further, I arrived at environmental toxins, more specifically from cosmetics. Dogs kiss their owners all the time, and they often seem to have a special penchant for hand cream or body lotion, so he might have ingested something this way. Being curious, I asked and found that the toxicity came from a dog shampoo that had been used on him as a puppy. No more information was needed, so I cleared the toxicity using a magnet on Temper himself. After the release, Temper, who had still been sitting next to me, trembling and panting, immediately laid down and stopped trembling, and the panting also subsided!

I asked if I could clear anything else in order to make him less sensitive to firecrackers in the future and was led to misalignments. His third lumbar vertebra was misaligned. There were no underlying reasons for the misalignment, but we needed to know more, so I continued testing and found that the misalignment had occurred at age four, while Temper had been running after a flying Frisbee and caught it midair. I also cleared this misalignment energetically, and later in the day, when hearing some more firecrackers, Temper remained lying and did not start to tremble again!

The next day, on New Year's Eve, Temper reacted with cautious curiosity to the increasingly frequent firecracker sounds. He looked up, went to the terrace door, and tried to figure out what was going on. After a while, he just returned to his normal routine, mostly ignoring the noise, and he slept through most of the fireworks around midnight. And on our New Year's Day walks he seemed completely unfazed by the occasional firecracker sound.

—Patricia F., Mannheim, Germany

This story proves once again that the holistic doctor's saying "Anything can cause anything" really holds true. A seemingly emotional issue (fear, panic) was caused—in this specific case—by an environmental toxin and facilitated by a misalignment, both from years before. Of course, other animals with similar symptoms might have completely different underlying causes, so always keep your mind open to all possibilities and trust in the process.

BEHAVIORAL CORRECTION

We often find that animals' bad behaviors are a result of their emotional baggage, and clearing those trapped emotions usually fixes the problem. In the following story, Jodie shares what happened after using the Body Code on a horse.

From Spooked to Winning Big

Cricket is a five-year-old Appaloosa horse who started spooking and bucking while being ridden. This behavior resulted in a serious injury to his owner, leaving him frightened to ride his horse. Eventually he called for an Emotion Code session. The results were remarkable. The owner took Cricket to a riding clinic and horse show the following day. He said that Cricket was a different animal. He was calm and relaxed and did everything he was supposed to do. The horse show was a huge success! Cricket and his owner earned two Grand Championship Awards and one Reserve Championship Award that weekend!

—Jodie P., New Jersey, United States

Many Body Code practitioners choose to work mostly on animals because success is usually immediate.

Depressed Animals

I chose to do energy work mainly on animals and have had a lot of success with animals that seem depressed and don't want affection from their owners. After releasing trapped emotions from them, the owners have stated that their animals began seeking attention from them once again.

—Jenny Marie G., Tennessee, United States

Another one of our practitioners sums up the wonder of helping animals.

No Placebo Effect with Animals

I think working with animals is the most enjoyable and enlightening task for me. Animals don't respond to placebos. They don't seem to care if you are new to the Body Code, and the results you witness from the animals are truly heartwarming.

—Guy M., Florida, United States

As you can see, animals are a joy to work with, and there are great rewards for both you and the animal when you engage in energy healing with them. Remember to get permission from the owner, and have fun!

28

WORKING WITH RELATIONSHIPS

If you fail to carry around with you a heart of gratitude for the love you've been so freely given, it is easy for you not to love others as you should.

—PAUL DAVID TRIPP

Without relationships, life would be bland and joy would be hard to come by. Being in partnership with another person can be the most rewarding and also the most challenging experience of our lives, especially if a deep commitment is in place, such as marriage. One of the great gifts of partnership is the sacred trust we place in the other to support us in becoming our best selves. This emotional and intellectual intimacy creates a vulnerability that can bless or hurt. When we are careful to honor the other and only use our inside knowledge to uplift and to bless, the relationship can thrive. But we all have relationships that are not always harmonious. Constant vigilance to repair damage, remove unhealthy patterns, and nurture each other is necessary.

Many people are in partnerships that are healthy and loving, yet the couple does not always share the same beliefs, nor are they always open to each other's ideas. Even when emotional or physical pain is present, and you feel you can help with the Body Code, let your partner choose whether or not he or she wants to participate. This generous wife got her reluctant husband's permission, and the Body Code made a difference.

A Reluctant Husband

My husband is not convinced of many of the things I believe and/or do, so when I mentioned doing Emotion Code sessions for him to release his Heart-Wall, I wasn't sure how he would respond. I was pleasantly surprised when he agreed for me to do sessions by proxy. It took five sessions, and after the first session, he noticed that his chest felt lighter. He is and has been under a lot of stress, so his body is on high alert all the time. For him to acknowledge he felt a weight come off his chest was huge. He is now more open to conversation, which is awesome. Now without a Heart-Wall, he worked on doing renovations while I was away for a month, which is an enormous step forward. He doesn't realize what the Body Code is nor acknowledge much change, but I sure do.

—Jennifer S., Nova Scotia, Canada

The Body Code can be a life-giving resource to strengthen each other and to demonstrate the loving commitment to help our partner's dreams come true. If someone has subconsciously built a Heart-Wall as a reaction to a bad relationship experience, or as a defense against further distress, much of that energy could be kept in the heart. Since a Heart-Wall is made of trapped emotional energy, that energy could radiate and have a negative effect not only on themselves, but on the people around them. Here are four different relationships from around the world that were transformed once the Heart-Wall was cleared.

I have been married for twenty-five years and never felt like I was fully connected to my husband. I felt distant, like there was a wall between his heart and mine. I could lay beside him at night and feel no connection to him at all. Since removing my Heart-Wall, well, what can I say? I feel it. . . . I feel love. . . . I feel whole and complete and happy. I have read all the how-to-be-happy books, done everything they said to do, but nothing ever changed for me. Thank you, Dr. Nelson. For the Emotion Code/Body Code is a real game changer!

—Amanda S., Queensland, Australia

The husband of my friend came to me for a session. He didn't want to tell his wife about the Heart-Wall we cleared, so I waited to see if my friend noticed any changes. She called me the next day saying, "I don't know what you did, but he has been *so loving.*" She said that she had never felt more loved in her marriage. All the wrinkles on his brow had eased away and he was smiling more. She even mentioned a couple of months later that she told him that he could thank me for saving their marriage.

—Joy P., London, United Kingdom

My marriage was saved from the brink of divorce because of my work with the Body Code. I had a huge Heart-Wall. Once removed, many aspects of my life improved, including my personal relationships and my health. Now I rarely have heart episodes where my blood pressure drops dangerously low, because my weak heart is regaining its strength. And I'm accomplishing all of my goals, including becoming a certified practitioner.

—Jerusalem D., New York, United States

For many years, I was upset with my husband. He was running our joint business and not listening to any of my suggestions on how to improve it. Over time I created a Heart-Wall that adversely affected our marriage. Since my work with the Emotion Code, over several sessions, our marriage was saved.

—Lynn H., Ontario, Canada

Feeling unappreciated and overlooked can be such a crushing state. Many of us struggle with this feeling in our work and public lives, but it can be even more frustrating when it happens in our personal relationships. Improving relationships can be as simple as a smile and a thank-you for a job well done. Kindness could conquer the world and has the potential to make it a much better place.

MOVING FORWARD FROM PAST RELATIONSHIPS

Past relationships can be haunting. Ghosts of feelings and trapped emotions can lurk in your subconscious. These negative thoughts can keep us on a roller coaster of emotional ups and downs.

The first thing you must do to rid yourself of these lingering thoughts and emotions and start feeling whole again after leaving past relationships is to identify the triggers. Do you get agitated after being around a certain person? Is there a specific kind of phrase, comment, or interaction that sets you off?

Often, these triggers have nothing to do with the current person or situation at all, but instead are a result of old imbalances from a past breakup or the deterioration of a relationship. For example, if you were in a verbally abusive relationship with a spouse who constantly put you down, a mere suggestion on how to do something as simple as folding clothes or washing dishes might elicit a strong reaction from you. You might begin to feel out of control from the baggage of your past relationships that lies just under the surface of your conscious mind.

One important thing to remember is that these triggers don't have to define who you are, how strong you can be, or what you can achieve. Triggers are your body's natural responses to past hurts, and their purpose is to let you know you have trapped emotions or other traumas waiting to be dealt with. Thankfully, the answers you need to deal with them are within you and are there for the asking.

Shaun shares his experience with his ex and how he never thought he could move on, but now he's found love again and is engaged.

Releasing the Past and Finding Love Again

Some four years ago, I had to leave a psychologically abusive relationship with my then wife. On top of the constant maltreatment that I'd been experiencing, including being degraded in front of my two young sons, I was faced with the choice of remaining with her and probably going insane after many episodes of depression, or leaving the relationship. I chose to leave. I realize, in retrospect, that I'd completely fallen apart, years into the marriage, due to having my mental, emotional, and physical energies continuously drained from me. While with my former wife, I couldn't see it happening, although close friends repeatedly told me. I couldn't hear them, understand them, or possibly I just did not want to. Essentially, I'd become a ghostly version of my previous self.

By happy and divine coincidences, my ambition to help others overcome their difficulties was sparked in a convoluted way. I found myself becoming more and more interested in energy healing work. Dr. Bradley Nelson's Emotion Code seemed to drop out of the clear blue sky, and suddenly everything about the enormous pains and difficulties I'd experienced made complete sense. After watching lots of videos about his work, theories, and principles, I began to experiment on friends and I started to get unexpectedly positive results. I decided to buy the book and take the EC practitioner course.

I put out a request for either an exchange or passing forward of treatment sessions, and Felix responded to offer his services. Since our sessions together, I've had some particularly touching experiences. A couple of particular issues that had been a "normal" part of my existence seem to have disappeared: the utter guilt and shame over my lack of finances, a constant draining stream of my energy toward my ex-wife.

I cannot explain how much enjoyment of life I feel now that I'm able to experience and express.

My new fiancée has also very happily remarked upon this several times. Bless you!

—Shaun D., Odense, Denmark

Trapped emotions can cause you to make wrong assumptions and misinterpret innocent remarks and behavior, ultimately short-circuiting your relationships.

When you share a life with someone, you share your energy. Sometimes that energy gets blocked and your relationship starts to fizzle. Using the Body Code, you and your partner may be able to help each other remove negative energies and live more openly and abundantly. You may find all sorts of underlying causes that block the success of your relationships. By removing them, you will be able to create the abundant and loving relationships you are meant to have. Remember that feeling you had when you first met? You could get that back!

HELPING OTHERS WITH THEIR RELATIONSHIPS

Not only can you use the Body Code to enhance your relationships, but you can help others with theirs. Everyone suffers from heartbreak at one time or another. As human beings with emotions, imperfections, and the need to be loved, none of us are immune. While the capacity for healing relationships may be inside you, sometimes a broken relationship can't be repaired. It's in times like these when it's critical to know how to heal heartbreak so you or others can move on and experience joy.

Healing from heartbreak can be a long process. If someone you're helping is dealing with emotional baggage or negative energy from past experiences or heartache, it could undermine the person's capacity for healing relationships or healing from heartbreak. While there is no single, correct method for healing from heartbreak, there are some things you can try in order to enable your innate ability to help other people recover from their losses. You can help them find, decode, and release trapped emotions or other negative energies with the Body Code. Getting rid of those issues may enable their minds, bodies, and spirits to recover. People have seen remarkable recovery from bad relationships, as Sheryl shares in the following story.

She Is Finally Free!

I have seen so many positive changes in the people I have worked with, but I will share this one experience. A lady was in a long-term relationship with a narcissist. She was sixty-two years old and, after twelve years of being beaten down, she was desperately seeking something or someone to help her. She heard about the Emotion Code and the Body Code from a mutual friend. She was skeptical but was willing to give it a try. Her friend had explained a little bit about energy work, and I directed her to watch some of Dr. Brad's videos on YouTube. In the interim, I did a proxy session for her. I found that she had many trapped emotions and negative energies related to her relationship. There were curses, negative entities, and cords. We cleared all of these imbalances, including her Heart-Wall.

After months of work and processing, I am happy to say that she is free! She has moved out, moved on, and now has a new happy life! She is looking forward to becoming a certified Emotion Code practitioner herself. The Emotion Code and the Body Code have changed her life! This is only one of the many miracles that I have seen with this amazing energy healing modality.

—Sheryl S., Florida, United States

Not only can you help others with their relationships, it works for repairing family connections as well. In the following story, Annabelle helped her husband heal his relationships with his ex and his sisters.

Beautiful Communication

My partner was in crisis with both his ex and his sisters, so I did a Body Code session on him. A few hours later his ex called and they communicated beautifully! Then his sisters called and were willing to talk. I attribute this shift to the Body Code session, as nothing else had changed.

—Annabelle M., Massachusetts, United States

Trapped emotions may play a part in an ongoing cycle of negativity that might compromise one's ability to build trust in a relationship. Trapped emotions such as resentment, anxiousness, abandonment, insecurity, feeling unsupported, jealousy, and others could make people more prone to feeling that way all the time . . . even in relationships.

Emotions have their own unique energy frequencies. When those feelings and their energies aren't fully processed by the body, they may become trapped.

When this happens, those emotions are felt much more easily than normal. Essentially, the part of the body where that energy is lodged is feeling that emotion all the time. Let's take jealousy, for example. If the energy frequency of jealousy is trapped in your body, you'd be prone to feeling jealous more easily, more of the time. How might that affect your ability to trust in a relationship? What if, like most people, you have a whole range of emotional baggage that is affecting your ability to function normally? In my experience, we all have inherited emotional baggage that is having its own effect on us, as Stephanie found in the following story.

Trust Regained

This program has changed my life. Releasing ancestral trauma has been important to me, as my family had a history of mother-daughter toxic relationships going back several generations. The improvement I noticed in my relationships has lit the fire under me to be able to help others in more ways than just telling everyone I know about it!

In fact, the relationship with my mom has improved so much that she is the one who purchased this program for me (on Mother's Day) in order to support my mission. My dad now keeps in touch weekly instead of months apart and has also shown much more support in my life in ways I never even expected. To someone with abandonment trauma and trust issues, that means the world.

I would love to share this gift and bless as many people as possible, because I can honestly say it's life changing.

—Stephanie S., Tennessee, United States

As grown-ups, we may have a hard time letting go of painful emotions associated with our parents from the days when we were growing up. Some will continue to experience strained relationships with their parents because of troubled times in their shared past.

Our parents may say or do things that trigger strong emotions in us. This can make family gatherings awkward and uncomfortable, or even lead to estrangement. We heal the hurts of the past so that we can restore relationships and move forward without regrets when we learn to identify and discover trapped emotions, the lingering, painful feelings many of us harbor from events in our past. This is important not only for our relationships but also our overall health and well-being.

29

CREATING A BETTER WORLD

Let us put our minds together and see what life we will make for our children.

—SITTING BULL

We are creators. All of us come into the world with a purpose and with the potential to do good. It is our choice to use the time we are given to serve, contribute, learn, and improve ourselves, or not. A key that I have learned in my life is that when our hearts are soft and open to the impressions of truth, we are blessed with more and more of them. Truth is like a stream continually flowing by us that we can dip into if we will but extend our cup to catch some of it.

Our Creator is aware of us and of every aspect of our lives. When you want to serve, and when you have light within because you have opened yourself to receiving light, you may choose to make it your purpose to bring joy or healing or wholeness to others, sometimes to those who are truly broken and suffering. It is up to you to use the gifts you have been given to create a better world. Whether your sphere of influence is small or large, there are those within your reach that need your help.

If you want a world of peace, love, creativity, and abundance, then you need to be engaged in its creation. Designing and manifesting the world is our birthright.

I believe this world will eventually be more than we can imagine, as we open our hearts to receive the truth and act upon what we feel and learn.

There has never been a time in the history of the world quite like this. There has never been so much truth and knowledge available to us, but on the other hand, there has never been such worldwide deception and division.

When we cannot tell what the truth is, when we cannot rely upon the opinions of others, we need to turn to the source of all truth. Our hearts must be soft enough and open enough to feel what is true. And the softer your heart, the more truth you will be given, until you know all of it.

So what do you feel? What do you know? What do you want to see? What do we, the people of this beautiful planet, want to change? What do we want to preserve and make better? What have we learned from the past and what are we learning from the current circumstances? What can we do to create more joy? And isn't joy what we all want to feel? What do we need to do to have it?

Questions are so important. Not only are they important as you use the Body Code to help you get to the root of your biggest health issues, your money problems, and your relationship difficulties, but they are important in every creative process you will ever be a part of. They are critical to creating your best life.

Life is an interesting thing. When you are born, suddenly you're here, without a stitch of clothing, without any recollection of where you were before this existence, without any idea of what you're doing here or why you came. You begin to figure out before long that you need love from others to survive, that you're dependent upon the care of others. And yet before many years have passed, you struggle for independence. Life has many stages and opportunities to grow and learn to understand where real happiness comes from.

I hope that by reading this book, you are beginning to understand the vast potential that the Body Code holds for you and for all of us. I foresee a day when no drug or remedy will be given and no treatment regimen started without first seeking help from the Divine and then consulting the database that is within each person.

This day is coming. It is no longer possible for humankind to ignore the deep intelligence within each of us that understands perfectly why we are sick and what we need to do to get well and be as healthy in mind, spirit, and body as we can be. With all that we are now learning and understanding, we get to be the creators of this new and better world.

A beautiful concept in the Jewish tradition is that of *tikkun olam.* It explains that when the

Creator made the world, He left it unfinished by design. He left the completion for us to finish deciding what it would become and how it would get there. A common but more modern understanding of this phrase is that we are in partnership with the Creator, and have the opportunity to take steps toward improving the state of the world and helping others. We can choose to make the world beautiful. We can choose to be healers instead of destroyers, peacemakers instead of troublemakers.

The power is within us to help bring about this new world, one heart and one person at a time.

YOUR UNIQUE GIFTS AND MISSION

Just as your life is full of experiences that no one else has had, your approach to this healing work will be uniquely yours.

Allow yourself to feel the deep gratitude that should be yours for participating in the sacred life stories of others. Share your gratitude often with those you work on. Their healing, releasing, and balancing is sacred work that will transform you as well. Always acknowledge the gift they are to you.

I hope these ideas prove to be worthwhile for you if you ever find that you are stuck. I know that these things have helped me when I have been unsure of what to do temporarily. In taking care of one another, it's our opportunity to ask the right questions and then see how the answers fit together. It really can feel like finding the pieces to a puzzle. When you have found the answers you need to help someone, it's always worth the effort.

I can't tell you how excited I am about the present age that we are living in. I believe that we are on the verge of a time when healers of all types will work together to the benefit of all. As we finally begin to wrap our heads around the true nature of our existence as energetic beings, and as we finally understand that the answers to our illnesses lie within our own subconscious minds, as we finally realize that we can access those answers simply and easily through these technologies, the world can't help but change for the better. The Emotion Code and the Body Code have already begun to play a role in bringing this new world into reality.

THE MEANING OF LIFE

One of my favorite cartoons on this topic has a guru on a mountaintop responding to a truth seeker by saying, "You'd better have a seat—people tend to fall down the mountain when I tell them the meaning of life!"

For some reason, I have been blessed with some profound spiritual experiences. I've learned for myself that we truly are all brothers and sisters in a most real sense, because I've learned for myself and know that we have a Father in Heaven, the Father of us all. Whether you refer to Him as "the Divine" or "Source Energy" or "Higher Power" or any other name, I think it's all the same. To call Him Father is more accurate in my view, and feels more personal and familial to me.

I've also learned for myself that we are strangers here in this world. In the words of William Wordsworth:

> *Our birth is but a sleep and a forgetting:*
> *The Soul that rises with us, our life's Star,*
> *Hath had elsewhere its setting,*
> *And cometh from afar:*
> *Not in entire forgetfulness,*
> *And not in utter nakedness,*
> *But trailing clouds of glory do we come*
> *From God, who is our home*

The best gift you could possibly give to yourself and to God is to consistently choose love, truth, forgiveness, and joy, to live a life filled with service, gratitude, and the highest good you can find, so that when you leave this life you will be comfortable returning home again, back to His presence, to your Father. Life is all about who we are becoming, ultimately. I think if we truly understood how important this is, we would probably "fall down the mountain" ourselves.

Many people have related to me how their ability to feel love as well as to give love has improved dramatically through the healing work that we have shared with them. Many people have even told us that for the first time in their lives, they are actually able to feel the love of the Higher Power for them, especially once their Heart-Walls were removed. I learned a powerful lesson about this love at Disneyland, of all places.

UNCONDITIONAL LOVE

When our children were young, we were fortunate to live only an hour away from Disneyland. We didn't have much extra money, so we didn't actually go there very often. But one day I found myself at Disneyland with a couple of my nieces and nephews. I had given in to their pleadings and, trying to be a good uncle, I agreed to take them to Disneyland. At a certain point during the day, while they were waiting in line to go on one of the rides, I took a short walk. As I walked along through the crowd, I began to notice the people around me. Some were tall, some short, some large, some small, some were good-looking, others not so much.

In general, I like people, but it occurred to me that none of these strangers held any real meaning for me. I didn't have any feelings about them one way or the other. I began to wonder what it must be like for our Father in Heaven, who, we are told, loves everyone unconditionally. In my mind, I said a silent prayer: "Father, help me to understand what it's like for you, to love all your children so much." I guess I didn't really expect an answer at that moment, and no answer came. I mentally shrugged my shoulders and went on with my day.

When I came home later, I was immediately besieged by my two youngest sons, Ian and Joseph, as well as their cousin Ciera, who began begging me to take them to Disneyland. There was no keeping a secret that I had taken some of the older kids, so how could I not take them? I somewhat reluctantly agreed to give up another day off and take them.

So the following Saturday I found myself at Disneyland again. At a certain point during the day, while the kids were waiting in line for a ride, I took a walk again. As I was meandering along, noticing the people around me, I had the same thought return to me.

These people seemed nice at a distance, but they held no meaning to me. I thought, "What must it be like for our Father . . ."

Suddenly my prayer was answered. Instantly, I was filled with an overwhelming, unconditional love for these people around me. I didn't know them, and it didn't matter! I was filled with a level of love that I have never felt before, an enormous, overwhelming, unconditional, and perfect love.

I glanced to my right and saw a crowd of at least two hundred people waiting in line for a ride. The love that filled my heart for every one of those strangers was so huge and so far outside of my normal experience that I felt a sudden moment of panic, and just as suddenly as it came, the experience was instantly over. I no longer felt the love for all of the unknown people that surrounded me. But I now knew that although they were strangers to me, they were not strangers to God.

I was given a short glimpse into the pure, immense love that our Father has for each of us. I know that He has unconditional love for you, whoever you are, whatever you have done or not done, whatever choices you have made or not made. He is unchangeable, His love for you is a constant in the universe; like gravity, it does not change, no matter what. I know that this is true.

It has been my goal, for many years, to serve that source of love. To do so requires being open and receptive to the influence and light that is there to bless us all, and in spite of our weaknesses, mistakes, and faults, to persevere.

As you journey through your life, seeking answers to your problems and helping others with theirs, I hope you will think of the Body Code and use it as a tool to help. I know it can uncover and bring to light the truth about your very nature, about the nature of the incredible body-temple you inhabit and its remarkable interface with your eternal mind, spirit, and heart. Remember to ask for help from above. When you do, the universe will open for you.

—Dr. Bradley Nelson
Saint George, Utah

APPENDIX 1
BODY CODE CERTIFICATION AND MORE

There are three parts to the Body Code:

1. The Body Code System App
   a. This mobile and desktop software is a patented mind-map interface between you and the subconscious mind, enabling you to drill down to any of thousands of underlying imbalances in seconds.
2. The Body Code System Method and Skills
   a. You can learn the basics of the Body Code System by participating in webinars, seminars, live events, and online courses available through DiscoverHealing.com.
3. The Body Code System Certifications
   a. Discover Healing offers in-depth online certification programs with video learning, mentoring, and practicums as the most comprehensive way to become skilled in the Body Code System. I host much of the training in an interactive teaching tool that enhances comprehension and retention.
   b. Certification is required to become a practitioner and to charge for services. In this way, we maintain standards and ongoing education for practitioners worldwide.

We currently offer four levels of online certification that build on one another, beginning with our prerequisite Level I, Emotion Code. Body Code Certification is Level II.

1. Level I Certification: Emotion Code
2. Level II Certification: Body Code
3. Level III Certification: Belief Code
4. Level IV Certification: Healing Mastery*

Our company is Discover Healing, Inc.

---

*Name subject to change

APPENDIX 2
LINKS AND RESOURCES

THE BODY CODE SYSTEM SOFTWARE

The Body Code System is fully realized in our mobile app of that name. It provides the complete tree structure of imbalances for you to navigate. As you drill down, layer by layer, to find the underlying imbalances, you are given definitions, descriptions, options, and direction. For this reason, extensive health education is not necessary—the information is provided for you. The app contains all of the functionality for all of our certification competencies—the Emotion Code, the Body Code, the Belief Code, and more.

Use this tool both online and offline on cell phones, tablets, and even desktop web browsers to identify and resolve imbalances of all kinds in the body and restore balance physically and emotionally.

It is available as a monthly subscription through our site at DiscoverHealing.com, as well as at the Apple App Store and Google Play Store, including an initial free trial period.

Start your free app trial by visiting discoverhealing.com/app. 

DISCOVERHEALING.COM

The official website for the Body Code System, including the Emotion Code, is DiscoverHealing .com. It provides the tool kit and knowledge so you can help people heal and thrive. I believe that this is your birthright: to know how to help yourself and your loved ones to discover and create the balance necessary for wellness, that all might live up to their full potential.

I created DiscoverHealing.com for the express purpose of making these powerful natural healing methods available to everyone.

- Learn more about energy healing.
- Watch videos about the Emotion Code, the Body Code, muscle testing, and more.
- Access videos, books, CDs, tools, and supplements.

- Ask questions and interact with other students.
- View our schedule of live and online events.
- Order copies of *The Emotion Code* and *The Body Code.*
- Find out about how to become a certified Emotion Code and Body Code practitioner.
- Purchase remote sessions from certified practitioners.
- Get listed as a certified practitioner for others to find and contact.
- Watch live webinars on the Emotion Code and the Body Code.

Take advantage of all the site has to offer by visiting DiscoverHealing.com. 

MY PERSONAL WEBSITE: DRBRADLEYNELSON.COM

Connect with me on my personal website at DrBradleyNelson.com, where I share more about my experiences, personal beliefs, photos, hobbies, and more.

My personal YouTube channel is at: youtube.com/drbradleynelson.

Subscribe to my YouTube channel and watch session demonstrations, and Q and A videos where I answer your questions and dive deeper into the Emotion Code and Body Code subjects, watch muscle-testing videos, and more.

THE EMOTION CODE BOOK

The first book I published is *The Emotion Code,* an essential part of the larger Body Code System. *The Emotion Code* book teaches you how to identify and release your trapped emotions, eliminating your "emotional baggage" and opening your heart and body to a productive and happy life. I highly recommend reading this book as part of your Body Code System tool kit.

Filled with real-world examples from many years of clinical practice, *The Emotion Code* is a distinct and authoritative work that has become a classic book on self-healing. The latest edition is expanded and includes a foreword by Tony Robbins. It is published by St. Martin's Press. Order your copy of *The Emotion Code* book by visiting discoverhealing.com/the-emotion-code/book, or online at Amazon.com and everywhere books are sold. It is also available as an audiobook at Audible.com.

E-MOTION, THE MOVIE

e-motion is a documentary (2014) that explores how human emotions affect the physiology of the human body and how negative emotions can be released, resulting in physical improvement. A team of emotion experts from around the world, including me, share their wisdom and methods to show humanity the path to health and enlightenment.

The trailer information says, "Imagine a world where everyone is manifesting from their heart the perfect creation that's inside each of us. Imagine a world where abundance, inner peace, longevity, and loving relationships abound. Imagine we are sacred, spiritual beings here for a much larger reason, serving a much higher purpose, a divine purpose. Imagine experts from around the world sharing their wisdom and negative emotion clearing techniques to light a new pathway for humanity." You can watch the *e-motion* movie by visiting e-motionthemovie .com.

SOCIAL MEDIA

Join our community on social media who are also learning about and using the Body Code System. Our Discover Healing team is on all the major channels, and we are grateful for your help in spreading the word about the Body Code System. Please use these tags when you post anything about the Body Code: #BodyCode, #BodyCodeStories. You will be helping us reach the world, and I'll be able to find your posts by searching on these hashtags. For more information and links to our social media channels, visit discoverhealing.com/social.

SHARE YOUR STORY

Our experiences bind us together, creating community, compassion, and wholeness when we share authentically. I hope you will tell us your stories of finding healing and purpose using the Body Code System. Please tag #BodyCodeStory in your posts, so we can share in your triumphs. If you would like to send me your story directly, please use the link on the website: discoverhealing.com/share-your-story/.

READ MORE STORIES

Get inspired by the thousands of stories on my website, submitted every day by people like yourself. Seemingly every kind of issue, concern, hope, and desire is represented. I share these stories to help us keep the faith of being able to make a real difference in the lives of our loved ones, and through the world.

Visit discoverhealing.com/testimonials for more true stories.

FREE MUSCLE-TESTING COURSE

Because I believe muscle testing is vital to your ability to quickly heal, and to find and release imbalances, I am giving away my online introductory course on the subject. Take advantage of this gift, and become skilled, so you can serve others.

Muscle testing can be used to tap into the subconscious mind to answer questions about physical, mental, and emotional well-being. It's a noninvasive method designed to determine the potential underlying causes of ailments and discomfort—everything from nutritional needs to trapped emotions.

For more information, visit discoverhealing.com/muscle-testing.

FIND A CERTIFIED PRACTITIONER

If you are interested in having a certified practitioner work with you using the Body Code remotely or in person, we have a growing community of people who can help, including our staff practitioners. For more information or to make an appointment, visit discoverhealing.com/practitioners for a global map of practitioners.

LANGUAGES

The Body Code System has books, seminars, and videos translated in many languages. For example, as of the printing of this book, *The Emotion Code* had been translated and printed in twenty different languages. The app can be found in English, German, and Spanish, with more languages coming. Find *The Emotion Code* and *The Body Code* in other languages by visiting discoverhealing.com/languages.

PUBLIC RELATIONS

I've been privileged to be able to teach these unique healing methods to audiences around the world, at live seminars and online as well. It's always exciting and rewarding for both me and the audience to see the immediate results that are obtainable in many cases with people who are suffering from all kinds of different issues. If you are interested in having me speak to your group or company or at a live event that you are involved with, please let us know.

FREQUENTLY ASKED QUESTIONS

If you have a question about the Emotion Code or the Body Code, chances are it has already been asked and answered. For the most up-to-date list of the most popular questions and answers regarding the work we're doing at Discover Healing, please see discoverhealing.com/faqs.

FOR MORE INFORMATION

If the FAQ web page didn't help, jump into our full support page, which houses our knowledge base at discoverhealing.com/support. You can see the questions others have asked, as well as ask any question you may have that has not yet been answered.

APPENDIX 3
DEFINITIONS

We touch on profound concepts throughout this book. Finding terms that everyone can agree with or even consider is difficult. In this appendix is an inadequate substitution list. I offer it in an attempt to create context for understanding why and how the Body Code System works. Thank you for your generosity in finding a way to put these concepts within a framework you can consider. These are my beliefs, and they work well together to enable positive transformations for anyone who wants to participate. As we learn more, models and concepts expand. May we never stop learning.

KEY TERM	ALTERNATIVE TERMS	DESCRIPTION
Angels	Spirit guides, guardian angels, departed loved ones, yet-to-be-born descendants	Angels entice us to do and feel things that bring us closer to the Creator. They are positive and of the light. They want to support us in our progress and joy.
Body	Physical body, body-temple	The body is the mortal temple that houses the spirit; it is our flesh and bones and is the physical medium through which we muscle-test to get answers.
Body energy fields	Biofield, chakras, electromagnetic field, plasma energy field	Energy fields that are generated by the physical body and are produced at the interface between the physical body and the spirit
Brain	Physical organ in the skull	The brain is the hardware interface for the physical body and the spirit.
Conscious mind	Intellect, the thinker, conscious awareness	The conscious mind is that part of us that contains what we think we know. It operates during waking hours.
Entities	Negative energies, ghosts, dark energies, unclean spirits, evil spirits, disembodied spirits, demons, etc.	Entities entice us to do and feel things that distance us from the Creator. They are negative and of the darkness. They want to cause unhappiness and stop our progress and control us. They may cause physical and mental/emotional symptoms such as depression, etc.
Higher Power	God, Lord, Jesus Christ, Almighty, Creator, Goddess, Allah, Messiah, Deity, the Divine, Redeemer, Supreme Being, Jehovah, Father God, etc.	Father of our spirits, and the all-powerful Creator and supreme ruler of the universe
Higher self, spirit body, soul, aura, chi, qi, ki, prana, eternal being, sentient energy	Being, a finer form of matter, blueprint for the physical body	The spirit is the part of ourselves that is eternal; it has no beginning and no end. It is organized intelligence, indestructible, innocent, and pure. In its desire to grow and progress, it takes on new capabilities, such as a physical body.
Subconscious mind and spirit	Unconscious awareness, the heart, the observer, the master computer, seat of the soul, core of our being, seat of love. While I see them as two separate aspects of the self, with distinct purposes, I use them interchangeably in this book for simplicity.	The subconscious mind is the vast majority of our mind that is always operating, that keeps the body working, remembers everything we've experienced, and is connected to all information everywhere. It is accessed through muscle testing.
Universal intelligence	Light, light of truth, the Light of Christ, morphic field, dark matter, cosmic, super conscious, immaterial realm, the quantum field, Buddha consciousness, etc.	The database of all that is; the truth, knowledge, and intelligence that fills the universe

GENERAL GLOSSARY

ASSOCIATED IMBALANCE: An imbalance that is either causing or is related to another imbalance. For example, "John's liver was imbalanced because of a trapped emotion."

BALANCE A healthy, normal state in which conditions are right for the physical body to recover, thrive, and create healing on its own.

DECODING The work of identifying an imbalance through a process of elimination and muscle testing. This step includes identifying the imbalance as well as any necessary details about it.

ENERGY The building blocks of everything in the universe. Everything is made of energy. Some energies are invisible, some energies are slowed down sufficiently in vibration to appear in the form of physical matter. All energy has a vibration, and all energy can be affected by other vibrations of other energies, positively or negatively.

ENERGY HEALING Any kind of work that attempts to create a more balanced state in the energy of the physical body and energy body, in order to empower physical recovery and increase both mental and emotional wellness.

GOVERNING MERIDIAN (ACUPUNCTURE MERIDIAN) A reservoir and river of energy in the body that is connected to the other meridians. Placing magnified intention into this meridian enables it to flow through the entire body instantly, completing the release of trapped emotions and other energetic imbalances.

IMBALANCE Anything that goes wrong in the physical body or energy body. Imbalances may be things that do not belong, things that the body lacks/needs, things that have moved out of place or have been interrupted. Imbalances are generally low-vibrational and are always disruptive to the normal, balanced state of the spirit or body or both. Imbalances frequently cause other types of imbalance in the body (e.g., a trapped emotion leading to kidney imbalance). These are called "associated imbalances" in the Body Code.

IMBALANCED (STATE) A state in which the physical body or energy body is overburdened by imbalances and energetic blockages. This may lead to trouble recovering and eventual malfunction, among myriad other symptoms.

INTENTION A focused state of mind set toward a specific goal. This may include the release or correction of an imbalance, along with any helpful actions for the individual to take, with the aim of restoring balance. When doing work with the Body Code, this is officially the last step in addressing any imbalance, but it's important to realize that intention to help and to heal is vital from the very beginning of a session.

MAGNETIC ENERGY A tool that amplifies or strengthens intention. This can be any strength or polarity magnet or your body's electromagnetic field (your hand).

MUSCLE TESTING A skill or art that enables communication with the subconscious mind. We can use it to discern slight changes in muscle strength when we ask the subconscious a yes or no question. A muscle will remain strong if the answer is affirmative, or yes. A muscle will test weaker for a few seconds if the answer is negative, or no.

NEGATIVE ENERGY Vibrations of energy that are inherently destructive, harmful, and/or imbalancing in some way.

OVERLOAD A temporary state in which muscle testing may be unclear or impossible. This may occur after the release of an intense imbalance or at the end of a session in which the person has already begun processing and cannot release anything further.

PHYSICAL BODY Made of energy in the form of matter, it can be affected by other vibrational frequencies. When imbalanced, the physical body may create symptoms to communicate that imbalance.

POSITIVE ENERGY Vibrations of energy that are inherently life-giving and balancing.

PROCESSING A state in which the energy body and physical body are shifting to process the release of one or more imbalances. Processing generally lasts one to three days and may create some mild fatigue or emotional sensitivity approximately 20 percent of the time.

PROXY A person who temporarily connects with the energy field / subconscious mind of a subject from a distance, so that imbalances may be located and removed from the subject.

RELEASE The process for removing an imbalance once it has been identified. Releasing requires three elements: intention, some other form of energy such as magnetic energy, and the governing meridian.

RESONANCE When two energies vibrate together at such a similar frequency as to become activated or triggered.

SPIRIT BODY The invisible spirit that animates the physical body. Also referred to as the qi, chi, ki, or prana. It is naturally very high-vibrational, but imbalances may interfere with this state.

SUBCONSCIOUS MIND That part of the brain and body that contains most of our overall intelligence. It is a massive database that can be queried to find answers about what the body and spirit need in order to find balance.

SUBJECT The person or animal who needs help and is being tested.

SURROGATE A person who temporarily accesses the energy field of another person or animal that is in close proximity, so imbalances can be identified and cleared from the subject.

SYMPTOM The body's way of communicating with us that it has one or more imbalances. Any imbalance can potentially contribute to any physical, mental, or emotional symptom.

TESTER The person performing the muscle testing.

VIBRATION / VIBRATION FREQUENCY Also known as molecular vibration, this refers to the constant and periodic motion of atoms in a molecule and all subatomic particles (energies). The frequency of the periodic motion is known as a vibrational frequency. The vibrational frequency of an energy will determine if it is positive or negative and what it feels and/or looks like. This applies to everything in the universe.

ACKNOWLEDGMENTS

My express thanks go out to those who have helped in the creation of this work.

Natalie Nelson, for her collaborative efforts helping to develop and refine this work over the years.

Josh Nelson, for his wonderful insights and contributions, and for being a great educator of our Body Code practitioners around the world.

Patti Rokus, for helping me organize a mountain of material and for helping me to get the book off the ground.

Jana Carter, for her superb help in the reviewing and editing process.

Gwen Hawkes, associate editor at St. Martin's Press, for being so patient with me.

My patients, for allowing me to be their friend and physician, and for allowing me to share their stories.

Our amazing practitioners around the world, for sharing their experiences.

My brother, Bruce Nelson Jr., my mentor and example in so many ways.

Tom Miller, my wonderful literary agent, for all his help in making this book beautiful.

Joel Fotinos, my publisher at St. Martin's Press, for helping make this book a great companion volume to *The Emotion Code*.

My wonderful colleagues at Discover Healing, for all their help in bringing this healing work to the world.

My wife, Jean, for her countless insights during the development of this work, for being my inspiration, my helper, and my best friend.

Finally, to the Creator for blessing me with the gifts I would need to accomplish this work, for making me an instrument of healing, and for guiding my life all along the way.

INDEX